D1273434

OXFORD MEDICAL PUBLICATIONS

5-Hydroxytryptamine in Psychiatry

5-Hydroxytryptamine in Psychiatry

A Spectrum of Ideas

Edited by

Merton Sandler
Alec Coppen
and
Sara Harnett

Oxford   New York   Tokyo
OXFORD UNIVERSITY PRESS
1991

Oxford University Press, Walton Street, Oxford OX2 6DP
Oxford New York Toronto
Delhi Bombay Calcutta Madras Karachi
Petaling Jaya Singapore Hong Kong Tokyo
Nairobi Dar es Salaam Cape Town
Melbourne Auckland
and associated companies in
Berlin Ibadan

Oxford is a trade mark of Oxford University Press

Published in the United States
by Oxford University Press, New York

British Library Cataloguing in Publication Data
5-Hydroxytryptamine in psychiatry.
1. Man. Psychoses. Drug therapy.
I. Sandler, Merton   II. Coppen, A. (Alec)   III. Harnett,
Sara
616.8918
ISBN 0–19–262011–8

Library of Congress Cataloging in Publication Data
5-hydroxytryptamine in psychiatry: a spectrum of ideas/edited by Merton Sandler,
Alec Coppen, and Sara Harnett.
Contains papers from the Collegium Internationale Neuro-
psychopharmacologicum Workshop, held Jan. 7–10, 1990, in San Juan,
Puerto Rico.
Includes index.
1. Serotonin–Congresses.   2. Mental illness–Physiological
aspects–Congresses.   3. Neuropsychiatry–Congresses.   I. Sandler,
Merton.   II. Coppen, Alec.   III. Harnett, Sara.   IV. Collegium
Internationale Neuro-psychopharmacologium. Workshops (1st : 1990 :
San Juan, P.R.)   V. International Union of Biochemistry.   VI. Ihwa
Yŏja Taehakkyo.
[DNLM: 1. Energy Metabolism–congresses.   2. Mitochondria–
metabolism–congresses.   3. Mitochondria–pathology–congresses.
QH603.M5 B615 1989]
RC 455.4.B5A13 1991   616.89'18—dc20   90-7859
ISBN 0–19–262011–8

Set by CentraCet, Cambridge
Printed in Great Britain by
Biddles Ltd, Guildford and Kings Lynn

Contents

Contents

Contributors

Anderson, I. M.
MRC Clinical Pharmacology Unit and University Department of Psychiatry, Littlemore Hospital, Oxford OX4 4XN, UK.

Arora, R. C.
Department of Psychiatry, School of Medicine, Case Western Reserve University, Cleveland, OH 44106, USA.

Belmaker, R. H. *
Psychiatry Research Unit, Division of Mental Health, Beer Sheva Mental Health Centre, P.O. Box 4600, Beer Sheva, Israel.

Bianchi, E.
Center of Neuropharmacology, Institute of Pharmacological Sciences, University of Milan, Italy.

Briley, M. *
Centre de Recherche Pierre Fabre, 17 Avenue Jean Moulin, 81100 Castres, France.

Brunello, N.
Centre of Neuropharmacology, Institute of Pharmacological Sciences, University of Milan, Italy.

Carlsson, A. *
Department of Pharmacology, University of Göteborg, P.O. Box 33031, S-40033 Göteborg, Sweden.

Carr, A. A.
Merrell Dow Research Institute, 2110 E. Galbraith Road, Cincinnati, OH 45215, USA.

Cheng, H. C.
Merrell Dow Research Institute, 2110 E. Galbraith Road, Cincinnati, OH 45215, USA.

Chopin, P.

Centre de Recherche Pierre Fabre, 17 Avenue Jean Moulin, 81100 Castres, France.

Coppen, A.*

MRC Neuropsychiatry Research Unit, Clinical Investigation Ward, Greenbank, West Park Hospital, Epsom, Surrey KT19 8PB, UK.

Cowen, P. J.*

MRC Clinical Pharmacology Unit and University Department of Psychiatry, Littlemore Hospital, Oxford OX4 4XN, UK.

Curzon, G.*

Institute of Neurology, Queen Square, London WC1N 3BG, UK.

Davis, R.

Department of Psychiatry and Human Behavior, Brown University, VA Medical Center, Providence, RI 02908, USA.

Deakin, J. F. W.*

Department of Psychiatry, Withington Hospital, West Didsbury, Manchester M20 8LR, UK.

Doogan, D.*

Pfizer Central Research, Sandwich, Kent CT13 9NG, UK.

Dudley, M. W.

Merrell Dow Research Institute, 2110 E. Galbraith Road, Cincinnati, OH 45215, USA.

Evenden, J.*

Astra Research Centre Sodertalje, S/15185 Sodertalje, Sweden.

Frazer, A.*

University of Pennsylvania School of Medicine, Veterans Administration Medical Center, University and Woodland Avenues, Philadelphia, PA 19104, USA.

Glover, V.*

Department of Chemical Pathology, Queen Charlotte's and Chelsea Hospital, Goldhawk Road, London W6 OXG, UK.

Gottfries, C. G.*

Department of Psychiatry and Neurochemistry, Gothenburg University, St Jörgen's Hospital, S-422 03 Hisings Backa, Sweden.

Guardiola-Lemaitre, B. *

IRIS et Compagnie–Developpement, 1 rue Carle Hébert, 92415 Courbevoie, France.

Guimaraes, F. S.

Department of Psychiatry, Withington Hospital, West Didsbury, Manchester M20 8LR, UK.

Hensman, R.

Department of Psychiatry, Withington Hospital, West Didsbury, Manchester M20 8LR, UK.

Insel, T. R. *

Laboratory of Clinical Science, National Institute of Mental Health, P.O. Box 289, Poolesville, MD 20837, USA.

Jarman, J.

Department of Chemical Pathology, Queen Charlotte's and Chelsea Hospital, Goldhawk Road, London W6 OXG, UK.

Kehne, J. H.

Merrell Dow Research Institute, 2110 E. Galbraith Road, Cincinnati, OH 45215, USA.

Kennett, G. A.

Beecham Pharmaceuticals, Research Division, Coldharbour Road, Harlow, Essex, CM19 5AD, UK.

Linnoila, M. *

Laboratory of Clinical Studies, DICBR, National Institute on Alcohol Abuse and Alcoholism, Bethesda, MD 20892, USA.

López-Ibor, Jr, J. J. *

Unit of Psychiatry, Ramón y Cajal Hospital, University of Alcalá de Henares, Av Nueva Zelanda 44, E-28035 Madrid, Spain.

Maître, L. *

Research Department, Pharmaceuticals Division, CIBA-GEIGY Ltd., CH-4002, Basle, Switzerland.

McIntyre, I. M.

Psychoendocrine Research Unit, Department of Psychiatry, University of Melbourne, Austin Hospital, Heidelberg, Victoria, Australia.

Meltzer, H. Y. *

Department of Psychiatry, School of Medicine, Case Western Reserve University, Cleveland, OH 44106, USA.

Mendlewicz, J. *

Hopital Erasme, Psychiatrie, Route de Lennik 808, 1070 Brussels, Belgium.

Moral, L.

Unit of Psychiatry, Ramón y Cajal Hospital, University of Alcalá de Henares, Av Nueva Zelanda 44, E-28035 Madrid, Spain.

Moreno, I.

Unit of Psychiatry, Ramón y Cajal Hospital, University of Alcalá de Henares, Av Nueva Zelanda 44, E-28035 Madrid, Spain.

Murphy, D. L. *

Laboratory of Clinical Science, National Institute of Mental Health, Bethesda, MD 20892, USA.

Oxenkrug, G. F. *

Department of Psychiatry and Human Behavior, Brown University, VA Medical Center, Providence, RI 02908, USA.

Palfreyman, M. G. *

Merrell Dow Research Institute, 2110 E. Galbraith Road, Cincinnati, OH 45215, USA.

Perez, J.

Centre of Neuropharmacology, Institute of Pharmacological Sciences, University of Milan, Italy.

Peroutka, S. J. *

Department of Neurology, Stanford University Medical Center, CA 94305, USA.

Racagni, G. *

Centre of Neuropharmacology, Institute of Pharmacological Sciences, University of Milan, Italy.

Ray, O. *

Vanderbilt University, Nashville, TN 37240, USA.

Requintina, P. J.

Department of Psychiatry and Human Behavior, Brown University, VA Medical Center, Providence, RI 02908, USA.

Robinson, D. S. *

Central Nervous System Research, Bristol-Myers Squibb Company, 5 Research Parkway, Wallingford, CT 06492, USA.

Sáiz-Ruiz, J.

Unit of Psychiatry, Ramón y Cajal Hospital, University of Alcalá de Henares, Av Nueva Zelanda 44, E-28035 Madrid, Spain.

Sandler, M.*

Department of Chemical Pathology, Queen Charlotte's and Chelsea Hospital, Goldhawk Road, London W6 OXG, UK.

Schmidt, A. W.

Department of Neurology, Stanford University Medical Center, CA 94305, USA.

Sorensen, S. M.

Merrell Dow Research Institute, 2110 E. Galbraith Road, Cincinnati, OH 45215, USA.

Sulser, F.*

Department of Pharmacology, Vanderbilt University School of Medicine, Nashville, TN 37232, USA.

Tinelli, D.

Centre of Neuropharmacology, Institute of Pharmacological Sciences, University of Milan, Italy.

Viñas, R.

Unit of Psychiatry, Ramón y Cajal Hospital, University of Alcalá de Henares, Av Nueva Zelanda 44, E-28035 Madrid, Spain.

Virkkunen, M.

Department of Psychiatry, University of Helsinki, Finland.

Waldmeier, P. C.

Research Department, Pharmaceuticals Division, CIBA-GEIGY, Ltd., CH-4002, Basle, Switzerland.

Wang, M.

Department of Psychiatry, Withington Hospital, West Didsbury, Manchester M20 8LR, UK.

Whitton, P.

School of Pharmacy, Brunswick Square, London WC1N 1AX, UK.

Youdim, M. B. H.*

Technion Faculty of Medicine, Rappaport Family Research Institute, Department of Pharmacology, Haifa, Israel.

* Participant in the Collegium Internationale Neuro-Psychopharmacologicum Workshop (San Juan, Puerto Rico, 7–10th January 1990).

1. Introduction

Merton Sandler

It is hard to believe that only ten years have gone by since Peroutka and Snyder's (1979) breakthrough in the 5-hydroxytryptamine (5-HT, serotonin) receptor field. There were good precedents with adrenoceptors and histamine receptors and it seemed sensible that multiple 5-HT receptors would also exist, but to find them one had to wait until the technology was right. Gaddum and Picarelli (1957) had already broken the ice, but with a combination of receptor binding technology and classical pharmacology over the past decade everything fell into place. Recently the molecular biology big guns have swung into action. One of the most striking papers to emerge during the past year was that of Julius *et al.* (1989) who transfected 5-HT$_{1C}$ receptors into rat fibroblasts where they are not normally present. They found they were dealing with a protooncogene, and when these altered fibroblasts were transplanted into the nude mouse they gave rise to tumour formation. The implications and ramifications of this type of work are substantial. Working in the rat, Nagatsu and his colleagues in Japan (Kohsaka *et al.* 1989) have been able to transfer the tyrosine hydroxylase cDNA into non-neuronal cells, for future use in intracerebral grafting. The need for caution in extrapolating such work to man cannot be overemphasized. On the other hand, the potential of this kind of approach is enormous. This is but one example of many that will be found within this volume of how the curtain is beginning to lift on many areas of biological psychiatry and, most particularly, on the subtle role of 5-HT.

References

Gaddum, J. H. and Picarelli, Z. P. (1957). Two kinds of tryptamine receptor. *British Journal of Pharmacology*, **12**, 323–8.

Julius, D., Livelli, T. J., Jessel, T. M., and Axel, R. (1989). Ectopic expression of the serotonin 1c receptor and the triggering of malignant transformation. *Science*, **244**, 1057–62.

Kohsaka, S., Uchida, K., Takamatsu, K., Toya, S., Kaneda, N., Nagatsu, T., and Tsukada, Y. (1989). Transfection of tyrosine hydroxylase cDNA into C-6 cells: application in the intracerebral grafting. *Journal of Neurochemistry*, **52**, Suppl., S135.

Peroutka, S. J. and Snyder, S. H. (1979). Multiple serotonin receptors: differential binding of [³H]5-hydroxytryptamine, [³H]lysergic acid diethylamide and [³H]spiroperidol. *Molecular Pharmacology*, **16**, 687–99.

2. An overview of 5-hydroxytryptamine receptor families

Stephen J. Peroutka and Anne W. Schmidt

Introduction

In the past decade, many 5-hydroxytryptamine (5-HT, serotonin) receptor subtypes have been characterized. Many of these subtypes were identified as a result of the development of potent and selective agonists and/or antagonists. More recently, molecular biological studies have identified numerous distinct amino acid sequences that appear to represent even more pharmacologically distinct receptor subtypes. This chapter summarizes the current status of 5-HT receptors using a framework in which those with similar characteristics are considered as a 'family' of receptors (Tables 2.1 and 2.2.).

The identification and characterization of receptor subtypes have significant clinical implications. Theoretically, each subtype provides a specific target site that can be pharmacologically manipulated. The goal of the basic scientific research is to identify the potential functional significance of each 5-HT receptor subtype.

The 5-HT$_1$ receptor family

The 5-HT$_1$ family of 5-HT receptors (Table 2.1) was first differentiated in 1979, when radioligand binding techniques were used to distinguish between two distinct subtypes of 5-HT recognition sites (Peroutka and Snyder 1979). 5-HT$_1$ binding sites were defined as having nanomolar affinity for 5-HT and were labelled with ^{3}H-5-HT. 5-HT$_{1A}$, 5-HT$_{1B}$, and 5-HT$_{1D}$ are distinct receptor subtypes that share certain characteristics and are members of the 5-HT$_1$ family (Gozlan *et al.* 1983; Hoyer *et al.* 1985; Heuring *et al.* 1987). The molecular biology, pharmacology, and biochemistry of the 5-HT$_{1C}$ receptor (Pazos *et al.* 1984; Yagaloff and Hartig 1985), initially classified as a 5-HT$_1$ subtype, suggest that it would be more appropriately placed in the 5-HT$_2$ family (see below).

Molecular biology

The first 5-HT receptor to be cloned successfully was the 5-HT$_{1A}$ receptor. The genomic clone, G-21, was identified by its cross reactivity with a

β-adrenergic receptor sequence (Fargin *et al.* 1988). Radioligand binding studies using membranes from cells that had been transfected with G-21 DNA revealed specific binding of ^{125}I-cyanopindolol, a radioligand which labels β-adrenergic and 5-HT$_{1A}$ receptors. The presence of 5-HT$_{1A}$ receptors was demonstrated by the specific binding of the selective 5-HT$_{1A}$ agonist ^{3}H-8-hydroxy-*N*,*N*-dipropyl-2-aminotetralin (^{3}H-8-OH-DPAT). Buspirone and 8-OH-DPAT potently inhibited ^{3}H-8-OH-DPAT binding to these transfected cells. The 5-HT$_{1A}$ receptor has seven membrane-spanning units, and the amino acid sequence of these domains shows the least variability in comparison with other cloned biogenic amine receptors. The third cytoplasmic loop shows the greatest variability in its amino acid sequence and is believed to interact with the G-protein.

Pharmacology

The 5-HT$_1$ receptors share nanomolar affinity for 5-HT and 5-carboxyamidotryptamine (5-CT) and micromolar affinity for ketanserin, mesulergine, and ICS 205-930 (Table 2.1). Radioligands, for example ^{3}H-OH-DPAT, which label 5-HT$_{1A}$ binding sites have been developed (Gozlan *et al.* 1983; Hoyer *et al.* 1985; Pedigo *et al.* 1981). The 5-HT$_{1A}$ receptor displays high and selective affinity for certain aminotetralins (for example, 8-OH-DPAT), pyrimidinylpiperazines (for example, ipsapirone and buspirone), and benzodioxanes (for example, WB 4101, spiroxatrine, MDL 72832, and flesinoxan). Autoradiography reveals a heterogeneous distribution of binding in the brain, with highest densities of the 5-HT$_{1A}$ site found in the CA1 region and dentate gyrus of the hippocampus and in the raphe nuclei (Hoyer *et al.* 1986). Many correlations have been established between the pharmacological characteristics of this binding site and specific effects of 5-HT. This has been possible because of the large number of agents which display potent and selective affinity for the 5-HT$_{1A}$ site (Peroutka 1988).

5-HT$_{1B}$ binding sites are pharmacologically distinct from 5-HT$_{1A}$ sites. ^{125}I-Cyanopindolol (Hoyer *et al.* 1985) and other radioligands can be used to label 5-HT$_{1B}$ binding sites in rat brain (Table 2.1). 5-HT$_{1B}$ receptors have high affinity for 5-HT, $(-)$-pindolol, and RU 24969, and relatively low affinity for buspirone and 8-OH-DPAT (Table 2.1). Autoradiography in rat brain with ^{3}H-5-HT reveals the highest density of binding sites with high affinity for 5-HT and RU 24969 in the globus pallidus, dorsal subiculum, and substantia nigra (Hoyer *et al.* 1986). The 5-HT$_{1B}$ receptor binding site appears to be species specific; radioligand binding studies have demonstrated 5-HT$_{1B}$ binding sites only in rat, mouse, and hamster brain, and not in guinea pig, cow, chicken, turtle, frog, or human brain membranes (Hoyer *et al.* 1986; Heuring *et al.* 1987).

The 5-HT$_{1D}$ site was identified initially in bovine brain membranes (Heuring and Peroutka 1987). 5-HT$_{1D}$ receptor binding sites display nanomolar affinity for 5-HT, 5-CT, 5-methoxytryptamine and metergoline (Table 2.1)

S. J. Peroutka and A. W. Schmidt

TABLE 2.1. *Characteristics of 5-HT receptor subtypes*

	5-HT$_1$ receptors		
	5-HT$_{1A}$	5-HT$_{1B}$	5-HT$_{1D}$
Molecular biology	Cloned	?	?
Radiolabelled by	^{3}H-5-HT ^{3}H-8-OH-DPAT ^{3}H-Ipsapirone ^{3}H-WB 4101 ^{3}H-Buspirone ^{3}H-PAPP ^{3}H-Spiroxatrine ^{125}I-BH-8-MeO-N-PAT	^{3}H-5-HT ^{125}I-CYP (Rat, mouse, and ?hamster only)	^{3}H-5-HT
High density regions	Raphe nuclei Hippocampus	Substantia nigra Globus pallidus	Basal ganglia
Potent pharmacological agents (< 10 nM): Selective	8-OH-DPAT Ipsapirone	None available	None available
Non-selective	5-HT 5-CT RU 24969 d-LSD (−)-Pindolol	5-HT 5-CT RU 24969 (−)-Pindolol	5-HT 5-CT Metergoline
Second messenger	Inhibition of adenylate cyclase	Inhibition of adenylate cyclase	Inhibition of adenylate cyclase
Membrane effects	Hyperpolarization via an opening of potassium channels	?	?
Other functional correlates	Basilar artery Hypotension Thermoregulation Sexual behaviour 5-HT syndrome	'Autoreceptor'	'Autoreceptor' ?Saphenous vein

8-OH-DPAT, 8-hydroxy-*N*,*N*-dipropyl-2-aminotetralin; 5-CT, 5-carboxyamidotryptamine; PAPP, *p*-aminophenylpiperazine; 8-MeO-N-PAT, 8-methoxy-*N*-propylaminotetralin; CYP, cyanopindolol; LSD, lysergic acid diethylamide.

TABLE 2.2. *Characteristics of 5-HT receptor subtypes*

	5-HT$_2$ receptors			5-HT$_3$ receptors
	5-HT$_{1C}$	5-HT$_{2A}$	5-HT$_{2B}$	
Molecular biology	Cloned	?	Cloned	?
Radiolabelled by	^{3}H-5-HT ^{3}H-Mesulergine ^{3}H-Mianserin ^{125}I-LSD ^{3}H-SCH 23390 ^{125}I-SCH 23892	^{3}H-DOB ^{77}Br-R(−)DOB ^{125}I-DOI ^{3}H-Ketanserin	^{3}H-Spiperone ^{3}H-Mesulergine ^{125}I-LSD ^{3}H-Ketanserin ^{3}H-Mianserin ^{125}I-Methyl-LSD ^{3}H-*N*-Methyl-spiperone	^{3}H-GR 65360 ^{3}H-ICS 205-930 ^{3}H-Quipazine ^{3}H-Zacopride ^{3}H-BRL 43694 ^{3}H-QICS 205-930
High density regions	Choroid plexus	Layer IV cortex	Layer IV cortex	Peripheral neurones Entorhinal cortex Area postrema
Potent pharmacological agents (< 10 nM): Selective	None available	DOB DOI	None available	GR 65630 Zacopride ICS 205-930 Granisetron Ondansetron
Non-selective	Mesulergine Metergoline Methysergide Mianserin	Mesulergine Metergoline Ketanserin Spiperone	Mesulergine Metergoline Methysergide Mianserin Ketanserin Spiperone	
Second messenger	PI turnover	?	PI turnover	?
Membrane effects	Depolarization via an opening of chloride channels	?	Depolarization	Depolarization
Other functional correlates	?	Vascular contractions Platelete shape changes Platelet aggregation Paw oedema Tryptamine seizures Head twitches	Transmitter release Von Bezold-Jarisch reflex	

DOB, 4-bromo-2, 5-dimethoxyamphetamine; DOI, 4-iodo-2, 5-dimethoxyamphetamine.

5-HT$_{1A}$ agents, such as 8-OH-DPAT, ipsapirone, and buspirone, display micromolar affinities for 5-HT$_{1D}$ sites. RU 24969 and (−)-pindolol are approximately two orders of magnitude less potent at these sites than at 5-HT$_{1B}$ binding sites. Agents which display nanomolar affinities for 5-HT$_{1C}$, 5-HT$_2$, and 5-HT$_3$ sites, such as mianserin, mesulergine, and ICS 205-930, respectively, are essentially inactive at 5-HT$_{1D}$ binding sites. Regional studies demonstrate that this class of site is most dense in basal ganglia but exists in all regions of bovine brain (Heuring and Peroutka 1987). The 5-HT$_{1D}$ binding site has also been identified and characterized in pig, calf, and human brain membranes. A recently described selective 5-HT$_{1D}$ receptor agent, sumatriptan (GR 43175), appears to have unique anti-migraine effects (McCarthy and Peroutka 1989; Doenicke et al. 1988).

Biochemistry

A characteristic shared by the 5-HT$_1$ receptor family is their linkage to the modulation of adenylate cyclase. Regulation of neurotransmitter binding by guanine nucleotides often reflects an association with an adenylate cyclase. For example, GTP and GDP, but not GMP, inhibit the binding of ^{3}H-8-OH-DPAT to 5-HT$_{1A}$ receptors in brain membranes (Gozlan et al. 1983). In addition, guanine nucleotides significantly reduce agonist potencies for ^{3}H-8-OH-DPAT-binding sites whereas antagonist potencies are not affected by the addition of nucleotides. 5-HT also inhibits forskolin-stimulated adenylate cyclase activity in rat and guinea pig hippocampal membranes (DeVivo and Maayani 1986; Bockaert et al. 1987). 8-OH-DPAT and d-lysergic acid diethylamide (d-LSD) are similar to 5-HT in their ability to inhibit adenylate cyclase activity, whereas spiperone is a competitive antagonist at this site. Ketanserin has no effect on 5-HT-induced inhibition of adenylate cyclase activity. This pharmacological profile is consistent with a 5-HT$_{1A}$ receptor.

The 5-HT$_{1B}$ receptor also mediates the inhibition of forskolin-stimulated adenylate cyclase. 5-HT, 5-CT, and RU 24969 inhibit forskolin-stimulated adenylate cyclase, whereas 8-OH-DPAT and ipsapirone are ineffective (Bouhelal et al. 1988). Cyanopindolol, propranolol, and metergoline reverse 5-HT inhibition of forskolin-stimulated adenylate cyclase, whereas spiperone, mesulergine, and ketanserin are ineffective. This pharmacological profile is consistent with a 5-HT$_{1B}$ receptor.

Finally, inhibition of forskolin-stimulated adenylate cyclase activity is also observed with the 5-HT$_{1D}$ receptor. 5-HT, 5-CT, and 5-methoxytryptamine, in the presence of GTP, inhibit forskolin-stimulated adenylate cyclase in calf substantia nigra, whereas 8-OH-DPAT has no effect (Schoeffter et al. 1988). Cyanopindolol, spiperone, and mianserin do not antagonize the effects of 5-HT. Methiothepin, a non-selective 5-HT antagonist, blocks 5-HT inhibition of forskolin-stimulated adenylate cyclase in calf substantia nigra. This pharmacological profile is consistent with the 5-HT$_{1D}$ receptor.

The 5-HT$_{1B}$ and 5-HT$_{1D}$ sites appear to be analogous receptors in different species. In addition to their pharmacological, anatomical, and biochemical similarities, both receptor subtypes appear to mediate the 5-HT autoreceptor in different species (Hoyer and Middlemiss 1989). These observations suggest that the 5-HT$_{1B}$ receptor is a relatively recent evolutionary descendant of the 5-HT$_{1D}$ receptor.

Physiology

The development and characterization of selective 5-HT$_{1A}$ agents has benefited neurophysiological analyses. For example, the 5-HT$_{1A}$ receptor appears to mediate the inhibition of cell firing in the raphe nuclei. 5-HT$_{1A}$-selective agonists, such as 8-OH-DPAT, buspirone, and ipsapirone, cause complete inhibition of dorsal raphe neuronal firing in the rat, whereas (−)-propranolol, a β-adrenergic agent which also displays affinity for the 5-HT$_{1A}$ receptor, reversibly blocks the inhibitory effects of ipsapirone and 8-OH-DPAT on raphe cell firing (Aghajanian *et al.* 1987). 5-HT$_{1A}$-selective agonists directly hyperpolarize hippocampal CA1 pyramidal cells by opening potassium channels via a pertussis toxin-sensitive G-protein (Andrade and Nicoll 1987). No data are available yet on the physiological properties of 5-HT$_{1B}$ or 5-HT$_{1D}$ receptors.

The 5-HT$_2$ receptor family

The 5-HT$_2$ receptors are similar in that they all display nanomolar affinity for 5-HT antagonists such as ketanserin, mesulergine, metergoline, and d-LSD. Molecular biological and pharmacological data suggest that subtypes exist within the 5-HT$_2$ receptor family. For example, 5-HT$_{1C}$ receptors are included in this family because they share molecular biological, pharmacological, and biochemical characteristics with other members.

Molecular biology

A functional 5-HT$_{1C}$ receptor cDNA was isolated using methods involving RNA expression vectors combined with a sensitive electrophysiological assay (Julius *et al.* 1988). ^{125}I-LSD was found to bind with high affinity to membranes from transfected mouse fibroblast cells. Mianserin and 5-HT potently (K_i values less than 20 nM) inhibited specific ^{125}I-LSD binding, whereas spiperone was a relatively weak competitor. This pharmacological profile is consistent with the 5-HT$_{1C}$ receptor. This receptor is encoded by a 460 amino acid sequence protein. *In situ* hybridization studies show that, as well as in choroid plexus, 5-HT$_{1C}$ receptor mRNA is found in basal ganglia, hypothalamus, hippocampus, and spinal cord (Julius *et al.* 1988).

5-HT$_2$ receptor cDNA was isolated from a cloned cDNA library using probes generated from the 5-HT$_{1C}$ receptor amino acid sequences 88–104 and 134–149 (Pritchett *et al.* 1988). The 5-HT$_2$ receptor is encoded by 449 amino acids. Fifty per cent of the amino acid sequence is identical to the sequence encoding the 5-HT$_{1C}$ receptor. Radioligand binding on membranes from a transfected mammalian cell line reveals high affinity binding with ^{3}H-spiperone. 5-HT antagonists such as ketanserin and mianserin potently (K_i values 1–2 nM) inhibit ^{3}H-spiperone binding to transfected cell membranes. The 5-HT$_{1A}$ agonist, 8-OH-DPAT, and the 5-HT$_3$ antagonist, MDL 72222, show low competitiveness against ^{3}H-spiperone binding. Kao *et al.* (1989) reported that the amino acid sequence encoding the human 5-HT$_2$ receptor differs from that encoding the rat 5-HT$_2$ receptor at 2–10 per cent of the amino acids. The possible pharmacological and functional significance of these differences remains unknown.

Pharmacology

The 5-HT$_{1C}$ receptor was discovered as a result of the autoradiographic analysis of 5-HT-binding site subtypes in pig choroid plexus and cortex (Pazos *et al.* 1984; Yagaloff and Hartig 1985). ^{3}H-5-HT, ^{3}H-mesulergine, ^{125}I-LSD or ^{3}H-SCH 23390 can be used to radiolabel the 5-HT$_{1C}$ receptor. The 5-HT$_{1C}$ binding site displays high affinity for 5-HT, methysergide, and mianserin and relatively low affinity for 8-OH-DPAT, RU 24969, and spiperone (Table 2.2).

The 5-HT$_2$ class of binding sites has been extensively analysed because of the availability of a large number of potent, selective antagonists (Leysen *et al.* 1978). Several radioligands, such as ^{3}H-spiperone, ^{3}H-LSD, ^{3}H-mianserin, ^{3}H-ketanserin, ^{3}H-mesulergine, ^{125}I-LSD, and N_1-methyl-2-^{125}I-LSD, can be used to label the 5-HT$_2$ binding site (Table 2.2). Serotonergic antagonists such as ketanserin, cinanserin, metergoline, and methiothepin display high affinity for the 5-HT$_2$ binding site whereas 5-HT and related tryptamines display markedly lower affinity (Table 2.2). 8-OH-DPAT, RU 24969, and 5-HT$_3$-selective agents display low affinity for this site. Autoradiography reveals high densities of 5-HT$_2$ receptor sites in the cerebral cortex and caudate, and all other brain regions have substantially fewer binding sites (Pazos and Palacios 1985).

Studies using ^{3}H-DOB (4-bromo-2,5-dimethoxyamphetamine) have provided data which suggest that there are distinct subtypes of the 5-HT$_2$ receptor binding site (Lyon *et al.* 1986). ^{77}Br-R-(−)-DOB-labelled sites comprise only 19 per cent of the density of 5-HT$_2$ sites in rat cortex and are not eliminated by the addition of 10^{-4} M GTP (Peroutka *et al.* 1988). 5-HT competition curves using ^{3}H-ketanserin in rat and human cortical membranes are shallow (Hill slopes = 0.67, 0.69, respectively). These data suggest that ^{3}H-ketanserin labels more than one population of 5-HT$_2$ receptor binding sites (Pierce and Peroutka 1989). 5-HT competition curves are steep in bovine cortical membranes (Hill slope = 0.97), indicating that a single site is labelled by ^{3}H-ketanserin. Moreover, no specific binding using ^{3}H-DOB can be detected in bovine membranes. The high affinity component of

^{3}H-ketanserin binding has been tentatively designated the 5-HT$_{2A}$ binding site (also labelled with ^{3}H-DOB or ^{77}Br-(−)-DOB in rat membranes). The subpopulation of 5-HT$_2$ binding sites labelled with low affinity by ^{3}H-ketanserin in rat, human, and bovine membranes is designated 5-HT$_{2B}$ (Pierce and Peroutka 1989). This 5-HT$_{2B}$ receptor binding site corresponds to the classical 5-HT$_2$ receptor described in earlier literature.

Biochemistry

The 5-HT$_2$ family of receptors is linked to the modulation of phosphoinositide (PI) turnover. 5-HT stimulates PI turnover in choroid plexus, an area of brain rich in 5-HT$_{1C}$ receptors (Sanders-Bush and Conn 1987). Mianserin, ketanserin, and spiperone inhibit the response with potencies that correlate with their binding affinities at the 5-HT$_{1C}$ receptor. Thus, 5-HT$_{1C}$ receptors in choroid plexus are likely to mediate the 5-HT-induced PI turnover (Sanders-Bush and Conn 1987).

5-HT-induced PI hydrolysis in rat cerebral cortex results from 5-HT$_2$ (5-HT$_{2B}$) receptor activation (Sanders-Bush and Conn 1987). 5-HT stimulates PI turnover with an EC$_{50}$ of 1 μM. Ketanserin and other 5-HT$_2$ antagonists potently block the response to 5-HT. The effects of 5-HT$_2$ antagonists on PI turnover in the rat cerebral cortex correlate well with their binding affinities at ^{3}H-ketanserin-labelled 5-HT$_2$ sites. Tissues in the periphery, such as the rat thoracic aorta, cultured bovine aortic smooth muscle cells, and platelets, contain a 5-HT receptor that appears to modulate PI turnover via the 5-HT$_2$ receptor. As yet, there are no data on possible biochemical correlates of putative 5-HT$_{2A}$ binding sites.

Physiology

Electrophysiological studies of *Xenopus* oocytes which express the 5-HT$_{1C}$ receptor reveal that application of 5-HT causes a detectable inward current. Activation of the 5-HT$_{1C}$ receptor liberates inositol phosphates that raise intracellular Ca^{2+} levels, leading to the opening of Ca^{2+}-dependent chloride channels (Lubbert *et al.* 1987). The pharmacological profile of this response suggests that the 5-HT$_{1C}$ receptor mediates this effect of 5-HT.

Two specific neurophysiological effects of 5-HT have been attributed to activation of the 5-HT$_2$ receptor (Aghajanian *et al.* 1987). In the facial motor nucleus, 5-HT facilitates the excitatory effects of glutamate. This effect is antagonized by 5-HT$_2$ antagonists such as methysergide, cyproheptadine, and cinanserin. On the other hand, Davies *et al.* (1987) demonstrated that 5-HT causes a slow depolarization of 68 per cent of cortical neurones. Ritanserin and cinanserin, selective 5-HT$_2$ receptor antagonists, block the depolarizing effects of 5-HT. These data suggest that the depolarizing effects of 5-HT on cortical pyramidal neurones and the facial motor nucleus appear to be mediated by 5-HT$_2$ receptors.

The 5-HT$_3$ receptor family

5-HT$_3$ receptors have been well characterized in the periphery where they mediate the excitatory effects of 5-HT. Ondansetron (formerly called GR 38032F), zacopride, ICS 205-930, and MDL 72222, potent and selective antagonists, block these effects. Heterogeneity may also exist within the 5-HT$_3$ family of receptors. At least three distinct subtypes have been hypothesized (Richardson *et al.* 1985), based on significant potency differences of selective 5-HT$_3$ antagonists in various physiological systems. However, a clear pharmacological differentiation of 5-HT$_3$ receptor subtypes within a single species is still lacking.

Molecular biology

No information is available yet on the molecular biology of 5-HT$_3$ receptors.

Pharmacology

5-HT$_3$ binding sites were identified first in rat brain using ^{3}H-GR 65630 (Kilpatrick *et al.* 1987), and a variety of radioligands have now been developed to label the 5-HT$_3$ sites (Table 2.1). 5-HT, 2-methyl-5-HT, and phenylbiguanide, agonists at 5-HT$_3$ receptors, display moderate affinity (average K_i value approximately 250 nM) for this site, whereas antagonists such as granisetron (formerly called BRL 43694), zacopride, and ICS 205-930 display potent affinity for this site (K_i values = 0.1–2.0 nM). Agents selective for 5-HT$_1$ and 5-HT$_2$ binding sites, such as 8-OH-DPAT, mesulergine, and ketanserin, have low affinity for 5-HT$_3$ binding sites in rat cortical membranes. Regional binding studies reveal the highest densities of 5-HT$_3$ binding sites in cortical areas (particularly entorhinal cortex) and in the area postrema.

Biochemistry

Stimulation of 5-HT$_3$ receptors appears to cause a release of dopamine from rat striatal slices (Blandina *et al.* 1988), an observation which is consistent with the behavioural finding that ondansetron inhibits dopamine-mediated hyperactivity in rats (Costall *et al.* 1987). Release studies using rat entorhinal cortex preloaded with ^{3}H-choline suggest that 5-HT$_3$ receptors mediate the inhibition of acetylcholine release (Barnes *et al.* 1989). 5-HT$_3$ agonists reduce acetylcholine release in cortex, whereas 5-HT$_3$ antagonists facilitate the release of acetylcholine. More biochemical data on 5-HT$_3$ receptors are likely to be collected in the near future.

Physiology

Depolarization by 5-HT in a number of postganglionic autonomic neurones causes a calcium-dependent release of neurotransmitter. Postganglionic autonomic neurones have been studied in a variety of systems, such as the isolated rabbit heart and the superior cervical ganglion in the rat (Fozard 1989).

Additionally, vagally mediated bradycardia (the von Bezold-Jarisch reflex) occurs when afferent neurones are depolarized in the right ventricle. 5-HT$_3$ agonists, such as 5-HT, 2-methyl-5-HT, and phenylbiguanide, elicit this response, whereas 5-HT$_3$ antagonists block the bradycardia.

Electrophysiological studies in cultured mouse hippocampal cells and certain mouse neuroblastoma cell lines appear to reveal that 5-HT$_3$ receptors mediate a rapid inward current. This response is blocked by ICS 205-930, whereas 2-methyl-5-HT acts as an agonist. Dopamine-induced membrane depolarizations in these cells are also blocked by ICS 205-930, but not by sulpiride (a dopamine$_2$ antagonist) (Neijt *et al.* 1988). These data suggest that 5-HT$_3$ receptors mediate this response also. Derkach *et al.* (1989) showed directly that 5-HT$_3$ receptors are ligand-gated cationic channels in excised membrane patches of guinea pig submucosal plexus neurones.

Other putative 5-HT receptors

The existence of a variety of other 5-HT receptor subtypes has been hypothesized. For example, Gershon and colleagues reported a receptor designated 5-HT$_{1P}$ in gut membranes (Mawe *et al.* 1986). The pharmacological profile of 5-HT$_{1P}$ sites is distinct from that of all other known 5-HT binding sites or receptor subtypes. Moreover, the pharmacological characteristics of this binding site correlate with the physiological effects of 5-HT in the gut (Mawe *et al.* 1986).

Bockaert and colleagues described a 'non-classical 5-HT$_4$' receptor that is positively coupled to adenylate cyclase (Dumuis *et al.* 1988). 5-HT stimulates cAMP production in a dose-dependent manner in cell cultures generated from mouse embryo colliculi. 5-Methoxytryptamine and 5-CT are full agonists, whereas tryptamine, bufotenine, and 2-methyl-5-HT are partial agonists. Spiperone, methiothepin, and ketanserin do not block the 5-HT-induced increases in cAMP levels, whereas ICS 205-930, but not MDL 72222, weakly but competitively blocks the effects of 5-HT (K_i = 997 nM). ICS 205-930 also competitively antagonizes the 5-HT-induced increase in cAMP levels in adult guinea pig hippocampal membranes (K_i = 454 nM). Further characterization of this site has revealed that 5-HT$_3$ antagonists of the benzamide chemical class (zacopride, cisapride, and metoclopramide) act as agonists to stimulate cAMP levels in mouse embryo colliculi cell cultures (Dumuis *et al.* 1989). This pharmacological profile is not consistent with any previously described 5-HT receptor family; further studies will determine whether it represents yet another major family.

Future trends

This review provides evidence from a variety of molecular, biochemical, and physiological studies to suggest that there are many 5-HT receptors. At present, the classification of 5-HT receptors into at least three major families appears to be the most relevant. Future progress will continue to depend upon the development of highly potent and selective agonists and antagonists for each 5-HT receptor subtype. Such progress is likely to elucidate the role of 5-HT in normal human physiology as well as in the pathophysiology of many human disorders.

Acknowledgements

We thank Mary Keller for editorial assistance. This work was supported in part by the Stanley Foundation and NIH Grants NS 12151-15 and NS 23560-03.

References

Aghajanian, G. K., Sprouse, J. S., and Rasmussen, K. (1987). Physiology of the midbrain serotonin system. In *Psychopharmacology: the third generation of progress*, (ed. H. Y. Meltzer), pp. 141–50. Raven Press, New York.

Andrade, R. and Nicoll, R. (1987). Pharmacologically distinct actions of serotonin on single pyramidal neurones of the rat hippocampus recorded *in vitro*. *Journal of Physiology*, **394**, 99–124.

Barnes, J. M., Barnes, N. M., Costall, B., Naylor, R. J., and Tyers, M. B. (1989). 5-HT$_3$ receptors mediate inhibition of acetylcholine release in cortical tissue. *Nature*, **388**, 762–3.

Blandina, P., Goldfarb, J., and Green, J. P. (1988). Activation of a 5-HT$_3$ receptor releases dopamine from rat striatal slice. *European Journal of Pharmacology*, **155**, 349–50.

Bockaert, J., Dumuis, A., Bouhelal, R., Sebben, M., and Cory, R. N. (1987). Piperazine derivatives including the putative anxiolytic drugs, buspirone and ipsapirone, are agonists at 5-HT$_{1A}$ receptors negatively coupled with adenylate cyclase in hippocampal neurons. *Naunyn-Schmiedeberg's Archives of Pharmacology*, **335**, 588–92.

Bouhelal, R., Smounya, L., and Bockaert, J. (1988). 5-HT$_{1B}$ receptors are negatively coupled with adenylate cyclase in rat substantia nigra. *European Journal of Pharmacology*, **151**, 189–96.

Costall, B., Domeney, A. M., Naylor, R. J., and Tyers, M. B. (1987). Effects of the 5-HT$_3$ receptor antagonist, GR 38032F, on raised dopaminergic activity in the mesolimbic system of the rat and marmoset brain. *British Journal of Pharmacology*, **92**, 881–94.

Davies, M. F., Diesz, R. A., Prince, D., and Peroutka, S. J. (1987). Two distinct effects of 5-hydroxytryptamine on single cortical neurons. *Brain Research*, **423**, 347–52.

Derkach, V., Surprenant, A., and North, R. A. (1989). 5-HT$_3$ receptors are membrane ion channels. *Nature*, **339**, 706–9.

DeVivo, M. and Maayani, S. (1986). Characterization of the 5-hydroxytryptamine$_{1A}$ receptor-mediated inhibition of forskolin-stimulated adenylate cyclase activity in guinea pig and rat hippocampal membranes. *Journal of Pharmacology and Experimental Therapeutics*, **238**, 248–53.

Doenicke, A., Brand, J., and Perrin, V. L. (1988). Possible benefit of GR43175, a novel 5-HT$_1$-like receptor agonist, for the acute treatment of severe migraine. *Lancet*, **i**, 1309–11.

Dumuis, A., Sebben, M., and Bockaert, J. (1988). A non-classical 5-hydroxytryptamine receptor positively coupled with adenylate cyclase in the central nervous system. *Molecular Pharmacology*, **34**, 880–7.

Dumuis, A., Sebben, M., and Bockaert, J. (1989). The gastrointestinal prokinetic benzamide derivatives are agonists at the non-classical 5-HT receptor (5-HT$_4$) positively coupled to adenylate cyclase in neurons. *Naunyn-Schmiedeberg's Archives of Pharmacology*, **340**, 403–10.

Fargin, A., Raymond, J. R., Lohse, M. J., Kobilka, B. K., Caron, M. G., and Lefkowitz, R. J. (1988). The genomic clone G-21 which resembles a β-adrenergic receptor sequence encodes the 5-HT$_{1A}$ receptor. *Nature*, **335**, 358–60.

Fozard, J. R. (1989). The development and early clinical evaluation of selective 5-HT$_3$-receptor antagonists. In *The peripheral actions of 5-hydroxytryptamine*, (ed. J. R. Fozard), pp. 354–76. Oxford University Press.

Gozlan, H., Mestikawy, S. E., Pichat, L., Glowinski, J., and Hamon, M. (1983). Identification of presynaptic serotonin autoreceptors using a new ligand: ^{3}H-PAT. *Nature*, **305**, 140–2.

Heuring, R. E. and Peroutka, S. J. (1987). Characterization of a novel ^{3}H-5-hydroxytryptamine binding site subtype in bovine brain membranes. *Journal of Neuroscience*, **7**, 894–903.

Heuring, R. E., Schlegel, J. R., and Peroutka, S. J. (1987). Species variations in RU 24969 interactions with non-5-HT$_{1A}$ binding sites. *European Journal of Pharmacology*, **12**, 279–82.

Hoyer, D. and Middlemiss, D. N. (1989). Species differences in the pharmacology of terminal 5-HT autoreceptors in mammalian brain. *Trends in Pharmacological Sciences*, **10**, 130–2.

Hoyer, D., Engel, G., and Kalkman, H. O. (1985). Molecular pharmacology of 5-HT$_1$ and 5-HT$_2$ recognition sites in rat and pig brain membranes: radioligand binding studies with [^{3}H]5-HT, [^{3}H]8-OH-DPAT, $(-)$-[^{125}I]iodocyanopindolol, [^{3}H]mesulergine and [^{3}H]ketanserin. *European Journal of Pharmacology*, **118**, 13–23.

Hoyer, D., Pazos, A., Probst, A., and Palacios, J. M. (1986). Serotonin receptors in the human brain. I. Characterization and autoradiographic localization of 5-HT$_{1A}$ recognition sites. Apparent absence of 5-HT$_{1B}$ recognition sites. *Brain Research*, **376**, 85–96.

Julius, D., MacDermott, A. B., Axel, R., and Jessel, T. (1988). Molecular characterization of a functional cDNA encoding the serotonin 1c receptor. *Science*, **241**, 558–64.

Kao, H. T., Olsen, M. A., and Hartig, P. R. (1989). Isolation and characterization of a human serotonin 5-HT$_2$ receptor clone. *Society for Neuroscience Abstracts*, **15**, 486.

Kilpatrick, G. J., Jones, B. J., and Tyers, M. B. (1987). Identification and distribution of 5-HT$_3$ receptors in rat brain using radioligand binding. *Nature*, **330**, 746–8.

Leysen, J. E., Niemegeers, C. J. E., Tollenaere, J. P., and Laduron, P. M. (1978). Serotonergic component of neuroleptic receptors. *Nature*, **272**, 168–71.

Lubbert, H., Snutch, T. P., Dascal, N., Lester, H. A., and Davidson, N. (1987). Rat brain 5-HT$_{1C}$ receptors are encoded by 5–6 kbase mRNA size class and are functionally expressed in injected Xenopus oocytes. *Journal of Neuroscience*, **7**, 1159–65.

Lyon, R. A., Davis, K. H., and Titeler, M. (1986). ^{3}H-DOB (4-bromo-2,5-dimethoxy-phenylisopropylamine) labels a guanyl nucleotide-sensitive state of cortical 5-HT$_2$ receptors. *Molecular Pharmacology*, **31**, 194–9.

Mawe, G. M., Branchek, T. A., and Gershon, M. D. (1986). Peripheral neural serotonin receptors: identification and characterization with specific antagonists and agonists. *Proceedings of the National Academy of Sciences USA*, **83**, 9799–803.

McCarthy, B. G. and Peroutka, S. J. (1989). Comparative neuropharmacology of dihydroergotamine and sumatriptan (GR 43175). *Headache*, **29**, 420–2.

Neijt, H. C., Karpf, A., Schoeffter, P., Engel, G., and Hoyer, D. (1988). Characterization of 5-HT$_3$ recognition sites in membranes of NG108-15 neuroblastoma-glioma cells with [^{3}H]ICS 205-930. *Naunyn-Schmiedeberg's Archives of Pharmacology*, **337**, 493–9.

Pazos, A. and Palacios, J. M. (1985). Quantitative auoradiographic mapping of serotonin receptors in the rat brain. I. Serotonin-1 receptors. *Brain Research*, **346**, 205–30.

Pazos, A., Hoyer, D., and Palacios, J. M. (1984). The binding of serotonergic ligands to the porcine choroid plexus: characterization of a new type of serotonin recognition site. *European Journal of Pharmacology*, **106**, 539–46.

Pedigo, N. W., Yamamura, H. I., and Nelson, D. L. (1981). Discrimination of multiple ^{3}H-5-hydroxytryptamine binding site by the neuroleptic spiperone in the rat brain. *Journal of Neurochemistry*, **36**, 220–26.

Peroutka, S. J. (1988). 5-Hydroxytryptamine receptor subtypes. *Annual Review of Neuroscience*, **11**, 45–60.

Peroutka, S. J. and Snyder, S. H. (1979). Multiple serotonin receptors: differential binding of ^{3}H-5-hydroxytryptamine, ^{3}H-lysergic acid diethylamide and ^{3}H-spiroperidol. *Molecular Pharmacology*, **16**, 687–9.

Peroutka, S. J., Hamik, A., Harrington, M. A., Hoffman, A. J., Mathis, C. A., Pierce, P. A., and Wang, S. S- H. (1988). (R)-(−)-[^{77}Br]4-Bromo-2,5-dimethoxy-amphetamine labels a novel 5-hydroxytryptamine binding site in brain membranes. *Molecular Pharmacology*, **34**, 537–42.

Pierce, P. A. and Peroutka, S. J. (1989). Hallucinogenic drug interactions with neurotransmitter receptor binding sites in human cortex. *Psychopharmacology*, **97**, 118–22.

Pritchett, D. B., Bach, A. W. J., Wozny, M., Taleb, O., Dal Toso, R., Shih, J. C., and Seeburg, P. H. (1988). Structure and functional expression of cloned rat serotonin 5-HT$_2$ receptor. *EMBO Journal*, **7**, 4135–40.

Richardson, B. P., Engel, G., Donatsch, P., and Stadler, P. A. (1985). Identification of serotonin M-receptor subtypes and their specific blockade by a new class of drugs. *Nature*, **316**, 126–31.

Sanders-Bush, E. and Conn, P. J. (1987). Neurochemistry of serotonin neuronal systems: consequences of serotonin receptor activation. In *Psychopharmacology: the third generation of progress*, (ed. H. Y. Meltzer), pp. 95–103. Raven Press, New York.

Schoeffter, P., Waeber, C., Palacios, J. M., and Hoyer, D. (1988). The 5-hydroxytryptamine 5-HT$_{1D}$ receptor subtype is negatively coupled to adenylate cyclase in calf substantia nigra. *Naunyn-Schmiedeberg's Archives of Pharmacology*, **10**, 130–2.

Yagaloff, K. A. and Hartig, P. R. (1985). ^{125}I-Lysergic acid diethylamide binds to a novel serotonergic site on rat choroid plexus epithelial cells. *Journal of Neuroscience*, **5**, 3178–83.

Discussion

SANDLER: Other 5-hydroxytryptamine (5-HT, serotonin) receptors have been described, including 5-HT_{1E}, 5-HT_4, and 5-HT_{1P}. Where does one stop?

PEROUTKA: The 5-HT_{1E} receptor binding site was reported by Leonhardt *et al.* (1989); when the 1A, 1B, 1C, and 1D binding sites are blocked a small amount of $^3\text{H-5-HT}$ binding remains. Only 5-HT is potent at the putative 5-HT_{1E} site. However, when a radiolabel is displaced with the 'cold' compound (for example, 5-HT versus $^3\text{H-5-HT}$) there is almost invariably a greater amount of displacement than is seen with other drugs. For example, lysergic acid diethylamide (LSD) displaces $^3\text{H-LSD}$ more than any other drug, but this appears to be simply an artefact of the binding studies. Therefore, the putative 5-HT_{1E} binding site may be a true receptor or may reflect an artefact of the radioligand techniques.

The 5-HT_{1R} receptor was described by David Nelson and colleagues. They found that the pharmacological properties of putative 5-HT_{1D} sites in rabbits are subtly different from those in cows (Xiong and Nelson 1989). It appears that 5-HT receptor subtypes may be subtly different in every species. For example, the human 5-HT_2 receptor gene differs from that in rats at only four amino acids in its transmembrane segment (Hartig 1989). Also, Hoyer *et al.* (1987) reported pharmacological differences between human and rat 5-HT_2 receptors; mesulergine is much more potent at 5-HT_2 sites in rats than in man. These species differences raise important questions. Should we be more cautious about looking at animal receptors in the future? Perhaps we shall have to use human cell lines which express human receptors.

The 5-HT_{1P} receptor is a gut receptor (Mawe *et al.* 1986) which may also be in brain. Frank Zemlan and colleagues have reported a 5-HT_{1S} receptor in the spinal cord. Again, this may or may not represent a new 5-HT receptor.

The best evidence for a new 5-HT receptor comes from Joel Bockaert's work on 5-HT_4, which is a well-characterized 5-HT receptor subtype that is positively coupled to adenylate cyclase (Dumuis *et al.* 1989) and is G-protein-linked. 5-HT is reasonably potent, substituted benzamides are moderately potent, but all other drugs are inactive at this site. Thus, just as with the 5-HT_{1D} receptor, we must wait until more selective agents are developed to sort out these subtypes.

INSEL: As this is such an ancient monoaminergic system, what receptors or proteins are available for binding in invertebrate species? Do we know what the ancestral receptor was?

PEROUTKA: That would be easy to study with available molecular biological techniques. We created a database containing the amino acid sequences of all the receptors that have been cloned. Some clear amino acid patterns are present in all the subtypes. These must be critical to the receptor function. Theoretically, any amino acid change may result in receptor diversity. We should be able to trace the evolution of these receptors in the near future. I am not sure that anyone is looking at lower organisms, but the technology is available.

RACAGNI: To improve our understanding of the function of the different receptors, we should study further the neuroanatomical distribution of the receptors, both at the pre- and post-synaptic levels and in the different brain areas. Do you have any data on that?

PEROUTKA: There have been extensive autoradiographical studies of human and rat brain (Pazos *et al.* 1987*a,b*). The measurement of mRNA expression levels is even more interesting. Expression of the 5-HT_{1C} receptor, for example, is much more widespread and dense throughout the brain than that of the 5-HT_2 receptor (Molineaux *et al.* 1989). This combination of autoradiography (showing where the receptors are) and molecular biology techniques (showing where the receptors are expressed) is a powerful anatomical approach.

MELTZER: You did not mention the possible implication of 5-HT_2 receptors in schizophrenia. It has been suggested that selective 5-HT_2 antagonists may be useful in negative symptoms, and that antagonism at 5-HT_2 rather than dopamine$_2$ (DA$_2$) receptors distinguishes atypical from typical drugs.

How much can we conclude from 'dirty' drugs, specifically mixed antagonists at various types of 5-HT receptors? There may be functional interaction between the subtypes; a drug which blocks 5-HT_{1A} and 5-HT_2 receptors at the same time will give a very misleading picture if there are synergistic or antagonistic actions betwen the two receptors. Given that all the available drugs are relatively non-specific, we could be mistaken in our estimates of the functional importance of these receptors until we understand these interactions.

PEROUTKA: That is a good point. There may be some optimal combination. Methysergide does many things besides antagonizing 5-HT_2 receptors. But chlorpromazine is fairly selective in blocking 5-HT_{1C} and 5-HT_2 receptors compared to other 5-HT receptor subtypes. It does, however, interact with many other non-5-HT receptors.

MELTZER: There is great emphasis on synergistic/antagonistic actions of DA$_1$ and DA$_2$ receptors, but relatively little work on this has been done in the serotonin field where there is ample opportunity for interaction.

PEROUTKA: That is probably because there are only two types of dopamine receptor, whereas there are seven or eight subtypes of 5-HT receptor, making it difficult to study synergism. We have found single neurones in layer IV cortex with both 5-HT_{1A} and 5-HT_2 receptors. That is clearly a place where synergistic receptor actions can affect the system. For example, LSD activates 5-HT_{1A} receptors, but is essentially a pure antagonist at 5-HT_2 receptors. Thus, this drug is activating a neurone via one 5-HT receptor subtype and blocking the effect of the natural transmitter on a second subtype.

SANDLER: Humphrey and his colleagues (see, for example, Humphrey *et al.* 1990) suggest that sumatriptan (GR 43175) has sites of action other than the 5-HT_{1D} site.

PEROUTKA: We have not determined exactly what sumatriptan does. It clearly acts at 5-HT_{1D} receptors in certain systems. The ergots and sumatriptan are equipotent clinically and their affinity for the 5-HT_{1D} receptor is identical (McCarthy and Peroutka 1989). It appears that they are similar in terms of anti-migraine efficacy, and only the 5-HT_{1D} site ties them together at the receptor level so far.

GLOVER: Are all the 5-HT receptors directly linked to 5-HT neurones, either pre- or post-synaptically? With regard to understanding the pathogenesis of migraine it is of interest to know whether the 5-HT could come from platelets and act on a receptor in blood vessels.

PEROUTKA: The 5-HT_{1A}, 5-HT_{1B}, 5-HT_{1D}, and 5-HT_3 receptors are on serotonergic terminals and are post-synaptic. The 5-HT_2 receptor is the only one that has not been shown to exist on 5-HT-containing neurones. The receptors are also located on platelets, blood vessels, and muscle.

GLOVER: What is their function when they are not linked to 5-HT neurones?

PEROUTKA: On platelets, they modulate platelet shape changes and aggregation; on muscle cells, they induce contraction or relaxation.

RACAGNI: Patients are given serotonergic drugs for varying lengths of time. Therefore, it is important to understand the adaptive changes of the receptors. In animal models these seem to differ from the classic response. After lesion of serotonergic neurones the classic increase of the 5-HT$_2$ receptors does not occur. On the other hand, when an antagonist is used there is a down-regulation of the receptor.

PEROUTKA: The classical idea is that antagonists should increase receptor density and agonists should decrease receptor density. That occurs in certain serotonergic systems, but it is not a rule.

EVENDEN: There seems to be a dissociation between the binding characteristics and functional effects of 8-hydroxy-N,N-dipropyl-2-aminotetralin (8-OH-DPAT), such as the 5-HT syndrome (forepaw treading and long body) and hypothermia. The functional effects show very rapid tolerance; there is considerable tolerance to the hypothermic effects of 8-OH-DPAT after only a single injection of a dose as low as 0.1 mg kg^{-1} (personal observation). In contrast, after one week of treatment (1.0 mg kg^{-1}, twice daily) there are no effects on pre- or post-synaptic 5-HT$_{1A}$ receptors or on 5-HT synthesis and turnover (Larsson *et al.* 1990). The 5-HT neurones and receptors appear to be resistant to change, whereas the behavioural effects change very rapidly.

SULSER: We have tended to emphasize only binding. Other receptor domains might be as important as the binding domains, if not more so. In β-adrenoceptors, for example, the intracytoplasmic loop 3 is essential in linking the receptor via the G-protein to the effector system (adenylate cyclase). Thus, changes in functional characteristics can be the consequences of changes in the efficacy of coupling of the receptors, with no change to the binding characteristics. We should learn not to look only at the binding of agonists or antagonists to the receptor. The functional domains of the receptor are more important because they determine the functional consequences of signal transduction.

PEROUTKA: Lithium is geared to modulate intracellular effects of drugs. However, from the pharmaceutical viewpoint, it is much easier to modulate the receptor than to modulate intracellular systems. We still have a long way to go at the receptor level. Despite the progress in the past decade, we are far from having selective tools for each of the 5-HT receptor subtypes, except the 5-HT$_3$ receptor, for which there are proven selective antagonists.

CARLSSON: 5-HT has very different affinities for the 5-HT$_1$ and 5-HT$_2$ receptors. How do you reconcile this with the possibility of both being synaptic? Should not the concentrations of the neurotransmitter in a synapse be similar in various parts of the brain? What are the currently accepted values for the affinity of 5-HT for the 5-HT$_1$ and the 5-HT$_2$ receptors?

PEROUTKA: The published values for the affinity of 5-HT for its putative receptors vary between 1 nM and 2800 nM. There is a clear spectrum of affinities in the order 5-HT$_{1A}$>5-HT$_{1B}$>5-HT$_{1D}$>5-HT$_{1C}$>5-HT$_3$>5-HT$_2$. 5-HT, in general, is present *in vivo* at nanomolar concentrations. I would speculate that the 5-HT$_1$ receptor family is a tonically active system. The 5-HT$_2$ and 5-HT$_3$ receptors, having lower affinities for 5-HT, may be classical synapse receptors involving vesicular release of 5-HT.

FRAZER: The difference in the affinity of 5-HT for the 5-HT$_1$ and the 5-HT$_2$ receptors may be more apparent than real; it may reflect the tools available when that work was done. ^{3}H-5-HT, which is an agonist, was used for the 5-HT$_1$ receptors, whereas spiperone, which is an antagonist, was used for the 5-HT$_2$ receptors. Consequently, the affinities of agonists for the 5-HT$_1$ receptors were for the 'ternary complex' or 'high affinity' state of that receptor, but the affinities of agonists for the 5-HT$_2$

receptor were for the low affinity state. Now that $5\text{-}HT_2$ agonists, such as 4-methyl-2, 5-dimethoxyamphetamine (DOM) or 4-iodo-2,5-dimethoxyamphetamine (DOI), have been developed, we see that 5-HT has an affinity of less than 10 nM when one labels with an agonist. Given that there are many affinity states, whether an agonist or antagonist radioligand is used can influence the apparent affinity of 5-HT for the receptor.

CARLSSON: From the physiological point of view, one should use 5-HT to determine affinity. In that case there is a difference.

PEROUTKA: Functionally, there is clearly a difference. $5\text{-}HT_{1A}$ receptor models are activated by nanomolar concentrations of 5-HT; $5\text{-}HT_2$ receptor models are activated by micromolar concentrations of 5-HT; and $5\text{-}HT_3$ models come in the mid-range.

FRAZER: I did not mean to imply that high affinity binding corresponds to functional effects. I wish to emphasize that binding data in isolation must be interpreted cautiously. Nevertheless, even at the functional level there might not be much difference—perhaps just several-fold—in 5-HT's potency to elicit $5\text{-}HT_1$ and $5\text{-}HT_2$-mediated responses. In general, it appears that EC_{50} values of 5-HT to elicit $5\text{-}HT_2$-mediated responses are in the micromolar range. However, this may reflect, in part, desensitization of this receptor during some assays, for example during one hour of transmitter action. In contrast, in a carefully controlled study using the isolated rabbit aorta, Clancy and Maayani (1985) found the EC_{50} value for 5-HT to elicit contraction (a $5\text{-}HT_2$ response) to be about 50 nM. This is about 40 times lower (i.e., higher affinity) than 5-HT's affinity for the $5\text{-}HT_2$ receptor as measured with labelled antagonists, and about 10 times greater (i.e., lower affinity) than that measured against labelled agonists. The EC_{50} of 5-HT in eliciting $5\text{-}HT_{1A}$-mediated responses, for example inhibition of adenylate cyclase, is about 50–100 nM, about 10–50 times higher (i.e., lower affinity) than its K_i value for this receptor when measured using a labelled agonist. Thus, although 5-HT may have somewhat greater potency at $5\text{-}HT_1$ than at $5\text{-}HT_2$ receptors, the difference may be less than an order of magnitude and not greater than two orders of magnitude as was originally surmised from binding data using radiolabelled antagonists for the $5\text{-}HT_2$ receptor and agonists for the $5\text{-}HT_1$ receptor.

CARLSSON: A related question is the so-called problem of mismatch. How does the distribution of post-synaptic receptors match with the occurrence of nerve terminals?

PEROUTKA: It matches poorly. It is difficult to find synapses. In layer IV of somatosensory cortex there are clearly receptors for 5-HT, but you do not see the true synaptic connections that are observed in other systems. I don't know what to make of that.

GLOVER: It is puzzling that the distribution of the $5\text{-}HT_2$ receptors is the least linked to synapses but their micromolar affinity would make them most suited to being post-synaptic.

Are there any data about endogenous factors other than 5-HT modulating any of the 5-HT receptors?

PEROUTKA: People have hypothesized that tryptamine, various tryptophols, and even different peptides may be endogenous modulators of 5-HT receptor subtypes. It is possible, but there is no hard evidence that such systems exist, except tryptamine-binding sites, which may or may not be related to 5-HT systems.

SANDLER: A new potent *agonist* at $5\text{-}HT_3$ sites, *m*-chlorophenylbiguanide, was reported recently (Kilpatrick *et al.* 1990).

PEROUTKA: That will be useful, but to date all available potent 5-HT$_3$ agents are antagonists.

DOOGAN: Is there any way of predicting whether a compound is an antagonist or an agonist?

PEROUTKA: We have hypotheses concerning 5-HT$_{1A}$ and 5-HT$_3$ receptors that need to be proved. We tend to think of a drug being either an agonist or an antagonist, but there is a clear spectrum. At least with the 5-HT$_{1A}$ receptor, there is a wide range of agonist activities. Is buspirone having a neuropsychiatric effect because it is a 30 per cent agonist? If you made a 50 per cent agonist, would it be better or worse? We should think in terms of percentage efficacies. At the 5-HT$_2$ receptor, 5-HT is 100 per cent; DOB and DOI are 50–80 per cent; and LSD is 10–30 per cent. Does the uniqueness of a drug effect come from its relative efficacy more than from its affinity? That is another area of research that is ripe for development.

DOOGAN: We are producing more specific drugs and discovering more receptors, but clinically we are lagging behind. We have shown improved efficacy with 5-HT specific drugs in obsessive-compulsive disorder and perhaps panic disorder, but we still produce the same levels of efficacy as 20 years ago with tricyclic antidepressants in anxiety and depression.

PEROUTKA: Although in some diseases we have not done much better in the past decade, we have improved significantly in many other areas.

GOTTFRIES: Do you have data on the sensitivity to ageing of the different receptors? Marcusson *et al.* (1987) found in post-mortem studies that after the age of 60 there is a slight decrease in 5-HT$_1$ receptors and a greater decrease in 5-HT$_2$ receptors. Ageing and dementia will be important aspects in this area in the 1990s.

PEROUTKA: We have not looked specifically at that. I agree that this will be an important matter in the future. As a neurologist, I like to think that we have degenerative diseases for every system: Parkinson's for dopamine; Shy Drager for adrenaline; Alzheimer's for acetylcholine. But what is the ageing disease for the serotonin system? There must be people who lose their 5-HT system disproportionately, just as people lose their dopamine systems.

PALFREYMAN: In lesion studies, if cholinergic neurotoxins are combined with serotonergic neurotoxins they produce dramatic effects on learning and memory in animals (Vanderwolf 1987). The potential of dual lesions should be pursued further.

OXENKRUG: I like the suggestion that we can expect a disease for every system. We might not live long enough to get the serotonin disease. In depression we might see something which we would all have if we lived to be more than 100.

PEROUTKA: But depression and sleep disturbances in the elderly are disproportionately common and we have not linked them clearly with any system. Also, they are reversible in a sense.

COWEN: The majority of 5-HT$_{1A}$ receptors are located post-synaptically. It seems that 5-HT$_{1A}$ receptor activation causes hyperpolarization, that is, an inhibition of cell firing. How does that fit with some of the functional effects of the 5-HT$_{1A}$ agonists, such as the 5-HT behavioural syndrome?

PEROUTKA: The system is so complex that it is impossible to make any inference on the net behavioural outcome of a neuronal membrane effect. I don't think there is a direct linkage between a single 5-HT receptor and a behaviour, except perhaps in the head twitch response. Otherwise, there are probably many other systems involved in 5-HT-mediated behaviours.

CARLSSON: I agree. Glutamate, the excitatory neurotransmitter, is necessary for induction of the akinesia seen in Parkinson's disease and after neuroleptic drugs

(Carlsson and Carlsson 1989), but by giving an antagonist to glutamate receptors you can induce movement again. That is a complicated system. In chains of GABA neurones, it makes a difference whether there is an odd or even number of neurones.

EVENDEN: Pharmacologists often talk as if there is one neurone, with all these receptors on it, rather than many different types of neurones, many of which are 5-HT mediated and interconnected with all other types of neurones. The simplistic idea of 'the 5-HT neurone' does not bear any relation to reality.

PEROUTKA: The system is clearly extremely complex. The β receptors on the heart provided a simple model system where one can truly measure drug–receptor interactions. This may have led people to think that there would be neuronal systems for which we would find one function. That is not the case.

SANDLER: How do you see this field progressing?

PEROUTKA: We should move away from animal receptors and prepare human cell lines that express receptors. The species differences are too dramatic for us to ignore. The drug companies that invested in the $5-HT_{1B}$ receptor probably wasted their money and effort. First we shall have to prove that human receptors expressed in cell lines are the same as those in the human brain. Then we shall have a renewable source.

Secondly, we continue to need better pharmacological tools to differentiate the subtypes. We are using computers to build the receptor structures, and we have hypotheses of where the receptors are linking with the drugs. Ultimately, we should be able to show a picture of the receptor and the exact location of the drug action.

PALFREYMAN: The available $5-HT_2$ antagonists have a fairly consistent effect on slow-wave sleep, both in animals and humans. Might some of the 'human pharmacology' seen with these drugs be a consequence of a more fundamental interaction, such as on sleep, which has an impact on behaviour at a later stage?

PEROUTKA: That is possible and needs to be investigated. Amitriptyline is probably one of the best prophylactic anti-migraine drugs. It is also very sedative and may simply be allowing patients to sleep well. For learning and memory disorders also one can argue that poor sleep might be the critical feature.

COPPEN: How do you forsee our progress in the study of human disease, for example depression? Once you have a specific agonist for human 5-HT receptors, how would you study its behavioural effect in humans?

PEROUTKA: First we would use animal models of depression, which exist but are not very good. Then we would move into humans. 3,4-Methylene dioxymethamphetamine (MDMA, Ecstasy) could be argued to have good antidepressant effects, but it is neurotoxic. Theoretically, that drug is having its acute antidepressant effect by a surge in the brain concentrations of 5-HT. A drug that could cause such a surge without being toxic might be a useful acute antidepressant.

COPPEN: Is there a way of evaluating 5-HT receptors in man?

PEROUTKA: We are trying to do that with positron emission tomography (PET).

MELTZER: We shall not appreciate the significance of these receptors until we study the drugs in man. For example, *m*-chlorophenylpiperazine (*m*-CPP) and MK 212 looked similar in *in vitro* binding studies but differ greatly in man. The clinical condition seems to influence strongly the effect of the drug.

The interaction between the pharmaceutical industry and academia is important here. Commercial potential *per se* may not justify proceeding with the studies to the point where the drug can safely be put in man, and yet the information is crucial for further research. Often development stops too early for us to be able to use the agents fully.

PEROUTKA: There has been much serendipitous progress in human 5-HT neuropharmacology. For example, the use of propranolol for migraine was discovered in angina patients. Also, nobody would have predicted Dennis Murphy's observations with migraine and *m*-CPP.

COPPEN: The history of the treatment of depression is a series of unexpected observations. However, it is more difficult now to make that sort of observation because research is controlled in a more rigid way.

PEROUTKA: That is simply because of the expense of bringing a drug to human use; drug regulatory trials require millions of dollars.

CARLSSON: The pharmaceutical industry spends too much time on animal models which have never been tested seriously. When we have a new pharmacological mechanism, it would be better to do the necessary safety studies and then move to man.

EVENDEN: Those of us working with animal models in the pharmaceutical industry have often believed the same thing. However, a drug company requires good reason to invest millions of dollars. If we have ten drugs with nice receptor profiles we cannot put several million dollars into each of them in the hope that one is a hit. Animal models provide a method of picking out drugs that are more likely to succeed. Unfortunately, because the animal models may not allow very good predictions, the process may be more random than one would like. Nevertheless, the function of animal models is to reduce the huge range of options for antidepressant or anti-anxiety drugs to a manageable number.

PALFREYMAN: The ability to follow up receptor or biochemical leads in man is important. If one can do this, the animal models of disease become less critical. For example, there is no easy animal or human test to validate the hypothesis that a drug will be useful against depression. However, if there was a test to see if a drug were, say, a 5-HT$_2$ antagonist in man and to study the tolerability, we would obtain quickly the impetus for further research.

One way of doing this might be to have a better handle on CNS activity with PET or SPECT (single-photon emission computed tomography) ligands. Another promising method is quantitative electroencephalography.

ROBINSON: The pharmaceutical industry is moving away from behavioural models; we are very influenced by receptor characteristics and molecular pharmacology.

CARLSSON: I was talking primarily about disease models. Animal experiments are extremely important at this time because binding data only tell us affinities. We have to discover whether a drug is an agonist or antagonist, and it is even more difficult to test the intrinsic efficacy. Many of the agonists are not full agonists; they might be agonists in one part of the brain and antagonists in another place. Animal experimentation is necessary to sort this out and to interpret feedback from the clinic.

References

Carlsson, M. and Carlsson, A. (1989). The NMDA antagonist MK-801 causes marked locomotor stimulation in monoamine-depleted mice. *Journal of Neural Transmission*, **75**, 221–6.

Clancy, B. and Maayani, S. (1985). 5-Hydroxytryptamine receptor in isolated rabbit aorta: characterization with tryptamine analogs. *Journal of Pharmacology and Experimental Therapeutics*, **233**, 761–9.

Dumuis, A., Sebben, M., and Bockaert, J. (1989). The gastrointestinal prokinetic benzamide derivatives are agonists at the non-classical 5-HT receptor (5-HT$_4$) positively coupled to adenylate cyclase in neurons. *Naunyn-Schmiedeberg's Archives of Pharmacology*, **340**, 403–10.

Hartig, P. R. (1989). Molecular biology of serotonin receptors: an overview. *Abstracts, American College of Neuropsychopharmacology*, **28**, 40.

Hoyer, D., Vos, P., Palacios, J. M., Engel, G., and Davies, H. (1987). [^{3}H]Ketanserin labels serotonin 5-HT$_2$ and alpha$_1$-adrenergic receptors in human brain cortex. *Journal of Cardiovascular Pharmacology*, **10**, S48–S50.

Humphrey, P. P. A., Feniuk, W., and Perren, M. J. (1990). 5-HT in migraine: evidence from 5-HT$_1$-like receptor agonists for a vascular aetiology. In *Migraine: a spectrum of ideas*, (ed. M. Sandler and G. Collins), pp. 147–68. Oxford University Press.

Kilpatrick, G. J., Butler A., Burridge, J., and Oxford A. W. (1990). *m*-Chlorophenyl-biguanide, a potent high affinity 5-HT$_3$ receptor agonist. *European Journal of Pharmacology*, **182**, 193–8.

Larsson, L-G., Renyi, L., Ross, S. B., Svensson, B., and Ängeby-Möller, K. (1990). Different effects on the functional pre- and post-synaptic 5-HT$_{1A}$ receptor responses by repeated treatments of rats with the 5-HT$_{1A}$ receptor agonist 8-OH-DPAT. *Neuropharmacology*, in press.

Leonhardt, S., Herrick-Davis, K., and Titeler, M. (1989). Detection of a novel serotonin receptor subtype (5-HT$_{1E}$) in human brain: interaction with a GTP-binding protein. *Journal of Neurochemistry*, **53**, 465–71.

Marcusson, J., Alafuzoff, I., Bäckström, I. T., Ericson, E., Gottfries, C. G., and Winblad, B. (1987). 5-Hydroxytryptamine-sensitive [^{3}H]imipramine binding of protein nature in the human brain. II. Effect of normal ageing and dementia disorders. *Brain Research*, **425**, 137–45.

Mawe, G. M., Branchek, T. A., and Gershon, M. D. (1986). Peripheral neural serotonin receptors: identification and characterization with specific antagonists and agonists. *Proceedings of the National Academy of Sciences USA*, **83**, 9799–803.

McCarthy, B. G. and Peroutka, A. J. (1989). Comparative neuropharmacology of dihydroergotamine and sumatriptan (GR 43175). *Headache*, **29**, 420–2.

Molineaux, S. M., Jessel, T. M., Axel, R., and Julius D. (1989). 5-HT$_{1C}$ receptor is a prominent serotonin receptor subtype in the central nervous system. *Proceedings of the National Academy of Sciences USA*, **86**, 6793–7.

Pazos, A., Probst, A., and Palacios, J. M. (1987*a*). Serotonin receptors in the human brain. III. Autoradiographic mapping of serotonin-1 receptors. *Neuroscience*, **21**, 97–122.

Pazos, A., Probst, A., and Palacios, J. M. (1987*b*). Serotonin receptors in the human brain. IV. Autoradiographic mapping of serotonin-2 receptors. *Neuroscience*, **21**, 123–39.

Vanderwolf, C. H. (1987). Near-total loss of 'learning' and 'memory' as a result of combined cholinergic and serotonergic blockade in the rat. *Behavioural Brain Research*, **23**, 43–57.

Xiong, W. and Nelson, D. L. (1989). Characterization of a [^{3}H]-5-hydroxytryptamine binding site in rabbit caudate nucleus that differs from the 5-HT$_{1A}$, 5-HT$_{1B}$, 5-HT$_{1C}$ and 5-HT$_{1D}$ subtypes. *Life Sciences*, **45**, 1433–42.

3. An overview of serotonin neurochemistry and neuroanatomy

Dennis L. Murphy

In the past decade, the predominant focus of basic science and clinical investigations of serotonergic neurotransmission has been the many serotonin (5-hydroxytryptamine, 5-HT) receptors and their signal transduction mechanisms. A survey of the papers presented at three major international symposia held in Florence, New York, and Maui in 1989, which were wholly devoted to serotonin, revealed that over 80 per cent of the papers concerned the explosion of new knowledge about serotonin receptor subtypes and receptor-selective drugs.

Fewer, and perhaps less remarkable, advances have occurred in other areas of investigation of serotonin neurochemistry. This literature is, nonetheless, voluminous, and this chapter can only highlight a few developments that seem of special relevance for consideration of the possible role of serotonergic neurotransmission in different neuropsychiatric disorders and their treatment. Some recent and other older, but still valuable, monographs and reviews should be consulted for coverage in depth of these and related issues (Barchas and Usdin 1973; Jacobs and Gelperin 1981; Ho *et al.* 1982; Osborne 1982; Green 1985; Baumgarten and Lachenmayer 1985; Kuhn *et al.* 1986; Osborne and Hamon 1988; Rech and Gudelsky 1988; Fozard 1989; Paoletti and Vanhoute 1990; Coccaro and Murphy 1990).

The 'model serotonin neurone' and serotonin neuroanatomy

Simple model diagrams of 'the serotonin neurone', as depicted in Fig. 3.1, display some important features of a neurone but need to be supplemented by much other information. As is well known, but nonetheless often underemphasized, conceptualizations based on such oversimplified diagrams can be seriously erroneous.

For example, recent developments in serotonin neuroanatomy and neurophysiology have clarified earlier data by suggesting that cell bodies and projections from different raphe nuclei have different characteristics. In serotonin projection areas of the rat brain, two major classes of 5-HT axon terminals are found. These differ in axon morphology, cells of origin, regional

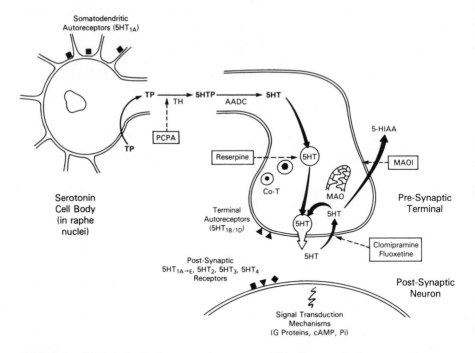

FIG. 3.1. Model of a brain serotonin neurone. This diagram depicts many elements common to serotonin neurones, but, in its necessary oversimplification, is also seriously misleading. There are, in fact, different types of serotonin neurones with different microanatomy, different co-transmitters (both neuropeptides and mono-amines), and different post-synaptic receptors on different target neurone cell bodies and terminals. TP, L-tryptophan; 5-HTP, 5-hydroxytryptophan; 5-HT, 5-hydroxy-tryptamine (serotonin); Co-T, co-transmitters and modulators, such as neuropeptides and monoamines other than serotonin; TH, tryptophan hydroxylase; AADC, L-amino acid decarboxylase; MAO, monoamine oxidase; MAOI, monoamine oxidase inhibitors; cAMP, cyclic adenosine monophosphate; Pi, phosphatidylinositol; PCPA, *para*-chlorophenylalanine.

distribution, and responses to neurotoxic and other drugs. Axons from the dorsal raphe nucleus (DRN), to the frontal cortex, for example, are very fine, with small varicosities, and are highly vulnerable to damage by *para*-chloroamphetamine, 3,4-methylene dioxyamphetamine (MDA), and 3,4-methylene dioxymethamphetamine (MDMA). In contrast, axons from the median raphe nucleus (MRN) to the parietal cortex, hippocampus, and lateral hypothalamus have large varicosities and are resistant to the neuro-toxic substituted amphetamines (Conrad *et al.* 1974; Moore and Halaris 1975; Kohler and Steinbusch 1982; Kosofsky and Molliver 1987; Molliver 1987; O'Hearn *et al.* 1988; Mamounas and Molliver 1988; Fritschy *et al.* 1988). Fine axonal projections from the DRN in layer Va of the rat somatosensory cortex are closely associated with a high density of 5-HT$_2$ binding sites in autoradiographical studies, suggesting that 5-HT$_2$ receptors may be selectively linked in this area to one type of serotonin neurone (Blue *et al.* 1988).

The evidence from neuroanatomical studies that there are different subclasses of serotonin neurones in brain is supported by some neurophysiological and neuropharmacological data. For example, the 5-HT$_{1A}$ partial agonists, 8-hydroxy-*N,N*-dipropyl-2-aminotetralin (8-OH-DPAT) or ipsapirone, are known to slow raphe serotonin neurone firing rates in a dose-dependent manner; however, the 8-OH-DPAT dose (ED$_{50}$) required to produce the slowing effect in the MRN is 30 times higher than that required for the same effect in the DRN (Sinton and Fallon 1988). Moreover, a range of doses of another serotonergic agent, trifluoromethylphenylpiperazine (TFMPP), yielded no consistent effects on cell firing rates in the DRN, but increased firing rates in the MRN in a dose-dependent manner (Sinton and Fallon 1988). The serotonin-selective tricyclic, clomipramine, affects serotonin turnover in the MRN more than in the DRN (Meek and Lofstrandh 1974).

In other experiments, direct application of 8-OH-DPAT or 5-HT to the MRN stimulated rat locomotor activity and exploratory behaviour, but similar results were not observed with applications to the DRN (Hillegaart *et al.* 1989; Carli and Samanin 1988; Hillegaart and Hjorth 1989). These results may be related to data from earlier studies indicating that electrolytic lesions of the MRN reduced 5-HT concentrations in the hippocampus by 82 per cent, while lesions of the DRN produced 5-HT reductions of only 10 per cent, although 5-HT reductions in the cortex and striatum (30–40 per cent) and hypothalamus (60 per cent) were similar after MRN and DRN lesions (Jacobs *et al.* 1974). Electrolytic lesions of the MRN, but not the DRN or control lesions in another brain area, produced sustained, 100 per cent increases in locomotor activity in rats; these changes were similar to those which followed lesions placed directly in the dorsal hippocampus, in agreement with the relative effects of MRN and DRN lesions on 5-HT concentrations in the hippocampus and a proposed role for modulation of locomotor activity by hippocampal 5-HT (Jacobs *et al.* 1974, 1975).

The extent to which these examples of differences in structure and function of the DRN and the MRN have implications for the other B1–B9 grouping of serotonin cell bodies in the raphe and non-raphe areas of the rodent brain is not yet clear, although there is considerable evidence that the descending and ascending projections from these different serotonergic cell body groups mediate different physiological and behavioural functions, and other evidence of functional differences among different ascending 5-HT projections (Consolazione and Cuello 1982; Azmitia 1987).

While evidence for multiple serotonin neuronal subsystems is accumulating from studies in rodents, less is known about primate, including human, brain serotonin subsystems. Some general similarities exist between rat and primate serotonin neuroanatomy, but there are some substantial differences (Azmitia

1987; Takeuchi 1988). In rats, the majority of serotonergic cell body groups are indeed in the raphe nuclei, with cells clustered tightly in the midline; in primates, relatively few cells lie directly in the midline—the cells are more scattered, with a paramedian organization. While the DRN is the most prominent nuclear group in the rat, the MRN equivalent in primates (the nucleus centralis superior, with its dorsalis portion) is larger and comprises the major group of ascending serotonin neurones. In primates, the dorsal raphe cortical tract contains more ascending fibres than the median forebrain bundle, the reverse of the situation in the rat. Also, there are more myelinated 5-HT fibres (approximately 25 per cent) in primates than in rats (< 1 per cent) (Azmitia 1987; Takeuchi 1988).

Further complexity involving co-transmitters, receptor localization, and serotonin metabolism

Co-localization of neuropeptides and other monoamines in serotonergic neurones

Rodent raphe nuclei contain, in addition to 5-HT, substance P (SP), thyrotropin-releasing hormone (TRH), leucine-enkephalin, methionine-enkephalin, and somatostatin; some of these peptides, including SP, TRH, and enkephalin, as well as γ-aminobutyric acid, coexist in the same cells with 5-HT (Johansson *et al.* 1981; Belin *et al.* 1983; Bowker *et al.* 1983).

The full significance of 5-HT and neuropeptide coexistence is not yet understood, but there appear to be subpopulations of 5-HT neurones which contain one or another neuropeptide. It has been suggested that the released co-transmitters might affect different target cells or modify the activities of the same target neurones in different fashions, including, perhaps, different effects at pre-synaptic and post-synaptic sites (Bowker *et al.* 1983). Under some circumstances, 5-HT and SP have been found to mutually reverse each other's excitatory effects, as studied using intracellular electrodes in the rat nucleus tractus solitarius (Jacquin *et al.* 1989).

In addition to neuropeptides, certain monoamines, including dopamine, tyramine, and adrenaline, can be accumulated in 5-HT-containing cells; likewise, 5-HT can be taken up, stored, and released from sympathetic nerves (Sah and Matsumoto 1987; Schmidt and Lovenberg 1985; Verbeuren 1989).

Quantitative estimates of elements of serotonin terminals in brain

Some attempts to obtain quantitative information on 5-HT concentrations in relation to numbers of serotonin terminals or varicosities and numbers of receptor binding sites may ultimately help us to unravel some of the complexities of serotonergic neurotransmission. However, some findings

TABLE 3.1. *Number of 5-HT axon terminals (varicosities) in rat brain estimated using 5-HT immunocytochemistry and electron microscopy in several sections*

Brain area	Density of varicosities per mm^3	Proportion of varicosities making a synaptic junction
Neocortex	5.8×10^6	30–40%
Neostriatum	2.6×10^6	~20%
Hippocampus	2.7×10^6	'Exceedingly low'

Adapted from Descarries (1990).

have raised new questions as well. Current estimates (Table 3.1) indicate similar numbers of 5-HT varicosities in three brain regions, but a considerable difference in the number of varicosities that appear to make synaptic junctional connections; most serotonergic varicosities do not make such connections (Descarries 1990). According to a series of papers (Audet *et al.* 1988, 1989; Doucet *et al.* 1988), rat cortex possesses approximately 500 000 5-HT terminals for each cell body in the dorsal and median raphe nucleus. There are approximately 200 5-HT terminals for each target cortical neurone, and one 5-HT terminal per 200 cortical neurone terminals. There are 2000–8000 5-HT$_2$ ([^{3}H]ketanserin) binding sites and 400–6200 uptake sites (labelled with [^{3}H]paroxetine or [^{3}H]cyanoimipramine) per each cortical 5-HT terminal. 5-HT concentrations in rat cortex varicosities are approximately 3 mM; similar concentrations were reported previously for 5-HT in human platelets, and 5-HT concentrations in platelet storage vesicles were estimated to be as high as 0.6 M (Costa *et al.* 1978).

Multiple synaptic and non-synaptic serotonergic terminals

Despite the fact that direct synaptic contacts may be the exception rather than the rule for 5-HT neurones (only 5 to 40 per cent of 5-HT varicosities appear to make synaptic junctions), there is evidence from studies of invertebrate (aplysia) serotonin neurones that when one serotonin neurone is stimulated it can evoke excitatory responses at some target cells and two different types of inhibitory responses at others (Gerschenfeld and Paupardin-Tritsch 1974). The serotonin uptake inhibitor, clomipramine, increased both the amplitude and duration of the excitatory post-synaptic potentials evoked by stimulation of the 5-HT neurone in aplysia, but failed to alter the amplitude of the inhibitory post-synaptic potentials; the enhancement was attributed to uptake blockade, whereas the failure to affect inhibitory responses was attributed to a 5-HT receptor-blocking action of the drug (Gerschenfeld *et al.* 1978). In another study using intracellular recording of rat single cortical pyramidal cells, evidence was found for two distinct, functional 5-HT receptors on the same cell (Davies *et al.* 1987). Activation

TABLE 3.2. *Regional localization of [³H]imipramine-, [³H]cyanoimipramine-, and [³H]paroxetine-binding sites in rat and human brain*

	Rats		Humans	
	[³H]IMI* (fmol mm⁻²)	[³H]CN-IMI[†] (fmol per mg protein)	[³H]IMI[§] (fmol per mg protein)	[³H]PAR[§] (fmol per mg protein)
Frontal cortex	0.052	610	371	307
Caudate	0.150	313	523	355
Hippocampus	0.192	–	453	–
Globus pallidus	0.198	441	502	235
Amygdala	0.257	–	491	–
Substantia nigra	0.434	2403	800	723
Median raphe	0.393	–	1560	1600
Dorsal raphe	0.660	3258	2400	1990

Adapted from: *Fuxe *et al*. 1983; [†]Kavachich *et al*. 1988; [§]Cortes *et al*. 1988.

of these two receptors by 5-HT produced opposing effects on membrane potentials and conductance. A depolarizing effect of 5-HT (probably produced by decreasing a resting K^+ conductance) was blocked by ritanserin and cinanserin. A hyperpolarizing effect of 5-HT associated with a state of increased conductance was insensitive to these 5-HT_2 antagonists, but could be mimicked by 8-OH-DPAT (Davies *et al*. 1987).

Serotonin transport and the tricyclic binding site

Much remains unknown about many aspects of the sequence of steps involved in serotonin re-uptake, which is the major mechanism for inactivating released serotonin. The release process itself also remains unclear. One issue has been clarified, however. It now appears that the tricyclic antidepressant-binding site, which was once thought to be a closely associated modulatory site, separate from the serotonin uptake site, is the same as the uptake site: [³H]paroxetine and other highly selective ligands for what was originally described as the [³H]imipramine-binding site bind directly and solely to the serotonin uptake site itself (Marcusson *et al*. 1988, 1989; Graham *et al*. 1989).

Significant progress has been made towards the purification of the serotonin uptake site (Graham and Langer 1988), but molecular biological studies have not yet been reported. Autoradiography using [³H]paroxetine and other ligands (Table 3.2) has revealed considerable diversity in the numbers of binding sites in different brain areas (Fuxe *et al*. 1983; Kovachich *et al*. 1988). Similar results have been obtained in human brain (Cortes *et al*. 1988; Plenge *et al*. 1990). Cortical areas contain relatively few sites, whereas the substantia nigra, among different projection areas, contains a relatively high number of sites. The raphe nuclei possess the highest density of sites, a finding interpreted as reflecting the possibility that the entire serotonin neurone— not only terminals but also the cell body dendrites and axons—possesses serotonin uptake capacity (Fuxe *et al.* 1983). That would seem to allow speculation about effects of uptake-inhibiting drugs directly on the 5-HT cell body as well as at terminals.

Synthetic and degradatory enzymes for serotonin

Tryptophan hydroxylase, the principal enzyme in serotonin synthesis, has been cloned and sequenced from preparations of rat and rabbit pineal bodies; the enzyme shows considerable homology with phenylalanine hydroxylase (58 per cent identity) and tyrosine hydroxylase (46 per cent identity), and has been mapped to the human chromosome 11 (Darmon *et al.* 1986, 1988; Grenett *et al.* 1987; Ledley *et al.* 1987).

Aromatic L-amino acid decarboxylase (AADC), which converts 5-hydroxytryptophan (5-HTP) to 5-HT, appears to be a single enzyme serving general decarboxylase functions in neuronal (brain, adrenal) and non-neuronal (liver, kidney) tissues; this conclusion is based on an aggregate of studies of immunological cross-reactivity, molecular size, and biochemical properties. Hybridization analysis using a cDNA probe complementary to bovine adrenal AADC mRNA indicated the presence of a single mRNA in these different tissues (Albert *et al.* 1987; Shirota and Fujisawa 1988). Southern blot analysis of bovine genomic DNA suggests that a single gene codes for AADC (Albert *et al.* 1987).

Monoamine oxidase (MAO), the principal degradatory enzyme for serotonin, exists in two forms, MAO-A and MAO-B. While serotonin is a better substrate for MAO-A than MAO-B, serotonin cell bodies in brain and in human platelets (which selectively take up and store serotonin) contain MAO-B either exclusively or predominately (Thorpe *et al.* 1987; Donnelly and Murphy 1977). Nonetheless, there is functional evidence that serotonergic synaptosomes preferentially deaminate 5-HT by MAO-A (Ross 1987). Both MAO-A and MAO-B have been sequenced and cloned, and it is now clear that they are encoded by separate genes located closely together on the short arm of the X-chromosome (Hsu *et al.* 1989). Humans with an X-chromosome deletion who lack both forms of MAO have markedly reduced urinary concentrations of deaminated noradrenaline metabolites, but, surprisingly, near normal urinary concentrations of the serotonin metabolite, 5-hydroxyindoleacetic acid (5-HIAA) (Sims *et al.* 1989*a*,*b*; Murphy *et al.* 1990).

Conclusions

There is now a considerable amount of detailed information indicating that there are not only many serotonin receptor subtypes but also many anatomical and functional brain serotonin subsystems. Activation of a given serotonin cell body may lead to very different consequences, depending upon the cell subtypes of origin, their projection networks, their co-transmitter peptides or other co-transmitters and, of course, the multiple pre- and post-synaptic receptors that the transmitter/co-transmitter complex may activate. This complexity of serotonergic subsystems has obvious implications for cautious interpretations of the meaning of any changes in global measures, such as 5-hydroxyindoleacetic acid or 5-HT in brain tissue, cerebrospinal fluid, or other body fluids, 5-HT receptor densities, or responses to 5-HT precursors, such as L-tryptophan. These may reflect the interactive consequences of many changes in the multiple serotonin subsystems.

References

Albert, V. R., Allen, J. M., and Joh, T. H. (1987). A single gene codes for aromatic L-amino acid decarboxylase in both neuronal and non-neuronal tissues. *Journal of Biological Chemistry*, **262**, 9404–11.

Audet, M. A., Doucet, G., Oleskevich, S., and Descarries, L. (1988). Quantified regional and laminar distribution of the noradrenaline innervation in the anterior half of the adult rat cerebral cortex. *Journal of Comparative Neurology*, **274**, 307–18.

Audet, M. A., Descarries, L., and Doucet, G. (1989). Quantified regional and laminar distribution of the serotonin innervation in the anterior half of adult rat cerebral cortex. *Journal of Chemical Neuroanatomy*, **2**, 29–44.

Azmitia, E. C. (1987). The CNS serotonergic system: progression toward a collaborative organization. In *Psychopharmacology: the third generation of progress*, (ed. H. Y. Meltzer), pp. 61–74. Raven Press, New York.

Barchas, J. and Usdin, E. (1973). *Serotonin and behaviour*. Academic Press, New York.

Baumgarten, H. G. and Lachenmayer, L. (1985). Anatomical features and physiological properties of central serotonin neurons. *Pharmacopsychiatry*, **18**, 180–7.

Belin, M. F., Nanopoulos, D., Didier, M., Aguera, M., Steinbusch, H., Verhofstad, A., *et al.* (1983). Immunohistochemical evidence for the presence of gamma-aminobutyric acid and serotonin in one nerve cell. A study on the raphe nuclei of the rat using antibodies to glutamate decarboxylase and serotonin. *Brain Research*, **275**, 329–39.

Blue, M. E., Yagaloff, K. A., Mamounas, L. A., Hartig, P. R., and Molliver, M. E. (1988). Correspondence between 5-HT2 receptors and serotonergic axons in rat neocortex. *Brain Research*, **453**, 315–28.

Bowker, R. M., Westlund, K. N., Sullivan, M. C., Wilber, J. F., and Coulter, J. D. (1983). Descending serotonergic, peptidergic and cholinergic pathways from the raphe nuclei: a multiple transmitter complex. *Brain Research*, **288**, 33–48.

Carli, M. and Samanin, R. (1988). Potential anxiolytic properties of 8-hydroxy-2-(di-N-propylamino)tetralin, a selective serotonin-1A receptor agonist. *Psychopharmacology*, **94**, 84–91.

Conrad, L. C., Leonard, C. M., and Pfaff, D. W. (1974). Connections of the median and dorsal raphe nuclei in the rat: an autoradiographic and degeneration study. *Journal of Comparative Neurology*, **156**, 179–205.

Coccaro, E. F. and Murphy, D. L. (1990). *Serotonin in major psychiatric disorders.* American Psychiatric Press, Washington DC.

Consolazione, A. and Cuello, A. C. (1982). CNS serotonin pathways. In *Biology of serotonergic transmission*, (ed. N. N. Osborne), pp. 29–61. Wiley, Chichester.

Cortes, R., Soriano, E., Pazos, A., Probst, A., and Palacios, J. M. (1988). Autoradiography of antidepressant binding sites in the human brain: localization using [³H]imipramine and [³H]paroxetine. *Neuroscience*, **27**, 473–96.

Costa, J. L., Stark, H., Shafer, B., Corash, L., Smith, M. A., and Murphy, D. L. (1978). Maximal packet size for serotonin in storage vesicles of intact human platelets. *Life Sciences*, **23**, 2193–7.

Darmon, M. C., Grima, B., Cash, C. D., Maitre, M., and Mallet, J. (1986). Isolation of a rat pineal gland cDNA clone homologous to tyrosine and phenylalanine hydroxylases. *FEBS Letters*, **206**, 43–6.

Darmon, M. C., Guibert, B., Leviel, V., Ehret, M., Maitre, M., and Mallet, J. (1988). Sequence of two mRNAs encoding active rat tryptophan hydroxylase. *Journal of Neurochemistry*, **51**, 312–16.

Davies, M. F., Deisz, R. A., Prince, D. A., and Peroutka, S. J. (1987). Two distinct effects of 5-hydroxytryptamine on single cortical neurons. *Brain Research*, **423**, 347–52.

Descarries, L. (1990). Morphology of central serotonin neurons. *Annals of the New York Academy of Science*, in press.

Donnelly, C. H. and Murphy, D. L. (1977). Substrate- and inhibitor-related characteristics of human platelet monoamine oxidase. *Biochemical Pharmacology*, **26**, 853–8.

Doucet, G., Descarries, L., Audet, M. A., Garcia, S., and Berger, B. (1988). Radioautographic method for quantifying regional monoamine innervations in the rat brain. Application to the cerebral cortex. *Brain Research*, **441**, 233–59.

Fozard, J. R. (1989). *The peripheral actions of 5-hydroxytryptamine.* Oxford University Press.

Fritschy, J. M., Lyons, W. E., Molliver, M. E., and Grzanna, R. (1988). Neurotoxic effects of p-chloroamphetamine on the serotoninergic innervation of the trigeminal motor nucleus: a retrograde transport study. *Brain Research*, **473**, 261–70.

Fuxe, K., Calza, L., Benfenati, F., Zini, I., and Agnati, L. F. (1983). Quantitative autoradiographic localization of [³H]imipramine binding sites in the brain of the rat: relationship to ascending 5-hydroxytryptamine neuron systems. *Proceedings of the National Academy of Sciences USA*, **80**, 3836–40.

Gerschenfeld, H. M. and Paupardin-Tritsch, D. (1974). On the transmitter function of 5-hydroxytryptamine at excitatory and inhibitory monosynaptic junctions. *Journal of Physiology*, **243**, 457–81.

Gerschenfeld, H. M., Hamon, M., and Paupardin-Tritsch, D. (1978). Release of endogenous serotonin from two identified serotonin-containing neurones and the physiological role of serotonin re-uptake. *Journal of Physiology*, **274**, 265–78.

Graham, D. and Langer, S. Z. (1988). The neuronal sodium-dependent serotonin transporter: studies with [3H]imipramine and [3H]paroxetine. In *Neuronal serotonin*, (ed. N. N. Osborne and M. Hamon), pp. 367–91. Wiley, Chichester.

Graham, D., Esnaud, H., Habert, E., and Langer, S. Z. (1989). A common binding site for tricyclic and nontricyclic 5-hydroxytryptamine uptake inhibitors at the substrate recognition site of the neuronal sodium-dependent 5-hydroxytryptamine transporter. *Biochemical Pharmacology*, **38**, 3819–26.

Green, A. R. (1985). *The neuropharmacology of serotonin.* Oxford University Press.

Grenett, H. E., Ledley, F. D., Reed, L. L., and Woo, S. L. (1987). Full-length cDNA for rabbit tryptophan hydroxylase: functional domains and evolution of aromatic amino acid hydroxylases. *Proceedings of National Academy of Sciences USA*, **84**, 5530–4.

Hillegaart, V. and Hjorth, S. (1989). Median raphe, but not dorsal raphe, application of the 5-HT1A agonist 8-OH-DPAT stimulates rat motor activity. *European Journal of Pharmacology*, **160**, 303–7.

Hillegaart, V., Ahlenius, S., and Larsson, K. (1989). Effects of local application of 5-HT into the median and dorsal raphe nuclei on male rat sexual and motor behaviour. *Behavioural Brain Research*, **33**, 279–86.

Ho, B. T., Schooler, J. C., and Usdin, E. (1982). *Serotonin in biological psychiatry*. Raven Press, New York.

Hsu, Y. P., Powell, J. F., Sims, K. B., and Breakefield, X. O. (1989). Molecular genetics of the monoamine oxidases. *Journal of Neurochemistry*, **53**, 12–18.

Jacobs, B. L. and Gelperin, A. (1981). *Serotonin neurotransmission and behaviour*. MIT Press, Cambridge, Massachussetts.

Jacobs, B. L., Wise, W. D., and Taylor, K. M. (1974). Differential behavioural and neurochemical effects following lesions of the dorsal or median raphe nuclei in rats. *Brain Research*, **79**, 353–61.

Jacobs, B. L., Trimbach, C., Eubanks, E. E., and Trulson, M. (1975). Hippocampal mediation of raphe lesion- and PCPA-induced hyperactivity in the rat. *Brain Research*, **94**, 253–61.

Jacquin, T., Denavit-Saubie, M., and Champagnat, J. (1989). Substance P and serotonin mutually reverse their excitatory effects in the rat nucleus tractus solitarius. *Brain Research*, **502**, 214–222.

Johansson, O., Hokfelt, T., Pernow, B., Jeffcoate, S. L., White, N., Steinbusch, H. W., *et al.* (1981). Immunohistochemical support for three putative transmitters in one neuron: coexistence of 5-hydroxytryptamine, substance P- and thyrotropin releasing hormone-like immunoreactivity in medullary neurons projecting to the spinal cord. *Neuroscience*, **6**, 1857–81.

Kohler, C. and Steinbusch, H. (1982). Identification of serotonin and non-serotonin-containing neurons of the mid-brain raphe projecting to the entorhinal area and the hippocampal formation. A combined immunohistochemical and fluorescent retrograde tracing study in the rat brain. *Neuroscience*, **7**, 951–75.

Kosofsky, B. E. and Molliver, M. E. (1987). The serotoninergic innervation of cerebral cortex: different classes of axon terminals arise from dorsal and median raphe nuclei. *Synapse*, **1**, 153–68.

Kovachich, G. B., Aronson, C. E., Brunswick, D. J., and Frazer, A. (1988). Quantitative autoradiography of serotonin uptake sites in rat brain using [^{3}H]cyanoimipramine. *Brain Research*, **454**, 78–88.

Kuhn, D. M., Wolf, W. A., and Youdim, M. B. H. (1986). Serotonin neurochemistry revisited: a new look at some old axioms. *Neurochemistry International*, **8**, 141–54.

Ledley, F. D., Grenett, H. E., Bartos, D. P., van Tuinen, P., Ledbetter, D. H., and Woo, S. L. (1987). Assignment of human tryptophan hydroxylase locus to chromosome 11: gene duplication and translocation in evolution of aromatic amino acid hydroxylases. *Somatic Cell and Molecular Genetics*, **13**, 575–80.

Mamounas, L. A. and Molliver, M. E. (1988). Evidence for dual serotonergic projections to neocortex: axons from the dorsal and median raphe muclei are differentially vulnerable to the neurotoxin p-chloroamphetamine (PCA). *Experimental Neurology*, **102**, 23–36.

Marcusson, J. O., Bergstrom, M., Eriksson, K., and Ross, S. B. (1988). Characterization of [3H]paroxetine binding in rat brain. *Journal of Neurochemistry*, **50**, 1783–90.

Marcusson, J. O., Andersson, A., and Backstrom, I. (1989). Drug inhibition indicates a single-site model of the 5-HT uptake site/antidepressant binding site in rat and human brain. *Psychopharmacology*, **99**, 17–21.

Meek, J. L. and Lofstrandh, S. (1976). Tryptophan hydroxylase in discrete brain nuclei: comparison of activity in vitro and in vivo. *European Journal of Pharmacology*, **37**, 377–80.

Molliver, M. E. (1987). Serotonergic neuronal systems: what their anatomic organization tells us about function. *Journal of Clinical Psychopharmacology*, **7**, Suppl. 6, 3S–23S.

Moore, R. Y. and Halaris, A. E. (1975). Hippocampal innervation by serotonin neurons of the midbrain raphe in the rat. *Journal of Comparative Neurology*, **164**, 171–83.

Murphy, D. L., Sims, K. B., Karoum, F., de la Chapelle, A., Norio, R., Sankila, E.-M., and Breakefield, X. O. (1990). Marked amine and amine metabolite changes in Norrie disease patients with an X-chromosomal deletion affecting monoamine oxidase. *Journal of Neurochemistry*, **54**, 242–7.

O'Hearn, E., Battaglia, G., DeSouza, E. B., Kuhar, M. J., and Molliver, M. E. (1988). Methylenedioxyamphetamine (MDA) and methylenedioxymethamphetamine (MDMA) cause selective ablation of serotonergic axon terminals in forebrain: immunocytochemical evidence for neurotoxicity. *Journal of Neuroscience*, **8**, 2788–803.

Osborne, N. N. (1982). *Biology of serotonergic transmission*. Wiley, Chichester.

Osborne, N. N. and Hamon, M. (1988). *Neuronal serotonin*. Wiley, Chichester.

Paoletti, R. and Vanhoute, P. M. (1990). *Serotonin from cell biology to pharmacology and therapeutics*. Kluwer, The Netherlands.

Plenge, P., Mellerup, E. T., and Laursen, H. (1990). Regional distribution of the serotonin transport complex in human brain, identified with 3H-paroxetine, 3H-citalopram and 3H-imipramine. *Progress in Neuropsychopharmacology and Biological Psychiatry*, **14**, 61–72.

Rech, R. H. and Gudelsky, G. A. (1988). *5-HT agonists as psychoactive drugs*, pp. 1–308. NNP Books, Ann Arbor, Michigan.

Ross, S. B. (1987). Distribution of the two forms of monoamine oxidase within monoaminergic neurons of the guinea pig brain. *Journal of Neurochemistry*, **48**, 609–14.

Sah, D. W. and Matsumoto, S. G. (1987). Evidence for serotonin synthesis, uptake, and release in dissociated rat sympathetic neurons in culture. *Journal of Neuroscience*, **7**, 391–9.

Schmidt, C. J. and Lovenberg, W. (1985). In vitro demonstration of dopamine uptake by neostriatal serotonergic neurons of the rat. *Neuroscience Letters*, **59**, 9–14.

Shirota, K. and Fujisawa, H. (1988). Purification and characterization of aromatic L-amino acid decarboxylase from rat kidney and monoclonal antibody to the enzyme. *Journal of Neurochemistry*, **51**, 426–34.

Sims, K. B., de la Chapelle, A., Norio, R., Sankila, E.-M., Hsu, Y.-P. P., Rinehart, W. B., Corey, T. J., Ozelius, L., Powell, J. F., Bruns, G., Gusella, J. F., Murphy, D. L., and Breakefield, X. O. (1989a). Monoamine oxidase deficiency in males with an X chromosome deletion. *Neuron*, **2**, 1069–76.

Sims, K. B., Ozelius, L., Corey, T., Rinehart, W. B., Liberfarb, R., Haines, J., *et al.* (1989*b*). Norrie disease gene is distinct from the monoamine oxidase genes. *American Journal of Human Genetics*, **45**, 424–34.

Sinton, C. M. and Fallon, S. L. (1988). Electrophysiological evidence for a functional differentiation between subtypes of the 5-HT1 receptor. *European Journal of Pharmacology*, **157**, 173–81.

Takeuchi, Y. (1988). Distribution of serotonin neurons in the mammalian brain. In *Neuronal serotonin*, (ed. N. N. Osborne and M. Hamon), pp. 25–56. John Wiley, Chichester.

Thorpe, L. W., Westlund, K. N., Kochersperger, L. M., Abell, C. W., and Denney, R. M. (1987). Immunocytochemical localization of monoamine oxidases A and B in human peripheral tissues and brain. *Journal of Histochemistry and Cytochemistry*, **35**, 23–32.

Verbeuren, T. J. (1989). Synthesis, storage, release, and metabolism of 5-hydroxy-tryptamine in peripheral tissues. In *The peripheral actions of 5-hydroxytryptamine*, (ed. J. R. Fozard), pp. 1–25. Oxford University Press.

Discussion

CURZON: Dr Murphy raised the question of when changes in the availability of tryptophan in the brain affect the availability of 5-hydroxytryptamine (5-HT, serotonin) to receptors. One circumstance in which this probably occurs is when 5-HT synthesis in rats is partially inhibited by *p*-CPA (*para*-chlorophenylalanine); the behavioural effects of tryptophan given then suggest that functional 5-HT is increased (Marsden and Curzon 1976). The therapeutic effect of increasing the availability of tryptophan to the brain in depression (Thomson *et al.* 1982, Moller *et al.* 1980) and neuroendocrine (Cowen and Charig 1987) and behavioural (Raleigh *et al.* 1988) effects of tryptophan provide evidence that is consistent with increased functional 5-HT in man and other primates. However, direct evidence from brain dialysis in rats is equivocal; dialysate 5-HT is reported to be increased (During *et al.* 1989; Carboni *et al.* 1989) and unaltered (Pei *et al.* 1989; Slight *et al.* 1988) by tryptophan administration. Furthermore, whether the relatively small brain trypto-phan changes which are likely to occur physiologically could affect 5-HT availability is another matter.

MURPHY: These are intriguing findings. The degree of saturation of tryptophan hydroxylase *in vivo* is debated. The state of the system is crucial. We don't know enough about the dietary and circadian status of the rats which might dampen the effect of tryptophan.

MELTZER: The other factors which determine how much tryptophan gets to the brain are the concentrations of the competing neutral amino acids and free-versus-bound tryptophan. In many of the systems I study, particularly neuroendocrine parame-ters, it is difficult to establish a functional effect of adding large concentrations of tryptophan.

MENDLEWICZ: Could tryptophan hydroxylase and phenylalanine hydroxylase origi-nate from the same family of ancestral genes?

MURPHY: The third enzyme, tyrosine hydroxylase, has been mapped to human chromosome 11, whereas phenylalanine hydroxylase is reported to be on chromo-some 12. One has to postulate that there were at least two different genetic steps leading to the different chromosome locations of these related enzymes.

LINNOILA: How confident are you that the *central* tryptophan hydroxylase has been cloned? There is clear hybridization in the pineal but I have not seen convincing hybridization in the brainstem. David Coldman and Jim Stohl have expressed the mouse tryptophan hydroxylase, which is different from the rat enzyme, in a tumour cell line. It hybridizes nicely in the pineal, but there is no detectable signal in the brainstem. The same has been observed at the National Institute of Mental Health with the enzyme from the ewe.

MURPHY: Tryptophan hydroxylase was cloned from pineal gland homogenates from rat and rabbit. Whether that is the tryptophan hydroxylase that is in brain or other tissues, or in other species, remains to be demonstrated.

LINNOILA: If *all* intraneuronal monoamine oxidase (MAO) within the serotonin neurones is of the B subtype, the intraneuronal soluble transmitter concentration may be significantly higher than it is in the catecholaminergic neurones, because there is a relatively low affinity enzyme metabolizing serotonin within the neurone. Could it be that the system needs a relatively small amount of the synthesizing enzyme, and therefore we cannot detect it?

MURPHY: There is evidence that MAO-A is present in serotonin synaptosomes. The early immunocytochemistry which suggested that serotonin neurones only contained MAO-B suffered from insensitivity. But, as you suggested, there may be different tryptophan hydroxylases.

MELTZER: Could you comment on the relationship between [^{3}H]paroxetine- and [^{3}H] imipramine-binding sites? It seems clear that paroxetine labels the transporter and that in platelets, the cortex, and the raphe, the numbers of both sites agree very closely. But in the globus pallidus, the number of paroxetine sites is 40 per cent that of the imipramine sites. In the caudate it is only about 60 per cent. Thus, there is still a possibility of many imipramine-binding sites, some of which are not the transporter.

MURPHY: Imipramine does bind to other sites besides the 5-HT transporter. Whether those sites are functionally important is debatable.

LINNOILA: It has been reported that in the brains of suicide victims there is no increase in the density of paroxetine-binding sites, but an increase in the number of imipramine-binding sites has been found. That also suggests a differential labelling with these two ligands.

MELTZER: I discuss this further in my chapter (Meltzer and Arora, this volume).

References

Carboni, E., Cadoni, C., Tanda, G. L., and DiChiara, G. (1989). Calcium-dependent, tetrodotoxin-sensitive stimulation of cortical serotonin release after a tryptophan load. *Journal of Neurochemistry*, **53**, 976–78.

Cowen, P. J. and Charig, E. M. (1987). Neuroendocrine responses to intravenous tryptophan in major depression. *Archives of General Psychiatry*, **44**, 958–66.

During, M. J., Freese, A., Heyes, M. P., Swartz, K. J., Markey, S. P., Roth, R. H., and Martin, J. B. (1989). Neuroactive metabolites of L-tryptophan, serotonin and quinolinic acid, in striatal extracellular fluid. Effect of tryptophan loading. *FEBS Letters*, **247**, 438–44.

Marsden, C. A. and Curzon, G. (1976). Studies on the behavioural effects of tryptophan and p-chlorophenylalanine. *Journal of Neurochemistry*, **15**, 165–71.

Meltzer, H. Y. and Arora, R. C. (1991). Platelet serotonin studies in affective disorders. In *5-hydroxytryptamine in psychiatry: a spectrum of ideas*, (ed. M. Sandler, A. Coppen, and S. Harnett), pp. 50–89. Oxford University Press.

Moller, S. E., Kirk, L., and Honore, P. (1980). Relationship between plasma ratio of tryptophan to competing amino acids and the response to L-tryptophan treatment in endogenously depressed patients. *Journal of Affective Disorders*, **2**, 47–59.

Pei, Q., Zetterstrom, T., and Fillenz, M. (1989). Measurement of extracellular 5-HT and 5-HIAA in hippocampus of freely moving rats using microdialysis: long term applications. *Neurochemistry International*, **15**, 503–9.

Raleigh, M. J., McGuire, M. T., and Brammer, G. L. (1988). Behavioural and cognitive effects of altered tryptophan and tyrosine supply. In *Amino acid availability and brain function in health and disease*, (ed. G. Huether), pp. 299–308. Springer-Verlag, Berlin.

Sleight, A. J., Marsden, C. A., Martin, K. F., and Palfreyman, M. G. (1988). Relationship between extracellular 5-hydroxytryptamine and behaviour following monoamine oxidase inhibition and L-tryptophan. *British Journal of Pharmacology*, **93**, 303–10.

Thomson, J., Rankin, H., Ashcroft, G. W., Yates, C. M., McQueen, J. K., and Cummings, S. W. (1982). The treatment of depression in general practice: a comparison of L-tryptophan, amitriptyline, and a combination of L-tryptophan and amitriptyline with placebo. *Psychological Medicine*, **12**, 741–51.

4. Milacemide: a neuropsychotropic glycine prodrug that potentiates serotonergic activity

Moussa B. H. Youdim

Milacemide is the first glycine prodrug (Cavalier *et al.* 1983; Christophe *et al.* 1983) which, unlike the inhibitory neurotransmitter, glycine (Cavalier *et al.* 1983), can readily cross the blood–brain barrier. In the brain, glycineamide and glycine are the major metabolites of milacemide (Christophe *et al.* 1983; Roba *et al.* 1986). Animal studies support the anticonvulsant activities of milacemide (Houtkooper *et al.* 1984; Albertson *et al.* 1984) and glycine (Cherubini *et al.* 1981; Seiler and Sarhan 1984). It is now apparent that the formation of glycine (Janssens de Varebeke *et al.* 1988, 1989) and the antiseizure action of milacemide (Youdim *et al.* 1988) are dependent on the activity of brain monoamine oxidase B (MAO-B), for which milacemide is a selective substrate *in vitro* and *in vivo* (Fig. 4.1) (Janssens de Varebeke *et al.* 1988). Thus, in hyperbaric oxygen-induced seizure, the selective MAO-B inhibition by L-deprenyl, rather than inhibition of MAO-A by clorgyline, prevents the milacemide-induced increase in seizure latency (Youdim *et al.* 1988). Therefore, milacemide's anticonvulsant property has been attributed to the formation of its major metabolites—pentanoic acid, glycineamide, and glycine—by the oxidative reaction of MAO-B (Youdim *et al.* 1988). Milacemide is also an enzyme-activated specific inhibitor of MAO-B. *In vitro* and *in vivo* studies confirm these findings (Janssens de Varebeke *et al.* 1989).

We have demonstrated another pharmacological property of milacemide— its ability to potentiate serotonin neurotransmission-dependent behaviour in rats in a dose-dependent fashion. The ability of milacemide to potentiate the serotonin (5-hydroxytryptamine, 5-HT) behavioural syndromes of head twitch and hyperactivity initiated by the putative 5-HT$_2$ receptor agonist, 5-methoxy-*N*,*N*-dimethyltryptamine (5-MeO-DMT), or 5-hydroxytryptophan (5-HTP) in mice and rats suggests a post-synaptically mediated event. Head twitching and hyperactivity, as measured in our study, are 5-HT$_2$ receptor-dependent behaviours (Youdim and Janssens de Varebeke 1990). The possibility that milacemide inhibits MAO-A and thereby raises the concentration of 5-HT can be discounted: *in vitro* and *in vivo* studies show limited inhibition of MAO-A by milacemide, even at high doses. Green and Youdim

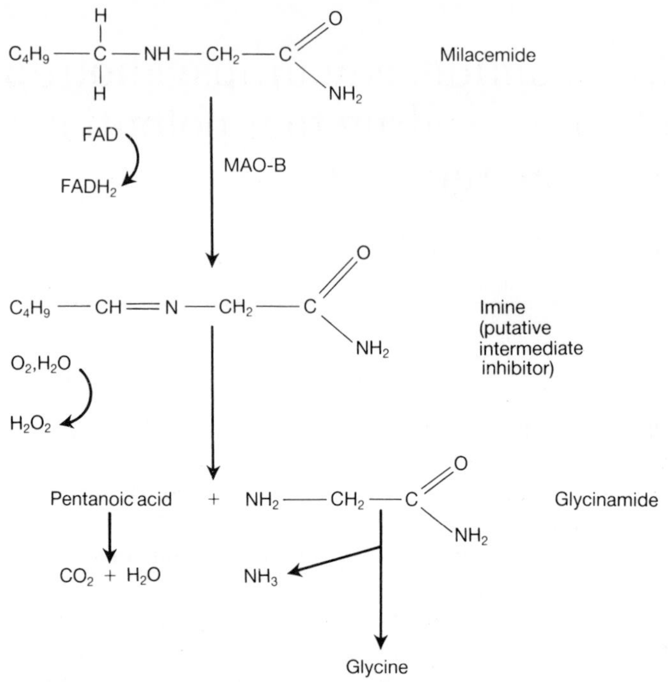

FIG. 4.1. The proposed reaction pathway for milacemide oxidation by monoamine oxidase B and inhibition of the enzyme.

(1975) demonstrated that more than 85 per cent inhibition of MAO-A and MAO-B is required for the increase of brain 5-HT and induction of 5-HT behavioural syndrome in tryptophan-treated rats. The fact that milacemide treatment alone, even at high doses (500 mg kg^{-1}), does not produce any overt 5-HT-dependent behaviour suggests that milacemide is not a 5-HT$_2$ receptor agonist. Binding studies with the post-synaptic 5-HT$_2$ receptor ligand, [^{3}H]ketanserin, have not revealed any significant interaction (unpublished data). Furthermore, in rats milacemide treatment does not change the concentrations of 5-HT and 5-hydroxyindoleacetic acid (5-HIAA) in the raphe nucleus and striatum; there is neither increased 5-HT release nor uptake inhibition. However, this study cannot exclude the possibility that milacemide increases 5-HT turnover.

There was a possibility that milacemide, being a selective MAO-B inhibitor (Janssens de Varebeke *et al.* 1989), might affect dopamine inactivation and release. The 5-HT behavioural syndrome, as induced by 5-HT precursor plus MAO inhibitor, or by 5-MeO-DMT, is thought to have a dopamine-dependent component (Green and Grahame-Smith 1976). Inhibition of dopamine synthesis by α-methyl-*p*-tyrosine or blockade of the dopamine$_2$

receptor by neuroleptics (chlorpromazine or haloperidol) prevents the 5-HT behavioural syndrome. However, an altered rat brain dopamine metabolism, via inhibition of MAO-B, can be discounted, because dopamine and its metabolites are unchanged in the striatum of rats treated with large doses of milacemide (Riederer *et al.* 1990). This finding contrasts with the ability of milacemide to increase dopamine, with a concomitant decrease of dihydroxy-phenylacetic and homovanillic acids, in the rhesus monkey striatum. Rhesus monkey brain is similar to human brain, in that, unlike in rat brain, the major form of MAO in the striatum is type B, for which dopamine is a substrate; selective MAO-B inhibitors alter dopamine's metabolism in human and monkey brains (Riederer and Youdim 1986).

The molecular mechanism by which milacemide enhances serotonergic activity remains unclear, but several findings support the possible involvement of the MAO-B activity known to be present in the 5-HT neurones of the brainstem (raphe nucleus) and spinal cord, and the formation of glycine from milacemide.

In mice and rats the insecticide 1,11-trichloro-2,2-bis(*p*-chloro-phenyl)ethane (PP-DDT) produces stimulus-sensitive myoclonus (Hwang and Van Woert 1978). Drugs that act as 5-HT agonists or that prolong the action of 5-HT in the brain, such as 5-HTP, monoamine oxidase inhibitors, quipazine, and fluoxetine, decrease the myoclonus induced by PP-DDT. In contrast, 5-HT antagonists increase the intensity of PP-DDT-induced myoclonus (Fahn *et al.* 1986). Behavioural and biochemical results suggest that PP-DDT-induced myoclonus does not result from a deficiency of central 5-HT (Truong *et al.* 1988*a*). However, increased 5-HT neuronal activity in brain does inhibit PP-DDT-induced myoclonus (see Fahn *et al.* 1986). In contrast, there is a reduction of brain glycine in PP-DDT-induced myoclonus (Truong *et al.* 1988*a,b*). Milacemide not only inhibits PP-DDT-induced myoclonus but also prevents the fall in brain glycine (Truong *et al.* 1988*b*). Furthermore, we have shown that whereas L-deprenyl (selective MAO-B inhibitor) potentiates PP-DDT-induced myoclonus, clorgyline inhibits it. These results can be explained by the inhibition by L-deprenyl of the conversion of milacemide to glycine by MAO-B, and the increase of brain glycine via the action of MAO-B in clorgyline-treated animals, as well as the elevation of brain 5-HT arising from selective inhibition of MAO-A by clorgyline (Youdim *et al.* 1990).

Serial transection experiments have shown that the complete serotonergic syndrome initiated in our experiments is mediated exclusively by neural mechanisms in the pons, medulla, and spinal cord (Riederer *et al.* 1990), where glycineamide and glycine accumulate during milacemide oxidation by MAO-B. The fact that when given alone milacemide is not a 5-HT agonist suggests that either milacemide or glycine can activate the glycinergic interneurones in these regions, which in turn is disinhibitory to post-synaptic 5-HT neurones. It remains to be seen whether other glycine prodrugs behave in a similar manner to milacemide or whether the potentiation of 5-HT behavioural syndrome is an intrinsic property of milacemide. Finally, consideration should also be given to the interaction of glycine, glycineamide, and pentanoic acid, formed from oxidation of milacemide by MAO-B, with the NMDA (*N*-methyl-D-aspartate) glutamate subtype receptor. Whether such an interaction would have a 5-HT post-synaptic disinhibitory potential remains to be investigated (Youdim 1989). Nevertheless, milacemide and its analogues have potential not only as tools to study 5-HT neurotransmission but also as drugs in the treatment of myoclonus, depressive illness, and even Parkinson's disease. The evidence for the latter has come from monkey studies where long-term treatment (6 months) with milacemide increases dopamine in the striatum. This has been attributed to milacemide's action as the most specific inhibitor of MAO-B so far described, as a consequence of it being a 'suicide' substrate.

References

Albertson, T. E., Stark, L. G., and Joy, R. M. (1984). The effects of a glycine derivative (CP 1552 S) on kindled seizures in rats. *Neuropharmacology*, **23**, 967–70.

Cavalier, R., Herin, M., and Franz, M. (1983). Metabolism of a new antiepileptic drug (milacemide) in the brain. *Archives of International Pharmacodynamics*, **270**, 169–70.

Cherubini, E., Bernardi, G., Stanzione, P., Marciani, M., and Mercuri, N. (1981). The action of glycine on rat epileptic foci. *Neuroscience Letters*, **21**, 93–7.

Christophe, J., Kutzner, R., Nguyen-Bui, N.D., Damien, C., Chatelain, P., and Gillet, C. (1983). Conversion of orally administered 2-n-pentylaminoacetamide into glycineamide and glycine in the rat brain. *Life Sciences*, **33**, 533–41.

Fahn, S., Marsden, D., and Van Woert, M. H. (1986). *Myoclonus*, Advances in Neurology, Vol. 43. Raven Press, New York.

Green, A. R. and Youdim, M. B. H. (1975). Effect of monoamine oxidase inhibition by clorgyline, deprenyl, and tranylcypromine on 5-hydroxytryptamine concentration in rat brain and hyperactivity following subsequent tryptophan administration. *British Journal of Pharmacology*, **55**, 415–22.

Green, A. R. and Grahame-Smith, D. G. (1976). The effect of drugs on the process regulating functional activity of brain 5-hydroxytryptamine. *Nature*, **260**, 487–91.

Houtkooper, M. A., Blom, G. F., Hoppener, R. J. E., Hulsman, J. R. A., Menardi, H., Meijer, J. W. A., and Van Oorschot, C. A. E. H. (1984). Double-blind study, milacemide (pentyl-glycine) in hospitalized therapy resistant patients with epilepsy. *Acta Neurologica Scandinavica*, **70**, 222–3.

Hwang, E. C. and Van Woert, M. H. (1978). PP'-DDT-induced neurotoxic syndrome: experimental myoclonus. *Neurology*, **10**, 1020–5.

Janssens de Varebeke P., Cavalier, P., David-Remacle, M., and Youdim, M. B. H. (1988). Formation of the neurotransmitter glycine from the anticonvulsant milacemide is mediated by brain monoamine oxidase B. *Journal of Neurochemistry*, **50**, 1011–16.

Janssens de Varebeke, P., Pauwells, G., Buyse, C., David-Remacle, M., Mey, J. D., Roba, J., and Youdim, M. B. H. (1989). The novel neuropsychotropic agent milacemide is a specific enzyme-activated inhibitor of brain monoamine oxidase B. *Journal of Neurochemistry*, **53**, 1109–16.

Riederer, P. and Youdim, M. B. H. (1986). Monoamine oxidase activity and monoamine metabolism in brains of Parkinsonian patients treated with l-deprenyl. *Journal of Neurochemistry*, **46**, 1359–65.

Riederer, P., Janssens de Varebeke, P., and Youdim, M. B. H. (1990). Increase of striatal dopamine with concomitant decreases of homovanillic acid and dihydroxy-phenylacetic acid in rhesus monkeys after milacemide treatment. *Neurochemistry International*, in press.

Roba, J., Cavalier, R., Cordi, A., Gorissen, H., Herin, M., Janssen de Varebeke, P., *et al.* (1986). Milacemide. In *New anticonvulsant drugs*, (ed. B. S. Meldrum and R. R. Porter), pp. 169–90. J. Libbey, London.

Seiler, N. and Sarhan, S. (1984). Synergistic anticonvulsant effects of GABA-T inhibitors and glycine. *Naunyn-Schmiedeberg's Archives of Pharmacology*, **323**, 49–57.

Truong, D. D., Diamon, B., Pezzoli, G., Mena, M. A., and Fahn, S. (1988*a*). Monoamine oxidase inhibitory properties of milacemide in rats. *Life Sciences*, **44**, 1059–66.

Truong, D. D., De Yebenes, J. G., Pezzoli, G., Jackson-Lewis, V., and Fahn, S. (1988*b*). Glycine involvement in DDT-induced myoclonus. *Movement Disorders*, **3**, 77–87.

Youdim, M. B. H. (1989). Monoamine oxidase (MAO) B: a unique neurotoxin and neurotransmitter producing enzyme. *Progress in Neuro-Psychopharmacology and Biological Psychiatry*, **13**, 363–71.

Youdim, M. B. H. and Janssens de Varebeke, P. (1990). Serotonin syndrome potentiating property of milacemide (2-n-pentylamino acetamide). Submitted.

Youdim, M. B. H., Kerem, D., and Duvdevani, Y. (1988). The glycine prodrug milacemide increases seizure threshold due to hyperbaric oxygen prevention by l-deprenyl. *European Journal of Pharmacology*, **150**, 381–4.

Youdim, M. B. H., Harkash, N., and Zinder, O. (1990). Anti-myoclonic activity of milacemide in PP-DDT treated rats. Submitted.

Discussion

INSEL: What is known about milacemide inhibition of monoamine oxidase B (MAO-B)?

YOUDIM: Milacemide is a suicide substrate; MAO-B converts it into an intermediate imine-like metabolite which inactivates the enzyme. This is similar to metabolism of N-methyl-4-phenyl-1,2,3,6-tetrahydropyridine (MPTP) by MAO-B. We have shown that chronic milacemide treatment increases brain dopamine with a concomitant decrease of homovanillic acid and DOPAC in monkey brains, as a result of MAO-B inhibition. Brain noradrenaline and 5-hydroxytryptamine (5-HT, serotonin) and their metabolites are unchanged (Janssens de Varebeke *et al.* 1990; Riederer *et al.* 1990).

BRILEY: Have you tried injecting glycine locally into the raphe?

YOUDIM: We have not, but many years ago it was shown that glycine inhibited convulsion. This was one reason for the interest in milacemide's anticonvulsant activity. The drug has been tested in Belgium and the USA and does have antidepressant activity, but there was a problem with liver toxicity. The antidepressant activity may arise from its serotonin-potentiating property.

MAÎTRE: Has milacemide proved to be an anti-epileptic in man?

YOUDIM: It is a poor anti-epileptic; the clinical trials have not been very positive. It is now being tried for antimyoclonus activity.

References

Janssens de Varebeke, P., Schallauer, E., Sofic, A., Rausch, W. D., Riederer, P., and Youdim, M. B. H. (1990). Milacemide, the selective substrate and enzyme-activated specific inhibitor of monoamine oxidase B, increases dopamine but not serotonin in caudate nucleus of Rhesus Monkey. *Neurochemistry International*, in press.

Riederer, P., Janssens de Varebeke, P., and Youdim, M. B. H. (1990). Increase of striatal dopamine with concomitant decreases of homovanillic acid and dihydroxyphenylacetic acid in rhesus monkeys after milacemide treatment. *Neurochemistry International*, in press.

5. The inactive enantiomer of a noradrenaline uptake blocker reduces 5-HT synthesis

Peter C. Waldmeier and Laurent Maître

Introduction

The enantiomers of the tetracyclic antidepressant oxaprotiline differ in their ability to inhibit noradrenaline (NA) uptake. While (+)-oxaprotiline (CGP 12104 A) is extraordinarily potent in this respect, the (−)-enantiomer (CGP 12103 A, levoprotiline) is virtually inactive *in vitro* and *in vivo*. Neither enantiomer has any effects on 5-hydroxytryptamine (5-HT, serotonin) uptake *in vitro* or *in vivo* (Waldmeier *et al.* 1982). Levoprotiline was originally tested clinically in depressed patients because this seemed to be an ideal way to test the catecholamine hypothesis of affective disorders. Contrary to the prediction by this hypothesis, the compound clearly showed antidepressant effects in patients (Schmauss *et al.* 1985, Wolfersdorf *et al.* 1988), which automatically raised the question of the mechanism of action. Levoprotiline has been found active in a number of behavioural tests for antidepressants: it was effective in the Porsolt swim test after chronic application; it enhanced the neurological syndrome induced by 5-hydroxytryptophan (5-HTP) and the stereotypies caused by apomorphine (Delini-Stula and Mogilnicka 1988, 1989); and after repeated treatment it also potentiated the effects of d-amphetamine and dopamine injected into the rat nucleus accumbens (Maj and Wedzony 1989). However, no biochemical correlate for these effects has been found as yet. Levoprotiline has little if any interaction with α_2- and β-noradrenergic, cholinergic, serotonergic (5-HT$_1$ subtypes, 5-HT$_2$), dopaminergic, GABA$_A$, benzodiazepine, adenosine, and opiate receptors. It is weakly α_1-noradrenolytic and moderately H$_1$-histaminolytic (Clinical orientation on CGP 12103A, the (−)-enantiomer of the antidepressant C 49802 B-Ba. CIBA-GEIGY Ltd., Basle, Switzerland, 1983).

In view of the enhancement by levoprotiline of the functional responsiveness towards 5-HTP reported by Delini-Stula and Mogilnicka (1989), it seemed of interest to investigate whether this compound also affects presynaptic parameters of 5-HT function. We therefore studied the effects of acute and repeated administration of levoprotiline on 5-HT synthesis, as measured by the accumulation of 5-HTP after central decarboxylase inhibition with NSD 1015.

Materials and methods

Female Tif:RAIF (SPF) rats (160–200 g; Tierfarm Sisseln, Switzerland) were used throughout. NSD 1015 (*m*-hydroxybenzylhydrazine × 2 HCl) was obtained from Janssen Chimica (Beerse, Belgium) and dissolved in H_2O. Levoprotiline, as the hydrochloride salt, was dissolved in H_2O in the experiment depicted in Fig. 5.1. Because of solubility problems at higher doses, polyethyleneglycol 400/H_2O 1:2 was used in the other experiments. α-Methyl-DOPA, a gift from Bayer AG, Leverkusen (Federal Republic of Germany), was dissolved in H_2O at slightly acidic pH (4.5). The accumulation of 5-HTP within 30 min after the intraperitoneal (i.p.) administration of 100 mg kg^{-1} NSD 1015 was determined by HPLC with coulometric detection, essentially as described previously (Waldmeier *et al.* 1988), except that *N*-methylserotonin was used as an internal standard. In the experiment with α-methyl-DOPA, α-methyldopamine (α-methyl-DA) was determined by the same procedure. The retention times were 11.4 min for 5-HTP, 17.2 min for α-methyl-DA, and 31.5 min for the internal standard.

Results

In rats treated with levoprotiline (10 mg kg^{-1} i.p.) twice daily (16.00 and 08.00) for one or ten days, statistically significant reductions of 5-HTP accumulation were observed in the striatum 2 and 24 h, but not 48 h, after the last administration. The same held true in the cortex 2 h after the last treatment; after 24 and 48 h only the acute effect was significant. A similar trend was also seen in the hippocampus; significant reductions of 5-HTP accumulation were seen only at 2 h after repeated and at 24 h after acute treatment (Fig. 5.1). The time course of the acute effect of levoprotiline was tested using the high dose of 100 mg kg^{-1} i.p., because the effects obtained with 10 mg kg^{-1} i.p. were relatively mild. As shown in Fig. 5.2, levoprotiline induced marked and significant ($p < 0.01$) decreases of 5-HTP accumulation, 40–50 per cent at their maxima, in striatum, hippocampus, and cortex. There was no noticeable difference in the extents of the reductions between the areas, as had already been suggested by the experiment depicted in Fig. 5.1. The effect was maximal between 2 and 4 h in all the areas and subsided within 24 h. In the cortex, but not in the other two areas, it was still significant ($p < 0.05$) after 16 h. Dose-response curves were generated after a single dose of levoprotiline or two consecutive doses administered 16h apart. Fig. 5.3 shows that while a reduction of 5-HTP accumulation of a similar magnitude as in the time course experiment was observed after a

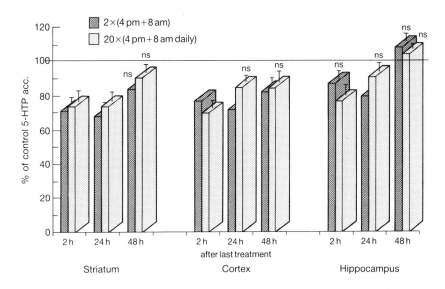

FIG. 5.1. Effect of acute and subchronic administration of levoprotiline on 5-hydroxytryptophan (5-HTP) accumulation after central decarboxylase inhibition in rat brain areas. Groups of seven or eight rats were treated twice daily for one or ten days with 10 mg kg^{-1} i.p. levoprotiline. They were decapitated 2, 24, and 48 h after the last treatment, having received 100 mg kg^{-1} i.p. decarboxylase inhibitor, NSD 1015, 30 min previously. Data refer to the amount of 5-HTP per g tissue $\pm$ S.E.M. as a percentage of that in controls. The absolute control values were (in ng g^{-1} per 30 min): striatum, 257 $\pm$ 8; cortex, 207 $\pm$ 6; hippocampus, 244 $\pm$ 16. ns indicates where the results were not significantly different from controls. All the other results were significant at at least the 5 per cent level (Dunnett's *t*-test).

single administration (left panel), the high dose (100 mg kg^{-1} i.p.) of levoprotiline was needed to produce the effect. After two consecutive doses, the dose-response relationship was shifted towards lower doses by a factor of about three (right panel).

The inhibitory effect of levoprotiline on 5-HTP accumulation after central decarboxylase inhibition might represent an artefact arising from an interference with the absorption, metabolism, distribution or action of the decarboxylase inhibitor, NSD 1015. To exclude this, groups of six to eight rats were treated with 100 mg kg^{-1} i.p. levoprotiline 3 h 55 min before subcutaneous administration of 100 mg kg^{-1} α-methyl-DOPA. Five minutes later, the animals received NSD 1015 (100 mg kg^{-1} i.p.). They were decapitated 60 or 120 min after this and α-methyl-DA was determined in the striatum, cortex, and hippocampus. The results in Table 5.1 clearly show that levoprotiline did not interfere with the action of the decarboxylase inhibitor.

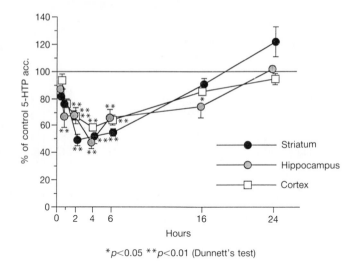

*p<0.05 **p<0.01 (Dunnett's test)

FIG. 5.2. Time course of the effect of a single dose of levoprotiline on 5-HTP accumulation after central decarboxylase inhibition in rat brain areas. Groups of six rats (controls $n = 12$) received 100 mg kg^{-1} i.p. levoprotiline. At various times thereafter, they received 100 mg kg^{-1} i.p. NSD 1015 and were decapitated 30 min later. Data refer to the amount of 5-HTP per g tissue ± S.E.M. as a percentage of control values. The absolute control values were (in ng g^{-1} per 30 min): striatum, 241 ± 20; cortex, 153 ± 5; hippocampus, 120 ± 11.

Discussion

Antidepressants that inhibit 5-HT uptake or monoamine oxidase (MAO) are known to reduce 5-HT synthesis. This has been ascribed to activation of a negative feedback mechanism by increased synaptic 5-HT, in the case of uptake inhibition, and direct product inhibition of tryptophan hydroxylase by increased cytoplasmic 5-HT, in the case of MAO inhibition. On the other hand, the specific noradrenaline uptake inhibitor desipramine has also been reported to reduce 5-HT synthesis after chronic administration at the same doses as those used here for levoprotiline. This effect was ascribed to its 5-HT antagonistic properties (Karoum *et al.* 1984), which are rather weak. Levoprotiline does not inhibit 5-HT uptake or MAO activity at doses more than an order of magnitude above those which were shown to reduce 5-HT synthesis in this study. As a 5-HT$_2$ receptor antagonist, it is about ten times less potent than desipramine, and both agents have virtually negligible anti-5-HT$_1$ receptor properties (H. Bittiger, personal communication).

   Thus, levoprotiline has none of the pharmacological properties that might explain the reduction of 5-HT synthesis. A possible artefact of the methodology—interference with the availability or action of the decarboxylase

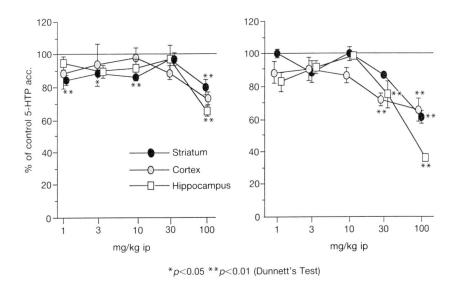

*p<0.05 **p<0.01 (Dunnett's Test)

FIG. 5.3. Dose-response relationships of the effect of a single dose and two consecutive doses of levoprotiline on 5-HTP accumulation after central decarboxylase inhibition. Groups of five or six rats received levoprotiline once (left panel) or twice, at 16.00 and 08.00 of the following day, (right panel). Ninety minutes after the last treatment, they received 100 mg kg⁻¹ i.p. NSD 1015 and were decapitated 30 min later. Data refer to the amount of 5-HTP per g tissue ± S.E.M. as a percentage of control values. The means of the absolute control values in the two experiments were (in ng g⁻¹ per 30 min): striatum, 248 and 251; cortex, 162 and 200; hippocampus, 211 and 255.

inhibitor, NSD 1015—has been excluded. A potential simple cause of this inhibitory effect on 5-HT synthesis—reduced cerebral tryptophan levels—was also excluded (results not shown). We are beginning to wonder whether this effect is an indirect consequence of an interference of some antidepressants with more fundamental process(es) of neuronal function, such as signal transduction. In this context it is interesting that antidepressant treatment increases the post-receptor-stimulated formation of cyclic AMP under certain circumstances (for a discussion see Newman and Lerer 1989). Enhancement of signal transduction might explain both the reduction in 5-HT synthesis and the increased functional responsiveness observed by Delini-Stula and Mogilnicka (1989) after administration of levoprotiline. Further studies are necessary to investigate this issue and to clarify whether the interference with 5-HT synthesis is a common feature of antidepressants, and particularly whether it is a feature of those which do not obviously

TABLE 5.1. *Absence of interference of levoprotiline with the inhibitory effect of NSD 1015 on decarboxylation*

	Min after NSD 1015	Striatum (ng g⁻¹)	Hippocampus (ng g⁻¹)	Cortex (ng g⁻¹)
Controls		<25	<25	<10
α-Methyl-DOPA	60	3208 ± 218	81 ± 3	83 ± 8
α-Methyl-DOPA	120	3888 ± 115	98 ± 2	90 ± 2
α-Methyl-DOPA +NSD 1015	60	130 ± 20	<25	<10
α-Methyl-DOPA + NSD 1015	120	210 ± 14	<25	<10
Levoprotiline + α-methyl-DOPA + NSD 1015	60	34 ± 5	<25	<10
Levoprotiline + α-methyl-DOPA + NSD 1015	120	179 ± 13	<25	<10

Groups of six to eight rats were treated with 100 mg kg⁻¹ i.p. levoprotiline 3 h 55 min before administration of 100 mg kg⁻¹ s.c. α-methyl-DOPA. 5 min later, the animals received 100 mg kg⁻¹ i.p. decarboxylase inhibitor, NSD 1015. They were decapitated 60 or 120 min after this and α-methyl-DA was determined in the tissue. Data are means ± S.E.M.

interfere with other aspects of 5-HT transmission, such as uptake, metabolism, and receptors.

Acknowledgements

The authors are indebted to Ms. A.-M. Buchle and Mr P. de Herdt for careful technical assistance.

References

Delini-Stula, A. and Mogilnicka, E. (1988). Single treatments with the antidepressant oxaprotiline and its (+) and (−) enantiomers increased behavioural responses to dopaminergic stimulation in the rat. *Journal of Neural Transmission*, **71**, 91–8.

Delini-Stula, A. and Mogilnicka, E. (1989). Rapid changes in functional responsiveness of the 5-HT system after single-dose and multiple-dose treatment with antidepressants: effect of maprotiline and oxaprotiline and its enantiomers. *Journal of Psychopharmacology*, **3**, 7–13.

Karoum, F., Korpi, E. R., Linnoila, M., Chuang, L.-W., and Wyatt, R. J. (1984).

Reduced metabolism and turnover rates of rat brain dopamine, norepinephrine and serotonin by chronic desipramine and zimelidine treatments. *European Journal of Pharmacology*, **100**, 137–44.

Maj, J. and Wedzony, K. (1989). The influence of oxaprotiline enantiomers given repeatedly on the behavioural effects of d-amphetamine and dopamine injected into the nucleus accumbens. *European Journal of Pharmacology*, **145**, 97–103.

Newman, M. E. and Lerer, B. (1989). Modulation of second messenger function in rat brain by in vivo alteration of receptor sensitivity: relevance to the mechanism of action of electroconvulsive therapy and antidepressants. *Progress in Neuro-Psychopharmacology and Biological Psychiatry*, **13**, 1–30.

Schmauss, M., Laakmann, G., Dieterle, D., Schmitz, R., and Wittmann, M. (1985). Clinical investigation on the importance of NE-reuptake inhibition for antidepressive efficacy: oxaprotiline versus its R-enantiomer CGP 12103 A. *Pharmacopsychiatry*, **18**, 86–7.

Waldmeier, P. C., Baumann, P. A., Hauser, K. Maître, L. and Storni, A. (1982). Oxaprotiline, a noradrenaline uptake inhibitor with an active and an inactive enantiomer. *Biochemical Pharmacology*, **31**, 2169–76.

Waldmeier, P. C., Williams, M., Baumann, P. A., Bischoff, S., Sills, M. A., and Neale, R. F. (1988). Interactions of isamoltane (CGP 361 A), an anxiolytic phenoxypropanolamine derivative, with 5-HT1 receptor subtypes in the rat brain. *Naunyn-Schmiedeberg's Archives of Pharmacology*, **337**, 609–20.

Wolfersdorf, M., Wendt, G., Binz, U., Steiner, B., and Hole, G. (1988). CGP 12103 A versus clomipramine in the treatment of depressed inpatients—results of a double-blind study. *Pharmacopsychiatry*, **21**, 203–7.

Discussion

CURZON: Levoprotiline decreases 5-hydroxytryptamine synthesis. Does it also decrease extraneuronal concentration of 5-HT in animal models? Another paradoxical antidepressant, tianeptine, unlike most other antidepressants, decreases brain dialysate 5-HT concentration (Sarna *et al.* 1989).

MAÎTRE: That is possible, but it has not been measured yet. We were surprised to see a biochemical effect of levoprotiline. If the drug is really an antidepressant, it is essential to know whether or not it interferes with biogenic amines in brain. We erroneously thought for a long time that it did not.

BRILEY: Does levoprotiline have any affinity for 5-HT receptors, particularly the 5-HT_{1B} or 5-HT_{1D} autoreceptors?

MAÎTRE: Up to 10 micromolar, it was inactive at 5-HT_{1B}, 5-HT_{1A}, 5-HT_{1D}, and 5-HT_2 receptors in radioligand binding assays.

Reference

Sarna, G. S., Whitton, P., O'Connell, M., and Curzon, G. (1989). Effect of tianeptine, a novel antidepressant, on potassium evoked 5-HT increases in the rat hippocampus as determined by in vivo dialysis. *Journal of Neuroscience Methods*, **29**, 285.

6. Platelet serotonin studies in affective disorders: evidence for a serotonergic abnormality?

Herbert Y. Meltzer and Ramesh C. Arora

Introduction

Various abnormalities of serotonergic processes have been demonstrated in patients with major depression or in post-mortem specimens from depressed patients or suicides (Meltzer and Lowy 1988). The most direct evidence of this type involves measurement of brain 5-hydroxytryptamine (5-HT, serotonin), its major metabolite 5-hydroxyindoleacetic acid (5-HIAA), or brain 5-HT receptor and [³H]imipramine-binding (IB) sites in suicides or deceased depressed patients. Less direct measures of serotonergic function in depression include studies of cerebrospinal fluid (CSF) 5-HIAA concentration, plasma tryptophan (free and total) in relation to the concentrations of large neutral amino acids, and the hormone and behavioural responses to challenges with tryptophan, 5-hydroxytryptophan (5-HTP), various direct 5-HT agonists, such as *meta*-chlorophenylpiperazine (*m*-CPP), buspirone, 6-chloro-2-[l-piperazinyl]pyrazine (MK 212) or fenfluramine, a 5-HT releaser. These studies have been reviewed elsewhere (Meltzer and Lowy 1988; Meltzer and Nash 1988). Perhaps the most indirect means of studying a possible disturbance of serotonergic mechanisms in depression involves the blood platelet, which is the subject of this review.

Although blood platelets lack the general characteristics of either 5-HT neurones or neurones with post-synaptic 5-HT receptors and are unable to synthesize 5-HT, they are able to take up, store, and release 5-HT via mechanisms that are sufficiently similar to those of 5-HT neurones to render the platelets interesting as a model for the 5-HT neurone (Pletscher 1968; Sneddon 1973; Stahl 1977). This has been particularly true for major depression because both the 5-HT active uptake site (Tuomisto and Tukiainen 1976) and the [³H]imipramine-binding (IB) site (Briley *et al.* 1980) were found to be abnormal in initial studies in unmedicated depressed patients. The finding of an increase in platelet 5-HT₂ binding sites in major depression (Biegon *et al.* 1987; Arora and Meltzer 1989*a*) further enhanced interest in the possible use of platelets to identify disturbances in serotonergic function that are present in the brain of some or all patients with major depression. It has also been suggested that measures of 5-HT uptake, ^{3}H-IB or 5-HT$_2$ binding sites in platelets might provide markers for major depression (i.e., biochemical abnormalities of sufficient sensitivity and specificity for major depression to be helpful for diagnostic purposes) or a means of studying the effects of antidepressant drugs on the 5-HT uptake or ^{3}H-IB site in man, with the hope that any observed effects could be generalized to brain.

Factors affecting 5-HT uptake and [^{3}H]imipramine binding in platelets

Before we review the data on platelet 5-HT uptake and ^{3}H-IB sites in major depression, we should consider some of the factors that affect the determination of these parameters. Among the major factors affecting platelet 5-HT uptake are: (a) platelet age and size (Arora and Meltzer 1982); (b) type of anticoagulant and plasma dilution (Malmgren *et al.* 1985); (c) separation of active and passive uptake by choice of a 0 °C or imipramine blank (Arora and Meltzer 1981); (d) circadian rhythms (Rausch *et al.* 1982; Arora *et al.* 1984*b*); (e) seasonal variation in 5-HT uptake (Swade and Coppen 1980; Arora *et al.* 1984*a*); and (f) duration of drug-free period (Ross *et al.* 1980; Ross and Aberg-Wistedt 1983). Some of these factors are discussed briefly here.

Platelet age and size

It is recognized that platelets are heterogeneous (Corash *et al.* 1977). The number of 5-HT uptake sites (V_{max}) is greater in larger, heavier platelets (which are younger) than in lighter, smaller platelets (which are older). Older platelets have higher K_m values (lower affinity) than lighter platelets (Arora and Meltzer 1982). Studies of 5-HT uptake in depression have used a variety of centrifugation speeds to isolate platelets, yielding mixtures of heavy and light platelets. The reported differences in K_m and V_{max} of 5-HT uptake between depressed patients and controls may arise partly from differences in the platelet subpopulations studied. A centrifugation procedure which obtains all the platelets should be used whenever possible.

Circadian rhythm

Rausch *et al.* (1982) reported that platelet 5-HT uptake studied between 07.00 and 16.00 varied in a similar fashion between depressed patients and controls. Healy *et al.* (1986) studied V_{max} in 20 controls and 28 unmedicated depressed patients at 06.30, 09.00, and 12.00. 5-HT uptake in the controls was greater at 06.30 and 09.00 than at 12.00. Depressed patients had lower 5-HT uptake rates than controls only at 06.30. There was no difference in

TABLE 6.1. *Seasonal variation of 5-HT uptake in normal controls and depressed patients*

Study	Normal controls			Depressed patients		
	K_m	V_{max}	Peak*	K_m	V_{max}	Peak*
Swade and Coppen (1980)	–	ND		–	Yes	Jan, Feb
Arora *et al.* (1984*a*)	ND	Yes	Apr, June	ND	Yes	Jan, Feb, May, Sept, Oct
Egrise *et al.* (1986)[§]	ND	Yes	July	ND	Yes	Nov
Malmgren *et al.* (1989)	Yes	Yes	July, Dec	Yes	Yes	Oct, Nov

–, no data; ND, no difference.
*For V_{max} only.
[§]Depressed patients were all in remission and taking drugs—amitriptyline (5), lithium (1), and amitriptyline + Li (1).

the values at the three time points in the unmedicated patients, but after treatment with various drugs a rhythm comparable to the controls was found only in those who responded to treatment. Healy *et al.* suggested that the observed abnormalities might be indicative of a circadian disturbance in depression. Variations in controls or patients in the K_m or V_{max} of platelet 5-HT uptake during the day have been reported by other authors (Oxenkrug *et al.* 1978; Wirz-Justice and Richter 1979; Arora *et al.* 1984*b*; Humphries *et al.* 1985; Modai *et al.* 1986; Jerushalmy *et al.* 1988) but sample sizes and sampling frequencies were small or only one concentration of 5-HT was used, which prevents firm conclusions about circadian variation as a relevant factor in platelet 5-HT uptake in depression. Replication of the interesting results of Healy *et al.* (1986) seems to be important. However, it is unlikely that this factor accounts for much of the variance between studies.

Seasonal variation
Seasonal variation in platelet 5-HT uptake has been reported by various authors (Table 6.1). Autumn-winter was most frequently reported to be the peak of platelet 5-HT uptake in depression whereas spring-summer appears to be when the uptake peaks in controls. Were this type of variation in 5-HT uptake to occur in brain, depressed patients might have relatively enhanced re-uptake (inactivation) during autumn-winter, which might account for some seasonal aspects of depression. Platelet 5-HT uptake, to our knowledge, has not been studied in patients with seasonal affective disorder *per se*.

Swade and Coppen (1980) found a significant bimonthly variation of 5-HT uptake (V_{max}) in depressed patients (lowest in summer) but not in controls. Arora *et al.* (1984*a*) found a difference throughout the year, but V_{max} was least in the autumn. Malmgren *et al.* (1989) found variations in K_m in controls during the first half of the year, with a nadir in March and peak in July but no variation in the second half of the year. V_{max} peaked in July and December. Seasonal variation in both K_m and V_{max} was also marked in the depressed patients. Depressed patients had lower V_{max} only in the summer. They, like Arora *et al.* (1984*a*), found that the difference in V_{max} between depressed patients and controls was largest in December. It is thus possible that any differences in platelet 5-HT uptake between depressed patients and controls may occur only during some seasons, that controls and patients must be studied simultaneously to establish group norms, and that platelet 5-HT uptake in a given patient must be adjusted for seasonal effects in a given region before it can be evaluated as possibly decreased. For these reasons, it is not possible to do a suitable meta-analysis with the available data.

Malmgren *et al.* (1989) speculated that seasonal variations in melatonin and 5-HT synthesis may be tied in with changes in brain 5-HT uptake which parallel those found in the platelet. This could be based on a common origin of platelets and brain (Campbell 1981) and reflect decreased serotonergic activity rather than enhanced serotonergic activity because of less re-uptake. If so, the abnormality in photoperiod-related changes in platelet 5-HT uptake may reflect a more generalized disturbance of this kind in depression.

Drug effects and the duration of wash-out

Tricyclic antidepressants generally block platelet 5-HT uptake by a competitive mechanism characterized by an increase in K_m with no change in V_{max} (Lingjaerde 1980). A few antidepressant drugs may act via a non-competitive mechanism leading to increased K_m and decreased V_{max}. Zimelidine treatment increases V_{max} (Lingjaerde 1980).

It is beyond the scope of this review to consider the effect of antidepressant treatments on platelet 5-HT uptake in detail. The relevant question is whether the wash-out period of 1–2 weeks used in most studies is sufficient for an unbiased assessment of uptake. Ross *et al.* (1980) and Ross and Aberg-Wistedt (1983) reported that 5-HT uptake in blood platelets of depressed patients returned to normal after two weeks of withdrawal from zimelidine and four weeks from clomipramine. They concluded that four weeks of wash-out were necessary before drawing blood from patients treated with clomipramine. However, Poirier *et al.* (1987) reported that after two weeks of wash-out after clomipramine treatment, 5-HT uptake returns to control values in blood platelets of normal controls, whereas with other drugs, for example maprotiline and amineptine, 5-HT uptake returns to control values after one week of withdrawal. Thus, the effects of treatment and wash-out differ among antidepressant drugs. Most studies have reported decreased V_{max} in

TABLE 6.2. *Drug-free period and* ^{14}C*-5-HT uptake in blood platelets of psychiatric patients*

Drug-free period (No. of days)	N	K_m (μM)	V_{max} (pmol per 10^7 platelets min^{-1})
1–6	97	0.47 ± 0.16*	10.6 ± 3.2
7–13	260	0.42 ± 0.14	10.4 ± 3.3
14 and over	52	0.42 ± 0.11	10.7 ± 3.1

± S.D.
*$p < 0.05$ compared to other two groups.

depressed patients, suggesting that they have probably included adequate wash-out periods, unless K_m and V_{max} can normalize at different rates when a drug effect on V_{max} has developed. We analysed our data on platelet 5-HT uptake in patients treated with various tricyclic antidepressants (mainly imipramine, desipramine, nortriptyline, and amitriptyline). Because there were relatively few patients for each drug, the data were pooled. K_m of 5-HT uptake was slightly greater in patients who were washed out for less than six days than in those with longer periods of wash-out (Table 6.2). There was no difference in V_{max} as a function of wash-out duration.

Comparison of platelet 5-HT uptake in depressed patients and normal controls

Tuomisto and Tukiainen (1976) compared 5-HT uptake kinetics in the blood platelets of depressed patients and age-matched normal controls. They reported significantly lower V_{max} (a measure of the number of sites) of 5-HT uptake in the depressed patients. There was no difference in K_m (inversely related to the affinity of 5-HT for the uptake sites) between controls and depressed patients. There have since been at least 32 published studies of 5-HT uptake in major depression (Table 6.3). Twenty-four of the 32 studies (75 per cent) reported significantly decreased V_{max} in patients with major depression. The sample sizes in these studies were generally quite small: fourteen studies had fewer than 15 depressed patients and only ten had more than 20, with the largest, Roy *et al.* (1987), having only 49 patients. In those studies which reported a decrease in V_{max}, the decrease ranged from 21 to 49 per cent, with a median of 33 per cent. The gross differences in methodology between studies and the lack of sufficient details for evaluation of critical factors in patient and control populations make it impossible to combine these studies for meta-analysis. The number of depressed patients whose V_{max} fell below the normal range was generally not reported. However, Wood *et al.* (1983) found no overlap in V_{max} between 15 depressed patients

TABLE 6.3. *5-HT uptake in blood platelets of depressed patients*

Study	N	K_m	V_{max}	Percentage change
Shaw *et al.* (1971)*	10	–	ND	
Hallstrom *et al.* (1976)**	11	–	decreased	
Tuomisto and Tukiainen (1976)	10	ND	decreased	−47
Coppen *et al.* (1978*a*)	13	ND	decreased	−30
Wirz-Justice and Pühringer (1978)*	11	–	ND	
Oxenkrug (1979)*	17	–	increased	+33
Tuomisto *et al.* (1979)	13	ND	decreased	−38
Scott *et al.* (1979)	25	ND	decreased	BP, −30
Coppen *et al.* (1980)	26	ND	decreased	−24
Mirkin and Coppen (1980)	8	ND	decreased	−48
Ross *et al.* (1980)*	18	–	ND	
Giret *et al.* (1980)	5 (3 on Li)	ND	decreased	
Ehsanullah (1980)**	19	ND	decreased	
Meltzer *et al.* (1981)	22	ND	decreased	UP, −27; BP, −49
Aberg-Wistedt *et al.* (1981)*	34	ND	decreased	−21
Raisman *et al.* (1982)	14	decreased	decreased	−39
Rausch *et al.* (1982)*	7	–	decreased	−30
Zemishlany *et al.* (1982)	10	ND	increased	BP, +48
Kaplan and Mann (1982)	16	increased	(trend decreased)	
Meltzer *et al.* (1982)	40	ND	decreased	−23
Wood *et al.* (1983)	15 (9 on TCA)	ND	decreased	−46
Stahl *et al.* (1983)	11	ND	decreased	BP, −27
Healy *et al.* (1983)	22	ND	decreased	−31[†]
Modai *et al.* (1984)	17	ND	decreased	UP, −26
		ND	increased	BP, +29
Healy *et al.* (1985)	37	ND	decreased	−48
Flasko *et al.* (1985)	16	ND	increased	+39, neurotic
Rausch *et al.* (1986)	16	ND	decreased	−21
Healy *et al.* (1986)	28	ND	decreased 06.30	−25
			trend 09.00	−8
Roy *et al.* (1987)	49	ND	ND	
Faludi *et al.* (1988)	14	decreased	decreased	−49
Pecknold *et al.* (1988)	17	ND	decreased	−39
Slotkin *et al.* (1989)***	30	–	decreased	

ND, no difference; TCA, tricyclic antidepressants; Li, lithium; UP, unipolar; BP, bipolar.
* Uptake determined at one concentration of ^{14}C-5-HT.
** Studied uptake at four concentrations of ^{14}C-5-HT.
*** Studied uptake at three concentrations of ^{14}C-5-HT.
[†] Only in responders.

TABLE 6.4.   *Platelet 5-HT uptake in normal controls, major affective disorders, and schizophrenia*

Group	N	K_m (μM)	V_{max} (pmol per 10^7 platelets min^{-1})
Normal controls	160	0.47 ± 0.13	12.5 ± 2.9
Major depression	133	0.44 ± 0.14	$10.1 \pm 2.9^*$
Unipolar	71	0.44 ± 0.15	$10.3 \pm 2.8^*$
Bipolar	39	0.45 ± 0.14	$8.6 \pm 2.8^*$
Psychotic	85	0.44 ± 0.16	$9.8 \pm 3.2^*$
Non-psychotic	48	0.44 ± 0.12	10.6 ± 2.6
Manic	57	0.46 ± 0.14	$10.5 \pm 2.5^*$
Schizophrenic	84	0.45 ± 0.13	10.9 ± 3.3

$\pm$ S.D.
$^*p <0.05$, significantly less than normals.

(six drug-free, nine on tricyclic antidepressants) and 10 controls. We found that 14 of 40 (35 per cent) depressed patients met this criteria. Because of this overlap, it is unlikely that V_{max} could be a biological marker.

A large-scale study which failed to find a decrease in V_{max} in depressed patients was that of Roy *et al.* (1987). This study included 32 unipolar patients, 6 bipolar depressives, and 11 with dysthymic disorder. No differences in V_{max} or K_m were noted between any of the subgroups. There are no obvious faults in the procedures used for diagnosis, the duration of wash-out, or the determination of K_m and V_{max}.

We studied platelet 5-HT uptake in 160 normal controls and 133 major depressive patients in Chicago between 1978 and 1985 (Table 6.4). There was no effect of age or sex on platelet 5-HT uptake. Hence, data from males and females were combined. V_{max} was significantly decreased with no change in K_m. The overall mean decrease in V_{max} was 19.2 per cent. Uptake was most decreased in bipolar depressed patients (31.2 per cent), compared to unipolar depressed (17.6 per cent). There was a slightly greater decrease in V_{max} in the psychotic depressed patients (21.6 per cent) than in the non-psychotic depressed (15.2 per cent), but this was not adjusted for the bipolar factor. The overlap in V_{max} between depressed patients and controls was marked. No differences in K_m were found.

These results were not replicated in a subsequent study, using the same methodology, in 42 normal controls and 45 unmedicated patients who met DSM-III or III-R criteria for major depression (V_{max} = 11.9 $\pm$ 2.7 and 11.2 $\pm$ 2.7 pmol per 10^7 platelets min^{-1}, respectively). However, 21 of the 45 depressed patients had a history of alcoholism: 14 of these had been abstinent for at least a year; seven for at least 3–4 weeks before the study. When the data from these patients were excluded, a significant ($p < 0.005$) decrease in V_{max} was observed in the 24 depressed patients with no history of alcohol dependence (9.9 ± 2.1 pmol per 10^7 platelets min^{-1}) compared to controls. It should be noted that V_{max} in 11 alcoholic patients in withdrawal without evidence of depression was 11.0 ± 2.6 pmol per 10^7 platelets min^{-1} compared to 12.5 ± 2.7 pmol per 10^7 platelets min^{-1} in 30 controls (R.C. Arora *et al.*, unpublished). These results suggest there could be a difference in V_{max} between depressed patients with and without a history of substance abuse. In addition, K_m was also significantly decreased in this group of depressed patients compared with normal controls (R. C. Arora and H. Y. Meltzer, unpublished). However, further study with a larger sample of patients with major depression and alcoholism is needed to confirm this finding.

There is some evidence for a relationship between V_{max} and the unipolar/bipolar division of major depression. Scott *et al.* (1979) and Stahl *et al.* (1983) both reported decreased V_{max} only in bipolar depressed patients, not in unipolar patients. Our studies (Meltzer *et al.* 1981, 1982, this report) found decreased V_{max} in both groups, but with significantly lower levels in bipolar patients. Roy *et al.* (1987) found no effect of polarity. On the other hand, Modai *et al.* (1984) found that bipolar depressed patients had increased V_{max} compared to controls and only unipolars had decreased V_{max}. There are a number of methodological problems with the latter study, for example use of too high a concentration of ^{14}C-5-HT.

There is conflicting evidence concerning V_{max} in psychotic depressives compared with non-psychotic depressives. Healy *et al.* (1986) reported decreased V_{max} in 20 non-psychotic depressives and not in eight psychotic depressives. We found that low V_{max} was related to paranoid psychotic symptoms ($\varrho = -0.31$, $n = 65$) rather than to mood congruent delusions. It is possible that Healy *et al.* (1986) studied only psychotic depressives with mood congruent delusions.

We found significant negative correlations between V_{max} and several aspects of depressive symptomatology (Table 6.5), including the Depression subscale of the *Schedule for Affective Disorders and Schizophrenia-Change* (SADS-C) and six of 16 subscale items, including suicidal ideation and insomnia. In a multivariate analysis, we found that V_{max}, after adjustment for K_m, was an even more powerful predictor of the SADS-C Depression scale rating (F = 6.899, df = 2,74, $p = 0.002$, standard beta weight for V_{max} = -3.71, $p < 0.0004$). Admission Hamilton Depression scale scores were less well related to V_{max} ($\varrho = -0.19$, $n = 91$, $p = 0.10$). However, the Hamilton Guilt and Work and Activities items were significantly negatively correlated with V_{max} (data not presented). We also found weak negative correlations between K_m and SADS-C total Depression scale score ($\varrho = -0.23$, $n = 91$, $p = 0.05$). Faludi *et al.* (1988), who reported markedly decreased V_{max} in 14 depressed patients, found no correlation between V_{max} or K_m and the total Hamilton Depression scale. No other study of platelet 5-HT uptake in major

TABLE 6.5.   *Correlation between psychopathology and 5-HT uptake*

Psychopathology	K_m rho	V_{max} rho
SADS-1 (Depression)	–	$-0.21, p=0.044, (94)$
SADS-C1 (Anxiety)	–	$-0.22, p=0.033, (94)$
SADS-C2 (Depression)	–	$-0.39, p=0.0001, (95)$
SADS-5 (Worrying)	–	$-0.37, p=0.0002, (95)$
SADS-9 (Suicidal)	–	$0.30, p=0.0035, (93)$
SADS-12 (Insomnia)	$-0.20, p=0.054, (93)$	$-0.33, p=0.011, (93)$
SADS-C2 (Depression)		
Psychotic	–	$-0.36, p=0.0028, (67)$
Non-psychotic	–	$-0.25, p=0.05, (47)$

( ), n

depression reported whether or not V_{max} was correlated with severity of depression.

There have been several studies of platelet 5-HT uptake in recovered depressed patients. Coppen *et al.* (1978*a*) found that platelet 5-HT uptake remained low after treatment with tricyclic antidepressants for six weeks and drug withdrawal for 15 days. Similar results were reported by Suranyi-Cadotte *et al.* (1985*b*). However, normalization of V_{max} was found after treatment with mianserin (Coppen *et al.* 1978*b*), imipramine (Tuomisto *et al.* 1979), trazodone and amitriptyline (Healy *et al.* 1983, 1985), nortriptyline (Meltzer *et al.* 1981), electroconvulsive therapy (ECT) (Healy *et al.* 1986), and lithium (Meltzer *et al.* 1983*a*). These results of Coppen *et al.* (1978*a*) and Suranyi-Cadotte *et al.* (1985*b*) suggest that V_{max} may be a trait marker for depression, but the effect of drug treatment to increase V_{max} must be considered.

Specificity of decreased platelet 5-HT uptake for major depressive disorder

Platelet 5-HT uptake has been studied in relatively few clinical populations other than major affective disorder. Schizophrenic patients were reported to have normal platelet 5-HT uptake (Meltzer *et al.* 1981; Stahl *et al.* 1983) whereas increased 5-HT uptake was reported in panic disorder (Norman *et al.* 1989). A slight decrease in V_{max} (18 per cent) was reported in a small group of adult male patients ($n = 15$) with episodic aggression (Brown *et al.* 1989). There was a significant negative correlation ($r = -0.62$) between the percentage of control value in platelet 5-HT uptake and Impulsivity but not Anger ratings. Decreased platelet 5-HT uptake has also been found in hypertension (Bhargava *et al.* 1979; Kamal *et al.* 1984). No significant differences were observed in premenstrual tension (Malmgren *et al.* 1987) or anorexia nervosa (Weizman *et al.* 1986*b*; Zemishlany *et al.* 1987). We have found no difference in platelet 5-HT uptake in alcoholism or obsessive-compulsive disorder (R. C. Arora *et al.*, unpublished data). It thus appears that decreased platelet 5-HT uptake may be reasonably specific for major depressive disorder.

Platelet 5-HT uptake as a marker for central serotonergic process

The question of whether decreased platelet 5-HT uptake in major depression is indicative of decreased 5-HT uptake in brain cannot be simply answered. The determination of ^{14}C-5-HT uptake in post-mortem tissue is not currently feasible because of the rapid post-mortem inactivation of the transporter. As will be discussed, [^{3}H]paroxetine binding may provide a measure of the density of 5-HT uptake sites but there are, as yet, no studies in major depression or suicide. There are studies of ^{3}H-IB in the brains of suicides or depressed patients which may provide some measure of 5-HT uptake sites, but the results are conflicting (Arora and Meltzer 1989*c*). There may be marked regional differences in the relative density of ^{3}H-IB sites in suicides compared to controls (Gross-Iseroff *et al.* 1989), making it even more hazardous to draw conclusions based on the platelet studies.

We have found another possible central correlate of platelet serotonin uptake. The cortisol response to 5-hydroxytryptophan is blocked by ritan-serin. Thus it is mediated by a 5-HT$_2$ or 5-HT$_{1C}$ receptor (J-C. Lee *et al.*, unpublished). This response may be increased in some depressed patients (Meltzer *et al.* 1984*c*). We measured platelet 5-HT uptake and the cortisol response to L-5-HTP (200 mg) in 51 depressed patients (26 unipolar, 13 bipolar, and 12 schizoaffective depressed, mainly affective). There was a significant positive correlation between K_m and the area under the 5-HTP-cortisol curve ($\varrho = 0.42$, $p = 0.01$). This correlation also held for all the subgroups of depression. There was a weaker correlation to V_{max} which disappeared after adjusting for K_m (H. Y. Meltzer *et al.*, unpublished). Thus, the lower the affinity for 5-HT (and hence the less the uptake) the greater the cortisol response to 5-HTP. Antidepressant drugs such as imipramine do not enhance this response (Meltzer *et al.* 1984*b*). Therefore, the conclusions to be drawn from this finding are very tentative.

Decreased platelet 5-HT uptake, then, may tell us nothing about brain 5-HT uptake. Decreased uptake in brain would contribute to enhanced serotonergic activity. This is not compatible with a simple 5-HT insufficiency theory of affective disorder. We suggested it could indicate that decreased uptake is a compensatory effort to overcome decreased 5-HT synthesis and release (Meltzer *et al.* 1981), which could explain the negative correlation with psychopathology. This would appear to be a very unlikely possibility. It is safest to conclude at this point that decreased platelet 5-HT occurs in some depressed patients, has no diagnostic significance, and is of unknown pathophysiological significance. At most, it provides some small additional evidence for a serotonergic disturbance in depression.

Cortisol, platelet 5-HT uptake, and imipramine binding

There is extensive evidence that adrenocorticoid secretion is increased in many patients with major depression. Lowering of platelet 5-HT uptake and IB may arise from the increased level of plasma cortisol. Meltzer *et al.* (1983*b*) reported that depressed patients who suppress cortisol secretion after dexamethasone have a strong trend towards lower 5-HT uptake (V_{max}), whereas those who do not suppress have higher levels of 5-HT uptake (V_{max}), suggesting that excessive corticosteroid stimulation may contribute to decreased V_{max} in platelets of depressed patients. However, Roy *et al.* (1987) did not find any correlation between 5-HT uptake and cortisol levels in depressed patients or normal controls at either 16.00 or 23.00 after a dexamethasone suppression test. They found a significant negative correlation between platelet IB (B_{max}) and plasma cortisol levels in depressed patients but not in normal controls, before (16.00) and after DST administration (23.00). Tukiainen (1981), Vermes *et al.* (1976), and Lee and Chan (1985) reported that corticosterone administration to adrenalectomized rats increases platelet 5-HT uptake. Administration of corticosterone to adrenalectomized rats was reported to decrease platelet and brain IB (Arora and Meltzer 1986). These results suggest that the effect of corticosteroids on platelet 5-HT uptake may arise, in part, from their effect on platelet IB as the IB site might inhibit 5-HT uptake. DeMet *et al.* (1989*b*) and Takeda *et al.* (1989) did not find any correlation between plasma cortisol and platelet IB in depressed patients.

Platelet 5-HT uptake: conclusions

Most studies of platelet 5-HT uptake in depression report a significant decrease in V_{max}. Significant correlations with depressive symptomatology, as well as with other biological parameters, for example the cortisol response to a 5-HTP challenge, have been found. However, study of platelet 5-HT uptake lacks specificity and sensitivity for clinical use on its own. Many of the positive studies were small scale, with possible artefacts because of methodological variance between groups. As will be discussed, no difference in [^{3}H]paroxetine-binding sites has been reported in the platelets of depressed patients and controls. As this measure should correlate closely to V_{max}, it appears that some other factors which affect V_{max}, for example endogenous ligands, may be responsible for some of the reported differences between depressed patients and controls. The presence of endogenous ligands which inhibit or stimulate platelet or brain ^{14}C-5-HT uptake and [3H]imipramine binding in human plasma and rodent brain has been reviewed by Barbaccia *et al.* (1988).

[3H]Imipramine-binding sites in human blood platelets

Langer and colleagues identified a high-affinity binding site for [3H]imipramine in brain and platelets ten years ago (Rehavi *et al.* 1980; Langer *et al.* 1980; Briley *et al.* 1979). The pharmacology of ^{3}H-IB in the brain and platelets is very similar to that of the inhibition of 5-HT transport into 5-HT nerve terminals and platelets (Langer *et al.* 1980; Paul *et al.* 1980). Some differences do exist, however (Langer and Schoemaker 1988). There is conclusive evidence that the ^{3}H-IB site is present on 5-HT neurones (Sette *et al.* 1981) and plays a critical role in modulating 5-HT uptake. There is controversy as to whether this site is separate but allosterically related to the 5-HT transporter (Briley *et al.* 1981; Langer and Raisman 1983) or is the transporter itself (Marcusson *et al.* 1986). The presence of an additional low affinity ^{3}H-IB site (Ieni *et al.* 1985) has been suggested at higher [3H]imipramine concentrations. However, Marcusson and Tiger (1988) reported the presence of a single saturable high-affinity ^{3}H-IB site using 5-HT to define non-specific ^{3}H-IB. Studies with [3H]paroxetine, a ligand with much greater affinity and specificity for the transporter than [3H]imipramine, suggest a single site for 5-HT uptake and antidepressant binding in rat and human brain (Marcusson *et al.* 1989). This conclusion is based on the similar pharmacology of both 5-HT and 5-HT uptake blockers against [3H]paroxetine binding (see Marcusson *et al.* 1989 for discussion).

Briley *et al.* (1980) were the first to report significantly lower density of ^{3}H-IB sites (B_{max}) in the blood platelets of unmedicated depressed patients compared to normal controls. There have since been at least 54 published studies of ^{3}H-IB in depressed patients (Table 6.6). Thirty-four of these reported a significant decrease in B_{max} of untreated depressed patients compared to normal controls, but many others found no difference (Table 6.7) and two found an increase (Mellerup *et al.* 1982, Carstens *et al.* 1988). The magnitude of the difference varied from 10–54 per cent, median 28 per cent. The number of depressed subjects ranged from 3–63, median 16. There were nine studies with more than 30 patients. In the 21 studies which found no difference or an increase in B_{max}, the sample size ranged from 7–55, median 28. Ten had 30 or more subjects. Although four studies (Baron *et al.* 1983; Hrdina *et al.* 1985; Carstens *et al.* 1988; Marazziti *et al.* 1988) reported significant difference in K_d, there is general agreement that K_d (affinity

TABLE 6.6. *Platelet imipramine binding in depression*

Study	N	K_d	B_{max}	Percentage change
Briley *et al.* (1980)	16	ND	Decreased	−54
Asarch *et al.* (1980)	22	ND	Decreased	−22
Paul *et al.* (1981)	14	ND	Decreased	−29
Raisman *et al.* (1981)	37	ND	Decreased	−48
Suranyi-Cadotte *et al.* (1982)	3	ND	Decreased	−53
Raisman *et al.* (1982)	14	ND	Decreased	−32
Mellerup *et al.* (1982)	19	ND	Increased	+18
Baron *et al.* (1983)	15	Decreased	Decreased	−22 ($p < 0.07$)
Wood *et al.* (1983)*	15	ND	Decreased	−21
Langer and Raisman (1983)	48	ND	Decreased	−43
Suranyi-Cadotte *et al.* (1983)	6	ND	Decreased	−44
Meltzer *et al.* (1984*a*)	11	ND	Decreased	−30
Suranyi-Cadotte *et al.* (1984)	10	ND	Decreased	−26
Lewis and McChesney (1985*a*)	45	ND	Decreased	−14
Tanimoto *et al.* (1985)**	19	–	Decreased	−29
Wägner *et al.* (1985)	63	ND	Decreased	−10
Arora *et al.* (1985)	50	ND	Decreased	−13
Schneider *et al.* (1985)	16	ND	Decreased	−20 (elderly depressed)
Suranyi-Cadotte *et al.* (1985*b*)	10	ND	Decreased	−25
Lewis and McChesney (1985*b*)†	6	ND	Decreased	−39
Nankai *et al.* (1986)	13	ND	Decreased	−23
Poirier *et al.* (1986)	17	ND	Decreased	−47
Baron *et al.* (1986)‡	33	ND	Decreased	−20 (only in BP)
Langer *et al.* (1986)	12	ND	Decreased	−50
Schneider *et al.* (1986)	15	ND	Decreased	−28 (with family history)
Innis *et al.* (1987)	9	ND	Decreased	−31
Roy *et al.* (1987)	32	ND	Decreased	−12 (only in females)
Pecknold *et al.* (1987)	17	ND	Decreased	−25
Marazziti *et al.* (1988*a*)	10	Decreased	Decreased	−42
Schneider *et al.* (1988*b*)§	18	ND	Decreased	−26 (elderly depressed)
Maj *et al.* (1988)	19	ND	Decreased	−25
Carstens *et al.* (1988)	22	Increased	Increased	+39
Nemeroff *et al.* (1988)	48	–	Decreased	−42
Takeda *et al.* (1989)	12	ND	Decreased	−14
Theodorou *et al.* (1989)	34	ND	Decreased	−13 (only in females)
Ambrosini *et al.* (1990)	10	ND	Decreased	−28

BP, bipolar depressed; ND, no difference.
* Patients ($n=9$) were taking tricyclic antidepressants at the time of study.
** At one concentration of [³H]imipramine.
† Patients were taking lithium and neuroleptics at the time of study.
‡ Patients were taking lithium carbonate at the time of study.
§ Patients ($n=6$) were on medication.

constant for [^{3}H]imipramine) does not differ between depressed patients and normal controls.

We determined platelet ^{3}H-IB in a large group of psychiatric patients and normal controls (Table 6.8). This includes previously reported subjects (Meltzer *et al.* 1984*a*). There was no sex effect on platelet ^{3}H-IB. Hence, data from males and females were combined. There was a significant correlation between age and B_{max} in all depressed ($\varrho = -0.28$, $n = 33$, $p < 0.05$) and manic patients ($\varrho = -0.44$, $n = 26$, $p < 0.05$), but not in normal controls. Therefore, age was covaried in the analysis of B_{max}. ANOVA (Analysis of Variance) with age as covariate showed that the B_{max} of only unipolar psychotic depressives was significantly less than that of normal controls. There was no difference in K_d between normal controls and depressed patients, and no difference in K_d or B_{max} between manic patients and normal controls. We have replicated the difference in B_{max} between depressed patients and controls since moving our laboratory to Case Western Reserve University, although B_{max} values in both groups were higher than those we previously determined. Thus, B_{max} in 25 normals and 12 unmedicated major depressions were 1388 ± 366 and 1186 ± 176 fmol per mg protein, respectively ($p < 0.05$). These values are approximately 50 per cent higher in both groups, possibly because of slight changes in methodology which will be described elsewhere.

Mellerup and Plenge (1988) reviewed the relationship between K_d values and the presence of lower ^{3}H-IB in the platelets of depressed patients. Lower K_d values were suggested to indicate optimal conditions for determining ^{3}H-IB. They themselves report a K_d of 0.6 nM. Most studies report K_d of approximately 1 nM or slightly higher, including those from the laboratories of Langer, Paul, and Arora and Meltzer. Mellerup and Plenge (1988) stated that of the 11 studies which they reviewed that report no significant difference in B_{max} values, six (55 per cent) had K_d below 1 nM, whereas only three of 19 studies (16 percent) which reported lower B_{max} in depression had K_d below 1 nM. They suggest that the studies which report high ^{3}H-IB generally do not use optimal conditions. However, a review of the data in their Table does not support this conclusion. Fourteen of the 30 studies reported no significant difference and of these nine (64 per cent) had K_d values $\geqslant 1.0$ nM. Fifteen reported lower B_{max} values in the depressed patients, and of these 11 (73 per cent) had K_d values $\geqslant 1.0$ nM. One study did not determine K_d.

Factors affecting determination of platelet [^{3}H]imipramine binding

There are a number of factors that may be relevant to the discrepancies between the studies which report lower B_{max} in depressed patients and those which do not. Among assay features that affect ^{3}H-IB are: (a) method of

TABLE 6.7.   *Platelet studies with no difference in imipramine binding (B_{max})*

Study	N
Berrittini *et al.* (1982)	12
Whitaker *et al.* (1984)	16
Tang and Morris (1985)	20
Hrdina *et al.* (1985)	20 but increased K_d
Gentsch *et al.* (1985)	55 psychiatric patients
Theodorou *et al.* (1985)	42
Braddock *et al.* (1986)	28
Horton *et al.* (1986)	47
Carstens *et al.* (1986)	29
Muscettola *et al.* (1986)	19
Egrise *et al.* (1986)	7
Roy *et al.* (1987)	43
Desmedt *et al.* (1987)	37
Kanof *et al.* (1987)	38
Georgotas *et al.* (1987)	23 elderly depressed
Bech *et al.* (1988)	30
Plenge *et al.* (1988)	46
Haug *et al.* (1988)	32
Gentsch *et al.* (1989)	19
Theodorou *et al.* (1989)	47

TABLE 6.8.   *Platelet imipramine binding in normal controls, major affective disorders, and schizophrenia*

Group	N	K_d (nM)	B_{max} (fmol per mg protein)
Normal controls	120	0.89 ± 0.28	914.4 ± 204.0
Depression patients	79	0.93 ± 0.42	827.3 ± 219.0
Unipolar	52	0.94 ± 0.45	812.2 ± 240.9
Bipolar	15	0.90 ± 0.39	852.9 ± 179.2
Pschotic	48	0.87 ± 0.33	808.2 ± 218.8*
Non-psychotic	31	1.02 ± 0.52	857.1 ± 219.6
Mania	36	0.90 ± 0.30	925.7 ± 292.4
Schizophrenia	51	0.99 ± 0.37	862.1 ± 245.2

± S.D.
*$p < 0.05$, significantly less than normal controls (ANOVA with age as covariate).

platelet isolation; (b) use of platelet membranes or whole platelets; (c) membrane protein concentration; (d) use of different concentrations of desipramine to define non-specific binding; (e) the range of [³H]imipramine concentrations used for the binding assay; (f) too short incubation time; and (g) presence of more than one binding site. Considerable differences in B_{max} in controls have been reported in various studies (Mellerup and Plenge 1988). Other factors affecting the density of ^{3}H-IB in platelets are: (a) subtype of depression; (b) ill versus recovered; (c) circadian rhythm; (d) seasonal variation; (e) contamination by prior drug treatment; (f) age; and (g) sex. It is beyond the scope of this chapter to consider these in detail (see, for example, Mellerup and Plenge 1988), but we shall consider some of the more relevant factors to illustrate the problems in determining the validity of such studies.

Effect of platelet population, protein concentration, and platelet membrane preparation

We (Arora and Meltzer 1984) reported significantly higher K_d and B_{max} of ^{3}H-IB in the younger, heavier platelets of normal controls. We (Arora *et al.* 1985) and Barkai *et al.* (1985) also reported that platelet ^{3}H-IB is affected by the amount of protein used in ^{3}H-IB assays. Wägner *et al.* (1985), Horton *et al.* (1986), Innis *et al.* (1987), and Theodorou *et al.* (1989) also confirmed the effect of protein concentration on the density of ^{3}H-IB. Friedl *et al.* (1983) reported that mechanical disruption of platelets does not completely lyse the platelets. Thus, membrane preparations contain varying amounts of intracellular protein. Consequently, considerable variation in B_{max} values in relation to total protein may be expected with membrane preparations. They suggested the use of intact platelets for determination of ^{3}H-IB. Most studies of platelet ^{3}H-IB have used isolated membranes. However, it seems unlikely that there would be a differential effect of membrane protein contamination by intracellular protein in patients and controls. Studies which used intact platelets also report a mixture of decreased or normal IB in depressed patients compared to controls.

Circadian rhythm of platelet ^{3}H-IB

Studies of circadian rhythms in platelet ^{3}H-IB are summarized in Table 6.9. Nankai *et al.* (1986) determined ^{3}H-IB in six normal controls every 6 hours throughout a 24 h period starting at 09.00. They found a significant circadian rhythm in B_{max}. The B_{max} at 21.00 and 03.00 was significantly lower than at 09.00. There was no difference in K_d. However, Baron *et al.* (1988), Gentsch *et al.* (1989), and Arora and Meltzer (unpublished observations) did not find any difference in K_d or B_{max} of platelet ^{3}H-IB determined at 08.00–10.00 and 15.00–16.00 in normal controls and depressed patients. As previously mentioned, possible endogenous ligands from brain (Barbaccia *et al.* 1983; Langer *et al.* 1984; Rehavi *et al.* 1985) and human plasma (Brusov *et al.* 1985; Barkai *et al.* 1986; Strijewski *et al.* 1988) which could affect ^{3}H-IB have been reported. The levels of these substances could fluctuate during the 24 h

TABLE 6.9. *Circadian rhythm of platelet ^{3}H-IB in normal controls and depressed patients*

Study	Normal controls	Depressed patients
Nankai *et al.* (1986)	Starting 09.00, every 6 h. Significant circadian variation: B_{max} 21.00–03.00 less than at 09.00	–
Baron *et al.* (1988)	ND: 09.00–11.00, 16.00–18.00	ND
Gentsch *et al.* (1989)	ND: 08.00, 15.00	ND
Arora and Meltzer (unpublished)	ND: 08.00–09.00, 16.00–16.30	–

ND, no difference

period, thereby affecting platelet ^{3}H-IB sites. However, studies with large groups of controls and more frequent intervals are needed to clarify the circadian hypothesis.

Seasonal variation of [^{3}H]imipramine binding

There have been eleven studies of seasonal variation in ^{3}H-IB in the blood platelets of normal controls or depressed patients (Tables 6.10 and 6.11). Six laboratories determined ^{3}H-IB in the blood platelets of the same subjects over time. There was no consensus for the month of lowest ^{3}H-IB. Three groups (Goziotis and Tang 1988; Egrise *et al.* 1983, 1986; Arora and Meltzer 1988) reported highest B_{max} in the blood platelets of normal controls in the month of September, one in February (DeMet *et al.* 1989*a*), and one in January (Whitaker *et al.* 1984). Galzin *et al.* (1986) did not find any significant variation throughout the 12-month period. Intraindividual variation is highlighted in the study of Goziotis and Tang (1988). These authors studied 12 normal controls at monthly intervals over nine months. The coefficients of variation ranged from 14.2 to 39.6 per cent. There was no clear-cut seasonal variation in this study nor in a study by Tang and Morris (1985) of different individuals over two years. They concluded that assay-based variance made determination of ^{3}H-IB unreliable. These results demonstrate the importance of measuring ^{3}H-IB in platelets from depressed patients and controls simultaneously. Four of six studies which compared different groups of depressed patients also found a seasonal variation in B_{max} (Table 6.11). Four of seven investigations of groups of controls studied throughout a 12-month period also found a seasonal variation. The lack of consensus among these groups as to the peaks and troughs indicates the problem with adjusting for seasonal

TABLE 6.10. *Seasonal variation of platelet imipramine binding in normal controls studied over time*

Study	K_d	B_{max}	Peak[+]
Egrise *et al.* (1983)	No	Yes	Sept
Whitaker *et al.* (1984)	No	Yes	Jan
Egrise *et al.* (1986)	No	Yes	Sept
Galzin *et al.* (1986)	No	No	
Arora and Meltzer (1988)*	No	Yes	Aug–Sept
Goziotis and Tang (1988)**	Yes	Yes	Sept
DeMet *et al.* (1989a)***	No	Yes	Feb 17

* Studied bimonthly.
** Nine-month (April to December) study using intact platelets.
*** Blood was drawn at six week intervals.
[+] Only for B_{max}.

TABLE 6.11. *Seasonal variation of platelet imipramine binding in normal controls and depressed patients*

Study	Normal controls		Depressed patients	
	K_d	B_{max}	K_d	B_{max}
Egrise *et al.* (1983)	No	Yes	No	Yes
Tang and Morris (1985)				
2-yr study (1983) 1st year	Yes	Yes	–	–
(1984) 2nd year	No	No	–	–
Egrise *et al.* (1986)	No	Yes	No	Yes*
Kanof *et al.* (1987)	No	No	No	No
Arora and Meltzer (1988)	Yes	No	No	Yes
Baron *et al.* (1988)	No	No	No	No
Theodorou *et al.* (1989)	–	Yes	–	Yes

* Patients were taking amitriptyline throughout the study period.

differences and the probable unreliability of existing assays over long periods of time.

Drug effects on ³H-IB and the duration of wash-out

The effect of treatment with antidepressant and other psychotropic drugs on ³H-IB of platelets has been extensively studied (see Langer and Schoemaker 1988 for review). Residual effects of such treatment on B_{max} or K_d must be considered as possible causes of the discrepancies between studies. Although there is no consensus about the duration of wash-out needed before drawing blood for ³H-IB studies, most studies were made after subjects were

TABLE 6.12. *Wash-out period and [³H]imipramine binding in the blood platelets of psychiatric patients*

Wash-out period (Days)	N	K_d (nM)	B_{max} (fmol per mg protein)
A. 1–6	36	1.10 ± 0.43*	819 ± 243**
B. 7–13	107	0.93 ± 0.44	900 ± 281
C. 14–21	24	1.04 ± 0.46	891 ± 320

* $t=2.02$, $p < 0.025$ compared to B.
** $t=1.512$, $0.1 > p > 0.05$ compared to B.

drug-free for at least seven days. Because the half-life of platelets is five to six days, seven days may not be sufficient. For example, Poirier *et al.* (1987) reported a significant decrease in B_{max} for healthy controls after one week of clomipramine treatment. This decrease in binding persisted for up to three weeks after the treatment. Theodorou *et al.* (1989) studied the effect of drug-free interval on platelet ³H-IB in major depressive patients. They did not find any difference in B_{max} in patients who were drug-free for 7–21 days and more than 22 days. K_d was, however, significantly lower in subjects with shorter antidepressant-free levels. In contrast, we found significantly higher K_d in subjects with a shorter drug-free interval (< 6 days) than patients with longer drug-free interval (< 15 days, 7–13 days). There was no significant effect of the duration of the drug-free period on B_{max} (Table 6.12). However, one should be cautious in interpreting these data, because the patients were treated with different types of antidepressants.

Relation between polarity, psychopathology, and ³H-IB in blood platelets of depressed patients

Imipramine binding studies were performed in the mixed population of unipolar, bipolar, psychotic, and non-psychotic patients or in the single population of depressed patients. Five studies have considered the effect of polarity on IB. Nankai *et al.* (1986) found low IB (B_{max}) in unipolar depressed patients, whereas Baron *et al.* (1986) reported low IB in only bipolar depressed patients who were treated with lithium. We (Meltzer *et al.* 1984a), Wägner *et al.* (1985), and Desmedt *et al.* (1987) found no difference between unipolar or bipolar depressed patients. Wägner *et al.* (1985) reported low IB in a population of unipolar and bipolar depressed patients, whereas Roy *et al.* (1987) reported only a trend for low IB in bipolar depressed patients. A detailed study with more unipolar and bipolar depressed patients is warranted.

Tanimoto *et al.* (1985) reported a significant negative correlation between B_{max} and Hamilton Depression rating score lower than twenty. None of the

TABLE 6.13. *Correlations between psychopathology and imipramine binding*

Psychopathology	K_d rho	B_{max} rho
Admission Hamilton Suicide	0.34, $p=0.0041$, (68)	–
SADS-C Worrying	–	0.26, $p=0.08$, (45)
SADS-C Psychic anxiety	–	0.36, $p=0.01$, (43)
SADS-C Insomnia	0.27, $p=0.06$, (45)	
SADS-C Thought disorder	–	0.29, $p=0.04$, (49)
SADS-Depression scale		
Psychotic	0.33, $p=0.051$ (36)	-0.35, $p=0.036$, (36)
Non-psychotic	–	0.38, $p=0.035$, (30)

( ), n

reported studies found any relation between binding and severity of depression. However, we found a significant positive correlation between K_d and Admission Hamilton Suicide rating score. B_{max} was correlated with four of six SADS-C scales examined (Table 6.13). The positive correlation between B_{max} and SADS-C subscales (Worrying, Psychic anxiety, and Thought disorder) implies that increased serotonin might promote these symptoms if the platelet IB reflects IB in the brain. The positive correlation between K_d and suicide is consistent with low 5-HT as a factor in suicide, because high K_d indicates low affinity for the endogenous imipramine-like compound which would mean less inhibition of 5-HT uptake. This correlation was positive and significant for most subgroups, especially psychotic depressed patients ($\varrho = 0.45$, $n = 25$, $p = 0.02$).

Because we found low IB (B_{max}) in the blood platelets of psychotic depressed patients, we divided our depressed patients in psychotic and non-psychotic groups and correlated B_{max} with the SADS-C depression scale (Table 6.13). B_{max} was negatively correlated ($p < 0.036$) with severity of depression in psychotic depressed patients and positively correlated in non-psychotic depressed patients. There was a trend towards positive correlation between K_d and severity of depression in psychotic depressed patients. There may be a significant negative correlation between binding and severity of depression in other binding studies but it is cancelled out by negative and positive correlation in psychotic and non-psychotic depressed patients. A negative correlation means that the greater the severity of depression, the lower the IB and vice-versa, which is consistent with the observations of Suranyi-Cadotte *et al.* (1985*a*), Hrdina *et al.* (1985), and Langer *et al.* (1986) that IB is a state-dependent marker for depression. However, study with a large group of psychotic depressed patients is needed to confirm this correlation.

[³H]Imipramine binding in platelets: state marker

Serotonin uptake sites are closely associated with the ³H-IB sites. As stated above, there are numerous reports of decreased ³H-IB (B_{max}) in the blood platelets of depressed patients compared to normal controls. Raisman *et al.* (1981) reported that ³H-IB (B_{max}) remained low even after recovery in a longitudinal study of depressed patients. Similar results were reported by Gay *et al.* (1983) and Baron *et al.* (1986). They suggested that ³H-IB may be a state-independent marker for depression. However, some studies (Suranyi-Cadotte *et al.* 1982, 1985*b*) have reported that the number of ³H-IB sites (B_{max}) returns to normal after recovery from depression. Lewis and McChesney (1985*a*) also reported that ³H-IB is low in the depressed phase and returns to normal in the manic phase of illness in bipolar depressed patients. They suggested that ³H-IB in platelets is a state marker for bipolar depression and not a trait marker for vulnerability. Langer *et al.* (1986) reported that B_{max} returns to normal levels in euthymic patients who were depressed. Marazziti *et al.* (1988*a*) found a significant correlation between binding parameters (K_d and B_{max}) and the improvement of clinical depression. These results suggest that ³H-IB may be a state-dependent marker for depression. We (Ambrosini *et al.* 1990) studied ³H-IB in normal children, depressed children and adolescents, and recovered children. B_{max}, which was low in the depressive phase, returns to normal in the recovery phase, suggesting that ³H-IB is a state-dependent marker for depression.

Platelet [³H]imipramine binding in other psychiatric disorders

Platelet ³H-IB has been studied in a large number of other disorders in which an abnormality of 5-HT has been postulated. B_{max} was found to be slightly but significantly decreased in 51 unmedicated schizophrenic patients (862 ± 245 fmol per mg protein) compared to 119 normal controls (916 ± 204 fmol per mg protein; $p < 0.05$; Arora *et al.* 1986). Similar results were obtained in a small series of neuroleptic-treated schizophrenic patients (Rotman *et al.* 1982). However, no differences in B_{max} of platelet ³H-IB were reported by Wood *et al.* (1983) or Weizman *et al.* (1987). These were both small studies that would have been unable to detect the size of the difference observed by Arora *et al.* (1986). Desmedt *et al.* (1987) actually found a higher B_{max} value in schizophrenic patients after adjusting for seasonal sampling time differences. Thus, there is no consensus on ³H-IB in schizophrenics.

Platelet ³H-IB has been studied in a variety of other psychiatric and neurological disorders. B_{max} has been reported to be normal in autism (Anderson *et al.* 1984; Weizman *et al.* 1987). Decreased B_{max} has been reported in anorexia nervosa (Weizman *et al.* 1986*b*) and obsessive-compulsive disorder (Weizman *et al.* 1986*a*; B. Bastani *et al.*, unpublished observations). Platelet ³H-IB was reported to be normal in three studies of Alzheimer's disease

(Suranyi-Cadotte *et al.* 1985*a*; Weizman *et al.* 1988; Arora *et al.*, unpublished observations). Schneider *et al.* (1988*a*) reported lower B_{max} only in Alzheimer's patients with agitation and delusions. Five studies reported no difference in B_{max} in patients with panic disorder (Innis *et al.* 1987; Nutt and Fraser 1987; Pecknold *et al.* 1987; Schneider *et al.* 1987; Uhde *et al.* 1987). However, Lewis *et al.* (1985*b*) and Marazziti *et al.* (1988*b*) reported a significant decrease in B_{max} in panic disorder patients.

Decreased B_{max} was reported in nine Parkinsonian patients compared with normal controls (Schneider *et al.* 1988*a*) as well as in 12 patients with Down's Syndrome (Tang *et al.* 1988). Magni *et al.* (1987) reported a 33 per cent decrease in B_{max} in patients with chronic pain. B_{max} increased to normal levels after treatment with mianserin which alleviated the pain. However, Mellerup *et al.* (1988) found no difference in psychogenic pain patients.

Decreased ^{3}H-IB has also been reported in enuretic children and adolescents (Weizman *et al.* 1985).

In view of the discrepancies about B_{max} in major depression, it is premature to conclude anything from these studies about the specificity of decreased B_{max} for major depression.

Platelet [^{3}H]imipramine binding in depression: discussion

Platelet ^{3}H-IB has attracted enormous interest as a possible index of serotonergic abnormalities in depression. In view of the reports of decreases in ^{3}H-IB in the frontal cortex of depressed patients (Stanley *et al.* 1982; Paul *et al.* 1984), which we, however, were unable to replicate (Arora and Meltzer 1989*c*), it is particularly important to establish whether ^{3}H-IB in platelets is decreased, at least in some depressed patients, at some phases of their illness. This could help to establish whether the platelet can be a marker for abnormalities in brain. Meticulous attention to drug-free states, diagnosis, simultaneous study of the control groups, assay reliability in the short and long term, and adequate size of all groups or subgroups will be needed to establish this point. Collaborative studies with many laboratories collecting and assaying samples seems unlikely to achieve the degree of rigour needed. As will be discussed, [^{3}H]paroxetine binding in platelets of depressed patients does not appear to be abnormal. This diminishes, but does not exclude, the possibility of an abnormality in ^{3}H-IB in platelets. The clinical significance of a decreased ^{3}H-IB in platelet or brain of depressed patients is difficult to predict. It might lead to increased uptake and hence decreased serotonergic activity.

[^{3}H]Paroxetine binding

Paroxetine is a potent and selective inhibitor of 5-HT uptake in platelets and brain (Buss-Lassen 1978). Specific binding of [^{3}H]paroxetine in rat brain has been characterized and found to be associated with the 5-HT transporter

(Habert *et al.* 1985; DeSouza and Kuyatt 1987; Marcusson *et al.* 1988, 1989). Studies by Scheffel and Hartig (1989) established that [^{3}H]paroxetine is a potent and selective agent for the *in vivo* labelling of cerebral 5-HT uptake sites. The B_{max} of [^{3}H]paroxetine-binding and ^{3}H-IB sites are comparable in normal human platelets; however, the K_d for [^{3}H]paroxetine was 0.08 nM, compared to 0.56 nM for [^{3}H]imipramine (Mellerup *et al.* 1983; Mellerup and Plenge 1986).

Galzin *et al.* (1988) determined [^{3}H]paroxetine binding in 16 depressed patients and 13 age-matched controls. There was no significant difference: 874 ± 44 fmol per mg protein in depressed patients and 895 ± 52 fmol per mg protein in controls. D'Haenen *et al.* (1988) also found no difference in K_d or B_{max} of platelet [^{3}H]paroxetine binding in 23 depressed patients and 23 controls. These authors suggested that [^{3}H]paroxetine is a more reliable ligand for studying the 5-HT transporter. In a continuing study, we have also found no difference in B_{max} or K_d between eight depressed patients and eight normal controls.

Replication of the results with [^{3}H]paroxetine by several more large-scale investigations would suggest that the reports of decreased platelet uptake sites and ^{3}H-IB sites in depression do not represent a real decrease in the density of 5-HT transporter sites in major depression. However, the results do not entirely exclude the possibility that other factors cause abnormalities in 5-HT uptake or ^{3}H-IB independent of changes in the transporter.

Platelet 5-HT$_2$ receptors

Serotonin-binding sites have been extensively studied in the central nervous system. On the basis of radioligand binding studies and autoradiographic analyses, 5-HT receptors have been subdivided into three major classes, 5-HT$_1$, 5-HT$_2$, and 5-HT$_3$ (Peroutka and Snyder 1979; Bradley *et al.* 1986). In platelets, two binding sites for 5-HT have been reliably identified—one associated with the 5-HT uptake site and the other with 5-HT-induced platelet shape change and aggregation (Drummond 1976). 5-HT-induced and -amplified aggregation is inhibited by ketanserin, a specific 5-HT$_2$ antagonist without any effect on 5-HT$_1$ binding sites (Leysen *et al.* 1981, 1982). The rank order of potencies for drug-induced inhibition of human blood platelet aggregation was highly correlated with that of [^{3}H]ketanserin binding to 5-HT$_2$ receptors in rat frontal cortex (DeClerck *et al.* 1984). McBride *et al.* (1987) also reported a significant correlation between 5-HT$_2$ binding using ^{125}I-labelled lysergic acid diethylamide (^{125}I-LSD) in normal human blood platelets and 5-HT-amplified aggregation response. It is thus believed that 5-HT-induced aggregation occurs via the 5-HT$_2$ receptor.

Studies using radioactive ligands to bind to 5-HT$_2$ receptors in human platelets are inconsistent and not yet fully developed. McBride *et al.* (1983), Cowen *et al.* (1987), and Elliott and Kent (1989) demonstrated a 5-HT$_2$

binding site on human blood platelets using ^{3}H-spiperone or ^{125}I-LSD. The binding of these ligands was significantly inhibited by 5-HT antagonists and the drug affinities were comparable to those reported for 5-HT$_2$ receptors in the frontal cortex of human brain, suggesting that platelet 5-HT$_2$ receptors are biochemically similar to those found in human frontal cortex. Geaney *et al.* (1984) demonstrated 5-HT$_2$ binding sites in human blood platelets using ^{3}H-LSD as the binding ligand. They found a significant correlation between the affinity of ^{3}H-5-HT$_2$ antagonists for ^{3}H-LSD-binding sites in human blood platelets and human frontal cortex as well as with the inhibition of 5-HT-induced shape change. The K_d (0.53 ± 0.02 nM) and B$_{max}$ (57.1 ± 5.6 fmol per mg protein) values for ^{3}H-LSD binding were similar to those reported by Elliott and Kent (1989) using ^{125}I-LSD as the ligand.

McBride *et al.* (1987), Cowen *et al.* (1987), Biegon *et al.* (1987), and we (Arora and Meltzer 1989*a*) studied 5-HT$_2$ binding in the blood platelets of unmedicated depressed patients and normal controls. Three of the four studies found increased 5-HT$_2$ binding (B$_{max}$) in depressed patients compared to normal controls. McBride *et al.* (1987) reported significantly increased 5-HT$_2$ binding in the platelets of depressed patients who made serious suicide attempts but not in the entire group of depressed patients, which consisted of 40 patients with major depression (24 with recent suicide attempts). There was no effect of age on K_d or B$_{max}$ in either group. The increase in B$_{max}$ was not due to any psychotropic drug effects because there was no difference in K_d or B$_{max}$ between unmedicated ($n = 6$) and previously medicated but currently drug-free patients ($n = 23$, Arora and Meltzer 1989*a*). There was no difference in K_d between normals and depressed patients in any of the above mentioned studies.

Increased 5-HT$_2$ binding (B$_{max}$) in depressed patients was also supported by the increased 5-HT$_2$ receptor functional response as measured by phosphoinositide turnover (Mikuni *et al.* 1989) and 5-HT-induced platelet aggregation (Brusov *et al.* 1989). However, Wood *et al.* (1985) found no difference in aggregation response to 5-HT in depressed patients compared to normal controls. Factors such as subtype of depression, duration of previous drug-free period, age and sex, and sample size may contribute to these discrepancies. In addition, the choice of ligand, the means of defining non-specific binding, and other aspects of the assay method may contribute to the observed discrepancies in binding assays.

We also studied 5-HT$_2$ binding in obsessive-compulsive disorder (OCD) and schizophrenic patients. Schizophrenic patients had not received any psychoactive drug for at least seven days before the study whereas OCD patients were drug-free for more than a month. There was no difference in K_d or B$_{max}$ between normal controls and OCD and schizophrenic patients (Table 6.14). These results suggest that 5-HT$_2$ binding is increased only in depressed patients. It is interesting to point out that most post-mortem studies have also reported an increase in 5-HT$_2$ receptor binding in the

TABLE 6.14. *5-HT$_2$ receptors as determined by ^{3}H-LSD binding in normal controls, major affective disorder, schizophrenia, and obsessive-compulsive disorder patients*

Group	N	K_d (nM)	B_{max} (fmol per mg protein)
Normal controls	32	0.76 ± 0.33	75.6 ± 20.6
Major depression	34	0.91 ± 0.58	99.6 ± 43.1*
Schizophrenia	28	0.67 ± 0.18	86.4 ± 18.5
Obsessive-compulsive disorder	16	0.73 ± 0.23	88.1 ± 16.9

$\pm$ S.D.
* $p < 0.05$ compared to normal controls.

frontal cortex of suicides (Stanley and Mann 1983; Mann *et al.* 1986; Arora and Meltzer 1989*b*) and depressed patients (McKeith *et al.* 1987). It is not known whether platelet 5-HT$_2$ and brain 5-HT$_2$ receptors are similarly regulated, for example by genetic, hormonal or environmental factors. If so, there could be a generalized up-regulation of 5-HT$_2$ receptors in some patients with major depression.

Summary and conclusion

This review considers four types of studies of platelet serotonergic measures in affective disorders: active 5-HT uptake, [^{3}H]imipramine binding, [^{3}H]paroxetine binding, and 5-HT$_2$ binding site or receptor studies. Two related measures—platelet 5-HT content and monoamine oxidase activity—are not considered.

For all these measures, except [^{3}H]paroxetine binding, the majority of the data support an abnormality in major depression. However, majority rule is not the most appropriate principle to apply. For those measures which have been most intensively studied, 5-HT uptake and ^{3}H-IB, it is apparent that assay conditions and secondary factors, such as previous drug treatment and circadian and seasonal rhythms, can influence significantly the outcome. Blinded, simultaneous study of patients and controls would be of great value in eliminating many systematic biases in the available literature.

The suggestion of comparable abnormalities in ^{3}H-IB and 5-HT$_2$ binding sites in platelets and brain of depressed patients encourages us to believe that the platelet can reflect abnormalities in brain. The platelet measure needs to be related to direct (e.g. positron emission tomography (PET) ligand studies) or indirect (e.g. CSF 5-HIAA, 5-HTP-induced cortisol response, behavioural ratings of depressive symptomatology) measures of brain serotonergic activity more rigorously than has been done so far.

After more than a decade of intensive work, it would be gratifying to be able to conclude that definitive answers are available as to platelet serotonergic abnormalities in affective disorders. Unfortunately, this is not the case. There is, however, clearly enough evidence with regard to all the measures to warrant further targeted research.

Acknowledgements

The research reported here was supported in part by USPHS MH41684, MH41594, GCRC MO1RR00080 and grants from the Cleveland Foundation and the John Pascal Sawyer Memorial Foundation. H.Y.M. is the recipient of a USPHS Research Scientist Award MH47808.

References

Aberg-Wistedt, A., Jostell, K.-G., Ross, S. B., and Westerlund, D. (1981). Effects of zimelidine and desipramine on serotonin and noradrenaline uptake mechanisms in relation to plasma concentrations and to therapeutic effects during treatment of depression. *Psychopharmacology*, **74**, 297–305.

Ambrosini, P. J., Metz, C., Arora, R. C., Lees, J-C., Kregel, L., and Meltzer, H. Y. (1990). Platelet imipramine binding in depressed children and adolescents. *Archives of General Psychiatry*, in press.

Anderson, G. M., Mendera, R. B., van Benthern, P. P.-G., Volkman, F. R., and Cohen, K. J. (1984). Platelet imipramine binding in autistic subjects. *Psychiatry Research*, **11**, 133–41.

Arora, R. C. and Meltzer, H. Y. (1981). A modified assay method for determining serotonin uptake in human platelets. *Clinica Chimica Acta*, **112**, 225–33.

Arora, R. C. and Meltzer H. Y. (1982). Serotonin uptake in subpopulations of normal human blood platelets. *Biological Psychiatry*, **17**, 1157–62.

Arora, R. C. and Meltzer, H. Y. (1984). Imipramine binding in subpopulations of normal human blood platelets. *Biological Psychiatry*, **19**, 257–62.

Arora, R. C. and Meltzer, H. Y. (1986). Effect of hypophysectomy, adrenalectomy and corticosterone on ^{3}H-imipramine binding in rat blood platelets and brain. *European Journal of Pharmacology*, **123**, 415–20.

Arora, R. C. and Meltzer, H. Y. (1988). Seasonal variation of imipramine binding in the blood platelets of normal controls and depressed patients. *Biological Psychiatry*, **23**, 217–26.

Arora, R. C. and Meltzer, H. Y. (1989a). Increased serotonin$_2$ (5-HT$_2$) receptor binding as measured by ^{3}H-lysergic acid diethylamide (^{3}H-LSD) in the blood platelets of depressed patients. *Life Sciences*, **44**, 725–34.

Arora, R. C. and Meltzer, H. Y. (1989b). Serotonergic measures in the brains of suicide victims: 5-HT$_2$ binding sites in the frontal cortex of suicide victims and control subjects. *American Journal of Psychiatry*, **146**, 730–6.

Arora, R. C. and Meltzer, H. Y. (1989c). [^{3}H]-imipramine binding in the frontal cortex of suicides. *Psychiatry Research*, **30**, 125–35.

Arora, R. C., Kregel, L., and Meltzer, H. Y. (1984a). Seasonal variation of serotonin uptake in normal controls and depressed patients. *Biological Psychiatry*, **19**, 795–804.

Arora, R. C., Kregel, L., and Meltzer, H. Y. (1984b). Circadian rhythm of serotonin uptake in the blood platelets of normal controls. *Biological Psychiatry*, **19**, 1579–84.

Arora, R. C., Wunnicke, V., and Meltzer, H. Y. (1985). Effect of protein concentration on kinetic constants (K_d and B_{max}) of ^{3}H-imipramine binding in blood platelets. *Biological Psychiatry*, **20**, 116–19.

Arora, R. C., Locascio, J. J., and Meltzer, H. Y. (1986). ^{3}H-Imipramine binding in blood platelets of schizophrenic patients. *Psychiatry Research*, **19**, 215–24.

Asarch, K. B., Shih, J.-C., and Kulcsar, A. (1980). Decreased ^{3}H-imipramine binding in depressed males and females. *Communications in Psychopharmacology*, **4**, 425–32.

Barbaccia, M., Brunello, N., Chuang, D. M., and Costa, E. (1983). On the mode of action of imipramine: relationship between serotonergic axon terminal function and down-regulation of β-adrenergic receptors. *Neuropharmacology*, **22**, 373–83.

Barbaccia, M., Costa, E., and Guidotti, A. (1988). Endogenous ligands for high-affinity recognition sites of psychotropic drugs. *Annual Review of Pharmacology and Toxicology*, **28**, 451–76.

Barkai, A. I., Kowalik, S., and Baron, M. (1985). Effect of membrane protein concentration on binding of ^{3}H-imipramine in human platelets. *Biological Psychiatry*, **20**, 215–19.

Barkai, A. I., Baron, M., Kowalik, S., and Cooper, T. B. (1986). Modification of ligand binding to membranes by a soluble acceptor. Alpha-l-acid glycoprotein attenuates ^{3}H-imipramine binding to cerebral membranes. *Biological Psychiatry*, **21**, 883–8.

Baron, M., Barkai, A., Gruen, R., Kowalik, S., and Quitkin, F. (1983). ^{3}H-imipramine platelet binding sites in unipolar depression. *Biological Psychiatry*, **18**, 1403–9.

Baron, M., Barkai, A., Gruen, R., Peselow, E., Fieve, R. R., and Quitkin, F. (1986). Platelet [^{3}H]imipramine binding in affective disorders: Trait versus state characteristics. *American Journal of Psychiatry*, **143**, 711–17.

Baron, M., Barkai, A., Kowalik, S., Fieve, R. R., Quitkin, F., and Gruen, R. (1988). Diurnal and circannual variation in platelet [^{3}H]imipramine binding: comparative data on normal and affectively ill subjects. *Neuropsychobiology*, **19**, 9–11.

Bech, P., Eplov, L., Gastpar, M., Gentsch, C., Mendlewicz, J., Plenge, P., *et al.* (1988). WHO pilot study on the validity of imipramine platelet receptor binding sites as a biological marker of endogenous depression. *Pharmacopsychiatry*, 147–150.

Berrettini, W. H., Nurnbergen, J. I., Post, R. M., and Gershon, E. S. (1982). Platelet ^{3}H-imipramine binding in euthymic bipolar patients. *Psychiatry Research*, **9**, 215–19.

Bhargava, K. P., Raina, N., Misra, N., Shanker, K., and Vrat, S. (1979). Uptake of serotonin by human platelets and its relevance to CNS involvement in hypertension. *Life Sciences*, **25**, 195–200.

Biegon, A., Weizman, A., Karp, L., Ram, A., Tiano, S., and Wolff, M. (1987). Serotonin 5-HT$_2$ receptor binding on blood platelets—a peripheral marker for depression? *Life Sciences*, **41**, 2485–92.

Braddock, L. E., Cowen, P. J., Elliott, J. M., Fraser, S., and Stump, K. (1986). Binding of yohimbine and imipramine to platelets in depressive illness. *Psychological Medicine*, **16**, 765–73.

Bradley, P. B., Angel, G., Feniuk, W., Fozard J. R., Humphrey, P. P. A.,

Middlemiss, D. N., *et al.* (1986). Proposals for the classification and nomenclature of functional receptors for 5-hydroxytryptamine. *Neuropharmacology*, **25**, 563–76.

Briley, M. S., Raisman, R., and Langer, S. Z., (1979). Human platelets possess high-affinity binding sites for ^{3}H-imipramine. *European Journal of Pharmacology*, **58**, 347–8.

Briley, M. S., Langer, S. Z., Raisman, R., Sechter, D., and Zarifian, E. (1980). Tritiated imipramine binding sites are decreased in platelets of untreated depressed patients. *Science*, **201**, 303–5.

Briley, M. S., Langer, S.Z., and Sette, M. (1981). Allosteric interaction between the ^{3}H-imipramine binding site and the serotonin uptake mechanism. *Proceedings of the British Pharmacological Society*, 817P–818P.

Brown, C. S., Kent, T. A., Bryant, S. G., Gevedon, R. M., Campbell, J. L., Felthous, A. R., *et al.* (1989). Blood platelets uptake of serotonin in episodic aggression. *Psychiatry Research*, **27**, 5–12.

Brusov, O. S., Formenko, A. M., and Katasonov, A. B. (1985). Human plasma inhibitors of platelet serotonin uptake and imipramine receptor binding: extraction and heterogeneity. *Biological Psychiatry*, **20**, 235–44.

Brusov, O. S., Beliaev, B. S., Katasonov, A. B., Zlobina, G. P., Factor, M. I., and Lideman, R. R. (1989). Does platelet serotonin receptor supersensitivity accompany endogenous depression? *Biological Psychiatry*, **25**, 375–81.

Buss-Lassen, J. (1978). Potent and long-lasting potentiation of two 5-hydroxytryptophan-induced effects in mice by three selective 5-HT uptake inhibitors. *European Journal of Pharmacology*, **47**, 351–8.

Campbell, I. C. (1981). Blood platelets and psychiatry. *British Journal of Psychiatry*, **138**, 78–80.

Carstens, M. E., Engelbrecht, A. H., Russell, V. A., Aalbers, C., Gagiano, C. A., Chalton, D. O., and Taljaard, J. J. F. (1986). Imipramine binding sites on platelets of patients with major depressive disorder. *Psychiatry Research*, **18**, 333–42.

Carstens, M. E., Engelbrecht, A. H., Russell, V. A., van Zyl, A. M., and Taljaard, J. J. F. (1988). Biological markers in juvenile depression. *Psychiatry Research*, **23**, 77–88.

Coppen, A., Swade, C., and Wood, K. (1978*a*). Platelet 5-hydroxytryptamine accumulation in depressive illness. *Clinica Chimica Acta*, **87**, 165–8.

Coppen, A., Ghose, K., Swade, C., and Wood, K. (1978*b*). Effect of mianserin hydrochloride on peripheral uptake mechanisms for noradrenaline and 5-hydroxytryptamine in man. *British Journal of Psychiatry*, **5**, 13S–17S.

Coppen, A., Swade, C., and Wood, K. (1980). Lithium restores abnormal platelet 5-HT transport in patients with affective disorders. *British Journal of Psychiatry*, **136**, 235–8.

Corash, L., Tan, H., and Gradnick, H. (1977). Heterogeneity of human whole blood platelet subpopulations. *Blood*, **49**, 71–87.

Cowen, P. J., Charig, E. M., Fraser, S., and Elliott, J. M. (1987). Platelet 5-HT receptor binding during depressive illness and tricyclic antidepressant treatment. *Journal of Affective Disorders*, **13**, 45–50.

DeClerck, F., Xhonneux, B., Leysen, J., and Janssen, P. A. J. (1984). Evidence for functional 5-HT$_2$ receptor sites on human blood platelets. *Biochemical Pharmacology*, **33**, 2807–11.

DeMet, E. M., Chicz-DeMet, A., and Fleischmann, J. (1989*a*). Seasonal rhythm of platelet ^{3}H-imipramine binding in normal controls. *Biological Psychiatry*, **26**, 489–95.

DeMet, E. M., Gerner, R. H., Bell, K. M., Kauffmann, C. D., Chicz-DeMet, A., and Warren, S. (1989*b*). Changes in platelet ³H-imipramine binding with chronic imipramine treatment are not state-dependent. *Biological Psychiatry*, **26**, 478–88.

Desmedt, D. H., Egrise, D., and Mendlewicz, J. (1987). Tritiated imipramine binding sites in affective disorders and schizophrenia influence of circannual variation. *Journal of Affective Disorders*, **12**, 193–8.

DeSouza, E. B. and Kuyatt, B. L. (1987). Autoradiographic localization of [³H]paroxetine-labeled serotonin uptake sites in rat brain. *Synapse*, **1**, 488–96.

D'Haenen, H., Waele, M. D., and Leysen, J.E. (1988). Platelet [³H]-paroxetine binding in depressed patients. *Psychiatry Research*, **26**, 11-17.

Drummond, A. H. (1976). Interactions of blood platelets with biogenic amines: uptake stimulation and receptor binding. In *Platelet in biology and pathology*, (ed. J. L. Gordon), pp. 203–239. North Holland Publishing, Amsterdam.

Egrise, D., Desmedt, D., Schoutens, A., and Mendlewicz, J. (1983). Circannual variations in the density of tritiated imipramine binding sites on blood platelets in man. *Neuropsychobiology*, **10**, 101–2.

Egrise, D., Rubinstein, M., Schoutens, A., Cantraine, F., and Mendlewicz, J. (1986). Seasonal variation of platelet serotonin uptake and ³H-imipramine binding in normal and depressed subjects. *Biological Psychiatry*, **21**, 283–92.

Ehsanullah, R. S. B. (1980). Uptake of 5-hydroxytryptamine and dopamine into platelets from depressed patients and normal subjects: influence of clomipramine, desmethylclomipramine and maprotiline. *Postgraduate Medical Journal*, **56**, Suppl. 1, 31–5.

Elliott, J. M. and Kent, A. (1989). Comparison of [¹²⁵I]iodo-lysergic acid diethylamide binding in human frontal cortex and platelet tissue. *Journal of Neurochemistry*, **53**, 191–6.

Faludi, G., Magyar, I., Tekes, K., Tothfalusi, L., and Magyar, L. (1988). Measurement of ³H-serotonin uptake in platelets of major depressive episodes. *Biological Psychiatry*, **23**, 833–6.

Flaskos, J., George, A. J., and Theophilopoulos, N. (1985). Platelet 5-HT uptake in obsessional neurosis and neurotic depression. *British Journal of Clinical Pharmacology*, **19**, 556P.

Friedl, W., Propping, P., and Weck, B. (1983). ³H-imipramine binding in platelets: influence of varying proportions of intact platelets in membrane preparations on binding. *Psychopharmacology*, **80**, 96–9.

Galzin, A. M., Loo, H., Sechter, D., and Langer, S. Z. (1986). Lack of seasonal variation in platelet [³H]imipramine binding in humans. *Biological Psychiatry*, **21**, 876–82.

Galzin, A. M., Poirier, M.-F., Loo, H., Sechter, D., Zarifian, E., and Langer, S. Z. (1988). [³H]Paroxetine binding from healthy volunteers and depressed patients. *British Journal of Pharmacology*, **93**, 12P.

Gay, C., Langer, S. Z., Loo, H., Raisman, R., Sechter, D., and Zarifian, E. (1983). ³H-imipramine binding in platelets—a state dependent or independent biological marker in depression. *British Journal of Pharmacology*, **78**, 57.

Geaney, D. P., Schachter, M., Elliott, J. M., and Grahame-Smith, D. G. (1984). Characterization of [³H]lysergic acid diethylamide binding to a 5-hydroxytryptamine receptor on human platelet membranes. *European Journal of Pharmacology*, **97**, 87–93.

Gentsch, C., Lichtsteiner, M., Gastpar, M., Gastpar, G., and Feer, H. (1985). ³H-imipramine binding sites in platelets of hospitalized psychiatric patients. *Psychiatry Research*, **14**, 177–87.

Gentsch, C., Lichtsteiner, M., Gastpar, M., Gastpar, G., and Feer, H. (1989). Platelet ^{3}H-imipramine binding sites in depressed patients and healthy controls: a comparison between morning and afternoon samples. *Journal of Affective Disorders*, **16**, 65–70.

Georgotas, A., Schweitzer, J., McCue, R. E., Armour, M., and Friedhoff, A. J. (1987). Clinical and treatment effects on ^{3}H-clonidine and ^{3}H-imipramine binding in elderly depressed patients. *Life Sciences*, **40**, 2137–43.

Giret, M., Launay, J. M., Dreux, C., Zarifian, E., Benyacoub, K., and Loo, H. (1980). Modifications of biochemical parameters in blood platelets of schizophrenic and depressive patients. *Neuropsychobiology*, **6**, 290–6.

Goziotis, A. and Tang, S. W. (1988). A longitudinal study of intact platelet ^{3}H-imipramine binding in 12 normal subjects. *Psychiatry Research*, **26**, 157–62.

Gross-Isseroff, R., Israeli, M., and Biegon, A. (1989). Autoradiographic analysis of initiated imipramine binding in the human brain post-mortem: effects of suicide. *Archives of General Psychiatry*, **46**, 237–41.

Habert, E., Graham, D., Tahraoui, L., Claustre, Y., and Langer, S. Z. (1985). Characterization of [^{3}H]paroxetine binding to rat cortical membranes. *European Journal of Pharmacology*, **118**, 107–14.

Hallstrom, C. O. S., Pare, C. M. B., Rees, W. L., Trenchard, A., and Turner, P. (1976). Platelet uptake of 5-HT and dopamine in depression. *Postgraduate Medical Journal*, **52**, 4044.

Haug, H. J., Fahndrich, E., Strauss, S., and Rommelspacher, H. (1988). Sleep deprivation and imipramine binding sites in depressed patients and healthy subjects. *Psychiatry Research*, **25**, 135–44.

Healy, D., Carney, P. A., and Leonard, B. E. (1983). Monoamine-related markers of depression: changes following treatment. *Journal of Psychiatric Research*, **17**, 251–60.

Healy, D., Carney, P. A., O'Halloran, A., and Leonard, B. E. (1985). Peripheral adrenoceptors and serotonin receptors in depression. *Journal of Affective Disorders*, **9**, 285–96.

Healy, D., O'Halloran, A., Carney, P. A., and Leonard, B. E. (1986). Variations in platelet 5-hydroxytryptamine in control and depressed populations. *Journal of Psychiatric Research*, **20**, 345–53.

Horton, R. W., Katona, L. L. E., Theodorou, A. E., Hale, A. S., Davies, S. L., Tunnicliffe, C., *et al.* (1986). Platelet radioligand binding and neuroendocrine challenge tests in depression. In *Antidepressant and receptor function*, Ciba Foundation Symposium 123, pp. 84–105. Wiley, Chichester.

Hrdina, P. D., Lapierre, Y. D., Horn, E. R., and Bakish, D. (1985). Platelet ^{3}H-imipramine binding: a possible predictor of response to antidepressant treatment. *Progress in Neuropsychopharmacology and Biological Psychiatry*, **9**, 619–23.

Humphries, L. L., Shirley, P., Allen, M., Codd, E. E., and Walker, R. F. (1985). Daily patterns of serotonin uptake in platelets from psychiatric patients and control volunteers. *Biological Psychiatry*, **20**, 1073–81.

Ieni, J. R., Zukin, S. R., and van Praag, H. M. (1985). Human platelets possess multiple [^{3}H]-imipramine binding sites. *European Journal of Pharmacology*, **106**, 669–72.

Innis, R. B., Charney, D. S., and Heninger, G. R. (1987). Differential ^{3}H-imipramine platelet binding in patients with panic disorder and depression. *Psychiatry Research*, **21**, 33–41.

Jerushalmy, Z., Modai, I., Chachkes, O., Mark, M., Valewski, A., Chachkes, M., and Tyano, S. (1988). Kinetic values of active serotonin transport by platelets of bipolar, unipolar and schizophrenic patients at 2 and 8 am. *Neuropsychobiology*, **20**, 57–61.

Kamal, L. A., Quan-Bui, K. H. L. B., and Mayer, P. (1984). Decreased uptake of ³H-serotonin and endogenous content of serotonin in blood platelets in hypertensive patients. *Hypertension*, **6**, 568–73.

Kanof, P. D., Coccaro, E. F., Johns, C. A., Siever, L. J., and Davis, K. L. (1987). Platelet [³H]imipramine binding in psychiatric disorders. *Biological Psychiatry*, **22**, 278–86.

Kaplan, R. D. and Mann, J. J. (1982). Altered platelet serotonin uptake kinetics in schizophrenia and depression. *Life Sciences*, **31**, 583–8.

Langer, S. Z. and Raisman, R. (1983). Binding of [³H]imipramine and [³H]desipramine as biochemical tools for studies in depression. *Neuropharmacology*, **22**, 407–13.

Langer, S. Z. and Schoemaker, H. (1988). Effects of antidepressants on monoamine transporters. *Progress in Neuro-Psychopharmacology and Biological Psychiatry*, **12**, 193–216.

Langer, S. Z., Briley, M. S., Raisman, R., Henry, J.-F., and Morselli, P. L. (1980). Specific ³H-imipramine binding in human platelets: influence of age and sex. *Naunyn-Schmiedeberg's Archives of Pharmacology*, **313**, 189–94.

Langer, S. Z. Raisman, R., Tahraoui, L., Scatton, B., Niddam, R., Lee, C. R., and Claustre, Y. (1984). Substituted tetrahydro-B-carbolines are possible candidates as endogenous ligand of the ³H-imipramine recognition site. *European Journal of Pharmacology*, **98**, 153–4.

Langer, S. Z., Sechter, D., Loo, H., Raisman, R., and Zarifian, E. (1986). Electroconvulsive shock therapy and maximum binding of platelet tritiated imipramine binding in depression. *Archives of General Psychiatry*, **43**, 949–52.

Lee, P. H. K. and Chan, M.-Y. (1985). Effect of steroids on the inhibition of platelet 5-HT uptake by desipramine and other antidepressants. *European Journal of Pharmacology*, **106**, 255–62.

Lewis, D. A. and McChesney, C. (1985*a*). Tritiated imipramine binding distinguishes among subtypes of depression. *Archives of General Psychiatry*, **42**, 485–8.

Lewis, D. A. and McChesney, C. (1985*b*). Tritiated imipramine binding to platelets in manic subjects. *Journal of Affective Disorders*, **9**, 207–11.

Lewis, D. A., Noyes, R., Coryell, W., and Clancy, J. (1985*b*). Tritiated imipramine binding to platelets is decreased in patients with agoraphobia. *Psychiatry Research*, **16**, 1–9.

Leysen, J. E., Awouters, F., Kennis, L., Laduron, P. M., Vanderberk, J., and Janssen, P. A. J. (1981). Receptor binding profile of R 41 468, a novel antagonist at 5-HT₂ receptors. *Life Sciences*, **28**, 1015–22.

Leysen, J. E., Niemegeers, C. J. E., Van Nueten, J. M., and Laduron, P. M. (1982). ³H-ketanserin (R 41 468), a selective ³H-ligand for serotonin₂ receptor binding sites. *Molecular Pharmacology*, **21**, 301–14.

Lingjaerde, O. (1980). Antidepressants and the serotonin uptake in platelets. *Acta Psychiatrica Scandanivica*, Suppl. 280, **61**, 111–18.

Magni, G., Andreoli, F., Arduino, C., Arsie, D., Ceccherelli, F., Ambrosio, F., *et al.* (1987). Modifications of [³H] imipramine binding sites in platelets of chronic pain patients treated with mianserin. *Pain*, **30**, 311–20.

Maj, M., Mastronardi, P., Cerreta, A., Romano, M., Mazzarella, B., and Kemali,

D. (1988). Changes in platelet ³H-imipramine binding in depressed patients receiving electroconvulsive shock therapy. *Biological Psychiatry*, **24**, 469–72.

Malmgren, R., Beving, H., and Olsson, P. (1985). Effects of different anticoagulants on human platelet size distribution and serotonin (5-HT) induced shape change and uptake kinetics. *Thrombosis Research*, **38**, 649–61.

Malmgren, R., Collins, A., and Nilsson, G.-G. (1987). Platelet serotonin uptake and effects of vitamin B_6-treatment in premenstrual tension. *Neuropsychobiology*, **18**, 83–8.

Malmgren, R., Aberg-Wistedt, A., and Martensson, B. (1989). Aberrant seasonal variations of platelet serotonin uptake in endogenous depression. *Biological Psychiatry*, **25**, 393–402.

Mann, J. J., Stanley, M., McBride, P. A., and McEwen, B. S. (1986). Increased serotonin₂ and β-adrenergic receptor binding in the frontal cortex of suicide victims. *Archives of General Psychiatry*, **43**, 954–9.

Marazziti, D., Perugi, G., Deltito, J., Lenzi, A., Maremmani, I., Placidi, G. F. and Cassano, G. B. (1988*a*). High-affinity ³H-imipramine binding sites: a possible state-dependent marker for depression. *Psychiatry Research*, **23**, 229–37.

Marazziti, D., Rotondo, A., Placidi, G. F., Perugi, G., Cassano, G. B., and Pacifier, G. M. (1988*b*). Imipramine binding in platelets of patients with panic disorder. *Pharmacological Psychiatry*, **21**, 47–9.

Marcusson, J. and Tiger, G. (1988). [³H]imipramine binding of protein nature in human platelets: inhibition by 5-hydroxytryptamine and 5-hydroxytryptamine uptake inhibitors. *Journal of Neurochemistry*, **50**, 1032–6.

Marcusson, J. O., Backtrom, I. T., and Ross, S. B. (1986). Single-site model of the neuronal 5-hydroxytryptamine uptake and imipramine-binding site. *Molecular Pharmacology*, **30**, 121–8.

Marcusson, J. O., Andersson, A., and Bäckstrom, I. (1989). Drug inhibition indicates a single-site model of the 5-HT uptake site/antidepressant binding site in rat and human brain. *Psychopharmacology*, **99**, 17–21

Marcusson, J. O., Bergstrom, M., Eriksson, K., and Ross, S. B. (1988). Characterization of [³H] paroxetine binding in rat brain. *Journal of Neurochemistry*, **50**, 1783–90.

McBride, P. A., Mann, J. J., McEwen, B., and Biegon, A. (1983). Characterization of serotonin binding sites on human platelets. *Life Sciences*, **33**, 2033–41.

McBride, P. A., Brown, R. P., Demeo, M., Keilp, J., Stanley, M., Mann, J. J., *et al.* (1987). Platelet 5-HT₂ receptors: depression and suicide. 140th Annual Meeting of American Psychiatric Association, Abstract p.104.

McBride, P. A., Mann, J. J., Polley, M. J., Wiley, A. J., and Sweeney, J. A. (1987). Assessment of binding indices and physiological responsiveness of the 5-HT₂ receptor on human platelets. *Life Sciences*, **40**, 1799–809.

McKeith, I. G., Marshall, E. F., Ferrier, I. N., Armstrong, M. M., Kennedy, W. N., Perry, R. H., *et al.* (1987). 5-HT receptor binding in postmortem brain from patients with affective disorders. *Journal of Affective Disorders*, **13**, 67–74.

Mellerup, E. T. and Plenge, P. (1986). High affinity binding of ³H-paroxetine and ³H-imipramine to rat neuronal membranes. *Psychopharmacology*, **89**, 436–9.

Mellerup, E. T. and Plenge, P. (1988). Imipramine binding in depression and other psychiatric conditions. *Acta Psychiatrica Scandanivica*, Suppl. **78**, 61–68.

Mellerup, E. T., Plenge, P., and Rosenberg, R. (1982). ³H-imipramine binding sites in platelets from psychiatric patients. *Psychiatry Research*, **7**, 221–7.

Mellerup, E. T., Plenge, P., and Engelstoft, M. (1983). High affinity binding of

^{3}H-paroxetine and ^{3}H-imipramine to human platelet membranes. *European Journal of Pharmacology*, **96**, 303–9.

Mellerup, E. T., Bech, P., Hansen, H. J., Langemark, M., Loldrup, D., and Plenge, P. (1988). Platelet ^{3}H-imipramine binding in psychogenic pain patients. *Psychiatry Research*, **26**, 149–56.

Meltzer, H. Y. and Arora, R. C. (1988). Genetic control of serotonin uptake in blood platelets: a twin study. *Psychiatry Research*, **24**, 263–69.

Meltzer, H. Y. and Lowy, M. T. (1988). The serotonin hypothesis of depression. In *Psychopharmacology: the third generation of progress*, (ed. H. Y. Meltzer), pp. 513–26. Raven Press, New York.

Meltzer, H. Y. and Nash, J. F. (1988). Serotonin and mood: neuroendocrine aspects. In *Current topics in neuroendocrinology*, (ed. D. Granten and D. Pfaff), Vol. 8, pp. 183–210. Springer-Verlag, Heidelberg.

Meltzer, H. Y., Arora, R. C., Baber, R., and Tricou, B. J. (1981). Serotonin uptake in blood platelets of psychiatric patients. *Archives of General Psychiatry*, **38**, 1322–6.

Meltzer, H. Y., Arora, R. C., and Song, P. (1982). Serotonin uptake in blood platelets as a biological marker for major depressive disorders. In *Biological markers in psychiatry and neurology*, (ed. E. Usdin and E. Costa), pp. 39–48. Pergamon Press, New York.

Meltzer, H. Y., Arora, R. C., and Goodnick, P. (1983a). Effect of lithium carbonate on serotonin uptake in blood platelets of patients with affective disorders. *Journal of Affective Disorders*, **5**, 215–21.

Meltzer, H. Y., Arora, R. C., Tricou, B. J., and Fang, V. S. (1983b). Serotonin uptake in blood platelets and the dexamethasone suppression test in depressed patients. *Psychiatry Research*, **8**, 41–47.

Meltzer, H. Y., Arora, R. C., Robertson, A., and Lowy, M. (1984a). Platelet ^{3}H-imipramine binding and platelet 5-HT uptake in affective disorders and schizophrenia. *Clinical Neuropharmacology*, **7**, 320–1.

Meltzer, H. Y., Lowy, M., Robertson, A., Goodnick, P., and Perline, R. (1984b). Effect of 5-hydroxytryptophan on serum cortisol levels in major affective disorders. III. Effect of antidepressants and lithium carbonate. *Archives of General Psychiatry*, **41**, 391–7.

Meltzer, H. Y., Umberkoman-Wiita, B., Robertson, A., Tricou, B. J., Lowy, M., and Perline, R. (1984c). Effect of 5-hydroxytryptophan on serum cortisol levels in the major affective disorders. I. Enhanced response in depression and mania. *Archives of General Psychiatry*, **41**, 366–74.

Mikuni, M., Kusumi, I., Kagaya, A., Yamamoto, H., Kuroda, Y., Nishikawa, T., and Takahashi, K. (1989). Responsiveness of serotonin-stimulated phosphoinositide hydrolysis is increased in platelets from unmedicated depressed patients. *Abstract, Society for Neuroscience*, p. 673.

Mirkin, A. M., and Coppen, A. (1980). Electrodermal activity in depression: clinical and biochemical correlates. *British Journal of Psychiatry*, **137**, 93–7.

Modai, I., Zemlishlany, Z., and Jerushalmy, Z. (1984). 5-Hydroxytryptamine uptake by blood platelets of unipolar and bipolar depressed patients. *Neuropsychobiology*, **12**, 93–5.

Modai, I., Malmgren, R., Asberg, M., and Irving, H. (1986). Circadian rhythm of serotonin transport in human platelets. *Psychopharmacology*, **88**, 493–5.

Muscettola, G., Lauro, A. D., and Giannini, C. P. (1986). Platelet ^{3}H-imipramine binding in bipolar patients. *Psychiatry Research*, **18**, 343–53.

Nankai, M., Yoshimoto, S., Narita, K., and Takahashi, R. (1986). Platelet [³H] imipramine binding in depressed patients and its circadian variations in healthy controls. *Journal of Affective Disorders*, **11**, 207–12.

Nemeroff, C. B., Knight, D. L., Krishnan, R. R., Slotkin, T. A., Bissette, G., Melville, M. L., and Blazer, D. G. (1988). Marked reduction in the number of platelet-tritiated imipramine binding sites in geriatric depression. *Archives of General Psychiatry*, **45**, 919–23.

Norman, T. R., Sartor, D. M., Judd, F. K., Burrows, G. O., Gregory, M. S., and McIntyre, I. M. (1989). Platelet serotonin uptake and ³H-imipramine binding in panic disorder. *Journal of Affective Disorders*, **17**, 77–81.

Nutt, D. J. and Fraser, S. (1987). Platelet binding studies in panic disorder. *Journal of Affective Disorders*, **21**, 7–11.

Oxenkrug, G. H. (1979). The content and uptake of 5-HT by blood platelets in depressive patients. *Journal of Neural Transmission*, **45**, 285–9.

Oxenkrug, G. H., Prakhje, I., and Mikhalenko, I. N. (1978). Disturbed circadian rhythm of 5-HT uptake by blood platelets in depressive psychosis. *Acta Nervosa Superior (Praha)*, **20**, 66–7.

Paul, S. M., Rehavi, M., Skolnick, P., and Goodwin, F. K. (1980). Demonstration of specific high affinity binding sites for [³H]imipramine on human platelets. *Life Sciences*, **26**, 953–9.

Paul, S. M., Rehavi, M., Skolnick, P., Ballenger, J. C., and Goodwin, F. K. (1981). Depressed patients have decreased binding of tritiated imipramine to platelet serotonin transporter. *Archives of General Psychiatry*, **38**, 1315–17.

Paul, S. M., Rehavi, M., Skolnick, P., and Goodwin, F.K. (1984). High affinity binding of antidepressants to a biogenic amine transport site in human brain and platelet, studies in depression. In *Neurobiology and mood disorders*, (ed. R. M. Post and J. C. Bellinger), pp. 845–53. Williams and Wilkins, Baltimore.

Pecknold, J. C., Chang, H., Fleury, D., Koszychi, D., Quirion, R., Nair, N. P. V., and Suranyi-Cadotte, B. (1987). Platelet imipramine binding in patients with panic disorder and major familial depression. *Journal of Psychiatric Research*, **21**, 319–26.

Pecknold, J. C., Suranyi-Cadotte, B., Chang, H., and Nair, N. P. V. (1988). Serotonin uptake in panic disorder and agoraphobia. *Neuropsychopharmacology*, **1**, 173–6.

Peroutka, S. J. and Snyder, S. H. (1979). Multiple serotonin receptors: differential binding of [³H]5-hydroxytryptamine, [³H]lysergic acid diethylamide and [³H]spiroperidol. *Molecular Pharmacology*, **16**, 687–99.

Plenge, P., Mellerup, E. T., and Gjerris, A. (1988). Imipramine binding in depressive patients diagnosed according to different criteria. *Acta Psychiatrica Scandanivica*, **78**, 156–61.

Pletscher, A. (1968). Metabolism, transfer and storage of 5–HT in blood platelets. *British Journal of Pharmacology*, **32**, 1–16.

Poirier, M.-F., Benkelfat, C., Loo, H., Sechter, D., Zarifian, E., Galzin, A.-M., and Langer, S.Z. (1986). Reduced B$_{max}$ of [³H]imipramine binding to platelets of depressed patients free of previous medication with 5-HT uptake inhibitors. *Psychopharmacology*, **89**, 450–61.

Poirier, M.-F., Galzin, A.-M., Loo, H., Pimoule, C., Segonzac, A., Benkelfat, C., *et al.* (1987). Changes in [³H]-5-HT uptake and [³H] imipramine binding in platelets after chlorimipramine in healthy volunteers: comparison with maprotiline and amineptine. *Biological Psychiatry*, **22**, 287–302.

Raisman, R., Sechter, D., Briley, M. S., Zarifian, E., and Langer, S. Z. (1981).

High affinity ³H-imipramine binding in platelets from untreated and treated depressed patients compared to healthy volunteers. *Psychopharmacology*, **75**, 368–71.

Raisman, R., Briley, M. S., Bouchami, F., Sechter, D., Zarifian, E., and Langer S. Z. (1982). ³H-imipramine binding and serotonin uptake in platelets from untreated depressed patients and control volunteers. *Psychopharmacology*, **77**, 332–5.

Rausch, J. L., Shah, N. S., Burch, E. A., and Donald, A. G. (1982). Platelet serotonin uptake in depressed patients: circadian effect. *Biological Psychiatry*, **17**, 121–3.

Rausch, J. L., Janowsky, D. S., Risch, S. C., and Huey, L Y. (1986). A kinetic analysis and replication of decreased platelet serotonin uptake in depressed patients. *Psychiatry Research*, **19**, 105–12.

Rehavi, M., Paul, S. M., Skolnick, P., and Goodwin, F. K. (1980). Demonstration of specific high affinity binding sites for [³H] imipramine in human brain. *Life Sciences*, **26**, 2273–9.

Rehavi, M., Ventura, I., and Sarne, Y. (1985). Demonstration of endogenous 'imipramine-like' materials in brain. *Life Sciences*, **36**, 687–93.

Ross, S. B. and Aberg-Wistedt, A. (1983). Inhibitors of serotonin and noradrenaline uptake in human plasma after withdrawal of zimelidine and clomipramine treatment. *Psychopharmacology*, **79**, 298–303.

Ross, S. B., Aperia, B., Beck-Friis, J., Jansa, S., Wetterberg, L., and Aberg, A. (1980). Inhibition of 5-hydroxytryptamine uptake in human platelets by antidepressant agents *in vivo*. *Psychopharmacology*, **67**, 1–7.

Rotman, A., Shatz, A., and Szekeley, G. A. (1982). Correlation between serotonin uptake and imipramine binding in schizophrenic patients. *Progress in Neuro-Psychopharmacology and Biological Psychiatry*, **6**, 57–61.

Roy, A., Everett, D., Pickar, D., and Paul, S. M. (1987). Platelet tritiated imipramine binding and serotonin uptake in depressed patients and controls. *Archives of General Psychiatry*, **44**, 320–7.

Scheffel, U. and Hartig, P. R. (1980). *In vivo* labeling of serotonin uptake sites with [³H]paroxetine. *Journal of Neurochemistry*, **52**, 1602–5.

Schneider, L. S., Severson, J. A. and Sloane, R. B. (1985). Platelet ³H-imipramine binding in depressed elderly patients. *Biological Psychiatry*, **20**, 1234–7.

Schneider, L. S., Fredrickson, E. R., Severson, J. A., and Sloane, R. B. (1986). ³H-imipramine binding in depressed elderly: relationship to family history and clinical response. *Psychiatry Research*, **19**, 257–66.

Schneider, L. S., Munjack, D., Severson, J. A., and Palmer, R. (1987). Platelet [³H]imipramine binding in generalized anxiety disorder, panic disorder and agoraphobia with panic attacks. *Biological Psychiatry*, **22**, 59–66.

Schneider, L. S., Chui, H. C., Severson, J. A., and Sloane, R. B. (1988a). Decreased platelet ³H-imipramine binding in Parkinson's disease. *Biological Psychiatry*, **24**, 348–51.

Schneider, L. S., Severson, J. A., Chui, H. C., Pollock, V. E., Sloane, R. B. and Frederickson, E. R. (1988b). Platelet tritiated imipramine binding and MAO activity in Alzheimer's disease patients with agitation and delusions. *Psychiatry Research*, **25**, 311–22.

Schneider, L. S., Severson, J. A., Sloane, R. B., and Fredrickson, E. R. (1988c). Decreased platelet ³H-imipramine binding in primary major depression compared with depression secondary to medical illness in elderly outpatients. *Journal of Affective Disorders*, **15**, 195–200.

Scott, M., Reading, H. W., and Loudon, J.B. (1979). Studies on human platelets in affective disorders. *Psychopharmacology*, **60**, 131–5.

Sette, M., Raisman, R., Briley, M., and Langer, S. Z. (1981). Localization of tricyclic antidepressant binding sites on serotonin nerve terminals in rat hypothalamus. *Journal of Neurochemistry*, **37**, 40–2.

Shaw, D. M., MacSweeney, D. A., Wollock, N., and Bevan-Jones, A. B. (1971). Uptake and release of ^{14}C-5-hydroxytryptamine by platelets in affective illness. *Journal of Neurological and Neurosurgical Psychiatry*, **34**, 224–5.

Slotkin, T. A., Whitmore, W. L., Barnes, G. A., Krishnan, K. R. R., Blazer, D. G., Knight, D. L., and Nemeroff, C. B. (1989). Reduced inhibitory effect of imipramine on radiolabeled serotonin uptake into platelets in geriatric depression. *Biological Psychiatry*, **25**, 687–91.

Sneddon, J. M. (1973). Blood platelets as a model for monoamine containing neurons. *Progress in Neurobiology*, **1**, 151–98.

Stahl, S. M. (1977). The human platelet: a diagnostic and research tool for the study of biogenic amines in psychiatric and neurologic disorder. *Archives of General Psychiatry*, **34**, 509–16.

Stahl, S. M., Woo, D. J., Mefford, I. N., Berger, P. A., and Ciaranello, R. D. (1983). Hyperserotonemia and platelet serotonin uptake and release in schizophrenia and affective disorders. *American Journal of Psychiatry*, **140**, 26–30.

Stanley, M. and Mann, J. J. (1983). Increased serotonin-2 binding sites in frontal cortex of suicide victims. *Lancet*, **i**, 214–16.

Stanley, M., Virgilio, J., and Gershon, S. (1982). Tritiated imipramine binding sites are decreased in the frontal cortex of suicides. *Science*, **216**, 1337–9.

Strijewski, A., Chudzik, J., and Tang, S. W. (1988). Inhibition of platelet [^{3}H]imipramine binding by human plasma protein fractions. *Life Sciences*, **42**, 1543–50.

Suranyi-Cadotte, B. E., Wood, P. L., Nair, N. P. V., and Schwartz, G. (1982). Normalization of platelet [^{3}H]imipramine binding in depressed patients during remission. *European Journal of Pharmacology*, **85**, 357–8.

Suranyi-Cadotte, B. E., Wood, P. L., Schwartz, G. and Nair, N. P. V. (1983). Altered platelet ^{3}H-imipramine binding in schizoaffective and depressive disorders. *Biological Psychiatry*, **18**, 923–7.

Suranyi-Cadotte, B. E., Quirion, R., McQuade, P., Nair, N. P. V., Schwartz, G., Mosticyan, S., and Wood, P. L. (1984). Platelet ^{3}H-imipramine binding: a state dependent marker in depression. *Progress in Neuro-Psychopharmacology and Biological Psychiatry*, **8**, 737–41.

Suranyi-Cadotte, B. E., Gauthier, S., Lafaille, F., DeFlores, S., Dam. T. V., Nair, N. P. V., and Quirion, R. (1985a). Platelet ^{3}H-imipramine binding distinguishes depression and Alzheimer dementia. *Life Sciences*, **37**, 2305–11.

Suranyi-Cadotte, B. E., Quirion, R., Nair, N. P. V., Lafaille, F., and Schwartz, G. (1985b). Imipramine treatment differentially affects platelet ^{3}H-imipramine binding and serotonin uptake in depressed patients. *Life Sciences*, **36**, 795–9.

Swade, C. and Coppen, A. (1980). Seasonal variations in biochemical factors related to depressive illness. *Journal of Affective Disorders*, **2**, 249–55.

Takeda, T., Harada, T., and Otsuki, S. (1989). Platelet ^{3}H-clonidine and ^{3}H-imipramine binding and plasma cortisol levels in depression. *Biological Psychiatry*, **26**, 52–60.

Tang, S. W. and Morris, J. M. (1985). Variation in human platelet ^{3}H-imipramine binding. *Psychiatry Research*, **16**, 141–6.

Tang, S. W., Berg, J. M., Bruni, J., and Davis, A. (1988). Decreased platelet ³H-imipramine binding in Down's Syndrome. *Psychiatry Research*, **24**, 67–70.

Tanimoto, K., Maeda, K., and Terada, K. (1985). Alteration of platelet [³H]imipramine binding in mildly depressed patients correlates with disease severity. *Biological Psychiatry*, **20**, 340–3.

Theodorou, A. E., Katona, C. L. E., Davies, S. L., Tunnicliffe, C., Hale, A. S., Horton, R. W., *et al.* (1985). Platelet alpha₂-noradrenergic and imipramine binding in depressed patients before and during treatment. *British Journal of Clinical Pharmacology*, **20**, 528P.

Theodorou, A. E., Katona, C. L. E., Davies, S. L., Hale, A. S., Kerry, S. M., Horton, R. W., *et al.* (1989). ³H-imipramine binding to freshly prepared membranes in depression. *Psychiatry Research*, **29**, 87–103.

Tuomisto, J. and Tukiainen, E. (1976). Decreased uptake of 5-hydroxytryptamine in blood platelets from depressed patients. *Nature*, **262**, 596–8.

Tuomisto, J., Tukiainen, E., and Ahlfors, U. G., (1979). Decreased uptake of 5-hydroxytryptamine in blood platelets from patients with endogenous depression. *Psychopharmacology*, **65**, 141–7.

Tukiainen, E. (1981). Effect of hypophysectomy and adrenalectomy on 5-hydroxytryptamine uptake by rat hypothalamic synaptosomes and blood platelets. *Acta Pharmacologica et Toxicologia*, **48**, 139–44.

Uhde, T. W., Berrettini, W. H., Roy-Byrne, P. P., Boulenger, J.-P., and Post, R. M. (1987). Platelet [³H]imipramine binding in patients with panic disorder. *Biological Psychiatry*, **22**, 52–8.

Vermes, I., Smelik, P. G., and Mulder, A. H. (1976). Effect of hypophysectomy, adrenalectomy and corticosterone treatment on uptake and release of putative central neurotransmitters by rat hypothalamic tissue in vitro. *Life Sciences*, **19**, 1719–26.

Wägner, A., Aberg-Wistedt, A., Asberg, M., Ekqvist, B., Martensson, B., and Montero, D. (1985). Lower ³H-imipramine binding in platelets from untreated depressed patients compared to healthy controls. *Psychiatry Research*, **16**, 131–9.

Weizman, A., Carel, C., Tyano, S., and Rehavi, M. (1985). Decreased high affinity ³H-imipramine binding in platelets of enuretic children and adolescents. *Psychiatry Research*, **14**, 39–46.

Weizman, A., Carmi, M., Hermesh, H., Shahar, A., Apter, A., Tyano, S., and Rehavi, M. (1986a). High affinity imipramine binding and serotonin uptake in platelets of eight adolescent and ten adult obsessive-compulsive patients. *American Journal of Psychiatry*, **143**, 335–9.

Weizman, R., Carmi, M., Tyano, S., Apter, A., and Rehavi, M. (1986b). High affinity ³H-imipramine binding and serotonin uptake to platelets of adolescent females suffering from anorexia nervosa. *Life Sciences*, **38**, 1235–42.

Weizman, A., Gonen, N., Tyano, S., Szekely, G.A., and Rehavi, M. (1987). Platelet [³H]imipramine binding in autism and schizophrenia. *Psychopharmacology*, **91**, 101–3.

Weizman, A., Dick, J., Mosek, A., Tyano, S., and Rehavi, M. (1988). Unaltered platelet [³H]imipramine binding in dementia of the Alzheimer's type. *Neuropsychobiology*, **19**, 69–72.

Whitaker, P. M., Warsh, J. J., Stancer, H. C., Persad, E., and Vint, C. K. (1984). Seasonal variation in platelet ³H-imipramine binding: comparable values in control and depressed populations. *Psychiatry Research*, **11**, 127–31.

Wirz-Justice, A. and Richter, R. (1979). Seasonality in biochemical determination: a source of variance and a clue to the temporal incidence of affective illness. *Psychiatry Research*, **1**, 53–60.

Wirz-Justice, A. and Pühringer, W. (1978). Seasonal incidence of an altered diurnal rhythm of platelet serotonin in unipolar depression. *Journal of Neural Transmission*, **42**, 45–53.

Wood, P. L., Suranyi-Cadotte, B. E., Nair, N. P. V., Lafaille, F., and Schwartz, G. Z. (1983). Lack of association between [³H]imipramine binding sites and uptake of serotonin in control, depressed and schizophrenic patients. *Neuropharmacology*, **22**, 1211–14.

Wood, K., Swade, C., Abou-Saleh, M. T., and Coppen, A. (1985). Apparent supersensitivity of platelet 5-HT receptors in lithium-treated patients. *Journal of Affective Disorders*, **8**, 69–72.

Zemishlany, Z., Munitz, H., Rotman, A., and Wijsenbeck, H. (1982). Increased uptake of serotonin by blood platelets from patients with bipolar primary affective disorder bipolar type. *Psychopharmacology*, **77**, 175–8.

Zemishlany, Z., Modai, I., Apter, A., Jerushalmy, Z., Samuel, E., and Tyano, S. (1987). Serotonin (5-HT) uptake by blood platelets in anorexia nervosa. *Acta Psychiatrica Scandanivica*, **75**, 127–30.

Discussion

COPPEN: Would you comment on the effects of lithium on serotonin (5-hydroxytryptamine, 5-HT) uptake? Lithium profoundly changes the course of affective disorders.

MELTZER: The data on the enhancement of serotonin uptake with lithium seem solid and there is convincing evidence that lithium acts, in part, via a variety of pre- and post-synaptic effects on the serotonergic system.

SANDLER: The serotonin transporter and its mechanisms remain mysterious, despite intensive study. Thirty years ago, we had a model which might throw some light on this (Pare *et al.* 1960). We studied a group of children with cerebral palsy who had very high concentrations of 5-HT in their platelets, higher even than the levels found in patients with carcinoid tumours. Techniques were not available at that time to measure 5-HT uptake, but it would be worthwhile to re-investigate not only platelet but cerebral uptake in this group, because it may well shed some light on the nature of their mental handicap.

MELTZER: Elevated serotonin in various types of mental retardation is one of the most robust findings in the literature, but this has not been pursued with modern techniques for studying platelets. Fenfluramine was studied as a treatment for autism, where platelet serotonin content is very high, but it was not effective.

BRILEY: You interpreted decreased serotonin uptake as meaning there is probably more serotonin left in the synapses. I have always interpreted the level of uptake as reflecting the density of innervation. Thus I would take a decrease in uptake to mean less innervation and thus less serotonin release.

MELTZER: I have considered the possibility that it could be a marker for weak serotonergic innervation. As I recall, others have suggested this based on findings from post-mortem studies of dementias. However, it is harder to argue for this idea on the basis of blood platelet studies, even though there is evidence of a common origin of central 5-HT neurones and platelets. There is no evidence for a difference in the total number of the platelets or concentrations of 5-HT in the platelets of depressed patients. So this does not argue for a 'weak' 5-HT system. If your interpretation is not correct, there still is the possibility of increased 5-HT at the synapse if there is a central decrease in 5-HT uptake in some depressed patients.

YOUDIM: Platelets are easy to obtain, but difficult to work with. Their age has a tremendous effect on their metabolic activity. Has that been investigated in these studies?

MELTZER: We obtained platelets via differential centrifugation to examine the differences in uptake and binding between young and old platelets and heavy and light platelets. Most people now use the Corash method for isolating 95 to 100 per cent of the platelets, so they are not dealing with subpopulations. Nobody has done a large-scale study of young versus old platelets.

YOUDIM: Most attention has been concentrated on 5-HT uptake and 5-HT receptors in platelets. Nobody has compared other receptor sites or other uptake systems on the platelet to see whether the defect is a selective effect on the 5-HT system.

OXENKRUG: We found a gender difference in serotonin uptake by blood platelets in depressed patients (Oxenkrug and Mikhalenko 1978). Have you seen that?

MELTZER: We always looked carefully, and we did not find a gender effect.

FRAZER: Is there any information about the other site to which [^{3}H]imipramine might be binding on the platelets? One could make a case that the serotonin transport site does not appear to be different to the main imipramine site, but that the second site may be where there is a difference if it is not an allosteric site on the serotonin transporter.

BRILEY: Very little has been done with that site. All we know is that it is sodium independent, and of micromolar affinity for most tricyclic antidepressants.

FRAZER: Are there enough counts left after blocking specific binding and re-uptake to do a pharmacological comparison?

BRILEY: You are down to the limits.

YOUDIM: Is the binding reversible or irreversible?

BRILEY: Reversible.

BELMAKER: Do you have heritability data on the binding and transport? If the lithium effect has enough variability, can you look at that as a marker? Does a large lithium enhancement of uptake predict a lithium response?

MELTZER: We did twin studies of both platelet uptake and imipramine binding. Uptake was heritable but the imipramine binding was not. We also had a problem of between-assay variance in this study. The same results for imipramine binding were reported by Friedl and Propping (1984). We found no relationship between the lithium-induced changes and uptake, but we have only looked *in vivo* at the chronic treatment.

YOUDIM: Did you look at release of serotonin from lithium-treated platelets? This is warranted because chronic lithium treatment in rats alters K^+-stimulated release of 5-HT from hippocampal slices.

MELTZER: That has not been explored.

PALFREYMAN: van Praag (van Praag *et al.* 1972, van Praag 1974) has suggested that there is a serotonin subgroup of depressives based on some 5-hydroxyindoleacetic acid studies in cerebrospinal fluid. Is there any evidence for a bimodal distribution in your platelet data?

MELTZER: The closest we would come to finding that split would be the psychotic bipolar depressives. One difference between the Chicago and Cleveland studies is that we had a high proportion of extremely sick bipolar psychotics in Chicago who seem to have a particular serotonin profile.

SULSER: Has anybody looked at the effect of stress and glucocorticoids on the regulation of 5-HT receptors and/or their function, either in platelets or in brain? β-adrenoceptor genes, for example, contain glucocorticoid responsive elements (GREs) in their promoter region and circulating glucocorticoids can change not only the receptor number but also the sensitivity to agonists.

MELTZER: We studied the effect of corticosterone treatment on platelet and brain imipramine binding in adrenalectomized rats (Arora and Meltzer 1986) and the correlation between V_{max} of 5-HT uptake and dexamethasone suppression in depressed patients (Meltzer *et al.* 1983). I don't know of any data on 5-HT receptors and adrenoceptors.

MURPHY: I have some relevant data about the imipramine- and paroxetine-binding site. The IC_{50} for inhibition of 5-HT uptake by imipramine is 150 nM, whereas the affinity of imipramine for the 5-HT$_2$ site is 80 nM. We know there are 5-HT$_2$ sites in platelets. Is imipramine perhaps binding to the 5-HT$_2$ site? Is that the difference between paroxetine and imipramine? Fluoxetine has considerably lower affinity for the 5-HT$_2$ site. I don't know about paroxetine.

PEROUTKA: The other possibility is that you are displacing the radioligand from non-specific binding sites, as we discussed earlier with the putative 5-HT$_{1E}$ binding site.

References

Arora, R. C. and Meltzer, H. Y. (1986). Effect of adrenalectomy and corticosterone on [^{3}H]imipramine binding in rat blood platelets and brain. *European Journal of Pharmacology,* **123**, 415–9.

Friedl, W. and Propping, P. (1984). ^{3}H-Imipramine binding in human platelets: a study in normal twins. *Psychiatry Research*, **11**, 279–85.

Meltzer, H. Y., Arora, R. C., Tricou, B. J., and Fang, V. S. (1983). Serotonin uptake in blood platelets and the dexamethasone suppression test in depressed patients. *Psychiatry Research*, **8**, 41–7.

Oxenkrug, G. F. and Mikhalenko, I. (1978). The ABO blood group distribution and rate of 5-HT uptake by blood platelets in depressives. *Activitas Nervosa Superior*, **20**, 256–7.

Pare, C. M. B., Sandler, M., and Stacey, R. S. (1960). 5-Hydroxyindoles in mental deficiency. *Journal of Neurology, Neurosurgery and Psychiatry*, **23**, 341–6.

van Praag, H. M. (1974). Therapy resistant depressions: biochemical and pharmacological consideration. *Psychotherapy and Psychosomatics*, **23**, 169–78.

van Praag, H. M., Korf, J., Dols, L. C. W., and Schut, T. (1972). A pilot study of the predictive value of the probenecid test in application of 5-hydroxytryptophan as an antidepressant. *Psychopharmacology*, **25**, 14–21.

7. The role of 5-HT in migraine: disentangling the links with depression

Vivette Glover, Joan Jarman, and Merton Sandler

Introduction

Some disturbance of the 5-hydroxytryptamine (5-HT, serotonin) system has been suggested to be present in a number of clinical conditions that often occur with differing degrees of overlap in affected subjects. Apart from depression, these include migraine, tension headache, and other pain syndromes. Thus, it is of interest to try to disentangle the pathology and treatment of these disorders; here, we focus on migraine and depression.

5-HT in migraine

It has long been known that the serotonergic system is disturbed during a migraine attack. There is an increased platelet aggregation (Hilton and Cummings 1972; Gawel *et al.* 1979) and a release of platelet 5-HT (Anthony *et al.* 1967). There is also an increase in urinary output of 5-hydroxyindole-acetic acid (5-HIAA) (Curran *et al.* 1965). Mean platelet monoamine oxidase levels are permanently low in migraine patients, especially males (Sandler *et al.* 1970; Glover *et al.* 1981). It has been suggested that a migraine attack is triggered by the fall in 5-HT, a speculation receiving some support from the claim that 5-hydroxytryptophan, the precursor of 5-HT, can alleviate the attack (Sicuteri 1972; Titus *et al.* 1986). There have been fewer studies of chronic daily headache (or severe tension headache), although Anthony and Lance (1989) have confirmed an earlier observation (Rolf *et al.* 1981) that affected patients have significantly lower mean platelet 5-HT content than controls. Thus, the questions of a link between chronic daily headache and migraine and the extent to which they possess a common pathogenesis involving low 5-HT have once again been raised.

The evidence for a role for 5-HT in migraine has been strengthened with the advent of certain new drugs, some acting on the central nervous system and some on vascular tissues: a model of the migraine process which involves both brain and extracerebral intracranial blood vessels has been developed

(Glover and Sandler 1989). It has been known for some years that several of the most effective prophylactic drugs for migraine, methysergide, cyproheptadine, and pizotifen, act on 5-HT receptors. With the recent delineation of 5-HT receptor subtypes, it now appears that they have selective nanomolar affinity for the 5-HT_2, 5-HT_{1A}, and 5-HT_{1C} receptors (Peroutka 1988a,b; Fozard 1990). A new drug that has aroused considerable interest is GR 43175 (sumatriptan), which rapidly aborts a migraine attack even after it has commenced (Doenicke *et al.* 1988). This drug acts as an agonist at certain 5-HT_1-like receptors located on blood vessels, including the basilar artery of primates (Connor *et al.* 1989). These receptors had been classified as the 5-HT_1 type as they respond to 5-HT itself with high affinity, but were thought to differ from the known subtypes of this receptor in other drug responses. However, Peroutka (p. 16, this volume) now reports that sumatriptan, like ergotamine, acts on 5-HT_{1D} receptors (Peroutka *et al.* 1989). Sumatriptan seems not to cross the blood–brain barrier (Humphrey *et al.* 1990), suggesting that at least part of the migraine cascade must occur extracerebrally, even if intracranially.

Another interesting drug is *m*-chlorophenylpiperazine (*m*-CPP). This is a somewhat non-specific agonist for central 5-HT receptors (pp. 203–6, this volume). It has been shown reproducibly to induce a migraine-type headache in sufferers already prone to migraine attacks (Brewerton *et al.* 1988). The headache typically develops several hours after administration of the drug and after plasma levels have fallen, suggesting that rebound or secondary receptor changes might be involved. It has long been known that reserpine, which depletes both 5-HT and catecholamines from their storage sites, can induce an attack in migraine-prone subjects, although not in others (Curzon *et al.* 1969). The *m*-CPP results add to this evidence for the involvement of monoamines, perhaps pointing more specifically to 5-HT.

Migraine attacks can be initiated by a variety of factors, stress being particularly often cited. A minority of patients believe red wine to be a trigger: in a controlled trial, this was confirmed for these patients, but not for others (Littlewood *et al.* 1988). Although mechanism is unclear, we have been able to show (unpublished) that red wine, but not white, or an equivalent dilution of ethanol, causes ^{14}C-5-HT to be released from platelets (Table 7.1). This effect cannot be accounted for by the tyramine content, which was low (1.9 mg l^{-1}). Thus, red wine, even at a dilution of one per cent, has a 5-HT-depleting action on platelets. This is similar to the action of reserpine, which may also trigger migraine attacks in susceptible subjects.

Links between migraine and depression

Several groups have produced substantial evidence from population studies for a link between migraine and depression, the most thorough investigation

TABLE 7.1.   *Effects of alcoholic beverages on platelet ^{14}C-5-HT release*

Beverage	Percentage of control value
Red wine (1/10)	142
Red wine (1/100)	126
Red wine extract*	150
Alcohol-free lager	98
Ethanol (1.2%)	96
Reserpine (10^{-6} M)	166

Platelets were preloaded with ^{14}C-5-HT by incubation in 0.6 μM for 5 min at 37 °C, and were then exposed to the releasing agent for 1 h. Concentrations given are those in assay incubation.
* Red wine extracted into ethyl acetate at pH 7.4 and reconstituted in buffer to original strength in assay.

TABLE 7.2.   *Platelet [^{3}H]imipramine binding (B_{max}) in migraine*

	n	Median value of B_{max} (range) (fmol per mg protein)
Controls	28	1668 (913–2860)
All migraine	40	1352 (559–4717)*
Migraine—no current depression	30	1327 (935–4717)*
Migraine—no history of major depression	7	1131 (1034–2321)
Migraine with history of major depression	7	1216 (559–4717)

* $p < 0.05$ compared with controls (Mann-Whitney U-test, two-tailed).

being by Merikangas *et al.* (1988). They studied patients with major depressive disorders, noticing a significant association between migraine and depression in both them and their relatives. Garvey *et al.* (1983) investigated the headache pattern of patients with major depressive disorders. They had a headache rate similar to controls during their non-depressed phases but this was increased during episodes of depression.

We used the *Schedule for Affective Disorders and Schizophrenia — Lifetime version* to obtain a more detailed psychiatric profile than had been obtained before of migrainous patients attending a specialist clinic (Jarman *et al.* 1990). More than half the patients had a lifetime history of some type of psychiatric illness. Major depression was the most common diagnosis (40 per cent) and, in all but one case, was of endogenous type. A history of anxiety disorder was the second most prevalent diagnosis (15 per cent).

Platelet [^{3}H]imipramine binding appears to be significantly decreased in migrainous patients (Geaney *et al.* 1984) and in at least some groups of depressed patients (Briley *et al.* 1980; Paul *et al.* 1981), although here the results have been conflicting (Kanof *et al.* 1987). We have confirmed the finding of a significantly low mean B_{max} in migraine (Table 7.2). This was

TABLE 7.3. *Tyramine test in migraine patients*

	n	Urinary excretion of tyramine-O-sulphate (mean ± S.D.) (mg per 3 h)
Controls	14	6.1 ± 1.7
All migraine	40	4.7 ± 1.7*
Migraine with a history of endogenous depression	15	3.8 ± 1.6 **,†
Migraine with no history of endogenous depression	25	5.2 ± 1.6

* p <0.02.
** p <0.001, compared with controls (Student's t-test, two-tailed).
† p <0.02, compared with no history of depression.

apparently independent of either present depressive state or a history of depression, suggesting that a low B_{max} for platelet imipramine binding is linked with migraine itself. The discrepant results in the literature with regard to depression may arise from the inclusion in the patient group of a varying proportion of headache sufferers, in view of the overlap between the two conditions.

The tyramine test is a well-established trait marker for endogenous depression, although its biochemical basis remains unclear. Low output of the tyramine sulphate conjugate after an oral tyramine load is a trait marker which distinguishes endogenous depression from that of the neurotic type (Hale *et al.* 1986) and also seems to correlate with a response to tricylic medication (Hale *et al.* 1989). Low tyramine sulphate output in migrainous patients was originally reported by our research group (Youdim *et al.* 1971), although in a later study (M. Sandler and S. Bonham Carter, unpublished) we were unable to replicate this finding. We have confirmed, however, that another group of migrainous patients do have a significantly lower output of tyramine sulphate than controls (Jarman *et al.* 1990). When this group was divided into those with a history of endogenous depression and those without, the reason for the earlier discrepancy became clear. Only the former showed significantly low values in this test (Table 7.3). Thus, low tyramine sulphate output is linked with endogenous depression which is, in turn, linked with migraine, but it does not appear to be a necessary feature of migraine *per se*.

The results of this study provide evidence against the idea that depression in these migrainous patients is secondary to their migraine; rather, they suggest that a particular disturbance of a biochemical system, most plausibly involving 5-HT, can predispose to both. There may be similar links to be disentangled with other pain syndromes which, in animals at least, have been shown to be linked with 5-HT depletion (Melzack and Wall 1988) and, like migraine and depression, can also respond to tricyclic medication (Feinmann 1985).

Acknowledgement

Joan Jarman was supported by the Migraine Trust.

References

Anthony, M. and Lance, J. W. (1989). Plasma serotonin in patients with chronic tension headaches. *Journal of Neurology, Neurosurgery and Psychiatry*, **52**, 182–4.

Anthony, M., Hinterberger, H. J., and Lance, J. W. (1967). Plasma serotonin in migraine stress. *Archives of Neurology*, **16**, 544–2.

Brewerton, T. D., Murphy, D. L., Mueller, E. A., and Jimerson, D. C. (1988). Induction of migrainelike headaches by the serotonin agonist m-cholorophenylpiperazine. *Clinical Pharmacology and Therapeutics*, **43**, 605–9.

Briley, M. S., Langer, S. Z., Raisman, R., Sechter, D., and Zarifian, E. (1980). ³H-Imipramine binding sites are decreased in platelets of untreated depressed patients. *Science*, **209**, 303–5.

Connor, H. E., Feniuk, W., and Humphrey, P. P. A. (1989). Characterization of 5-HT receptors mediating contraction of canine and primate basilar artery by use of GR 43175, a selective 5-HT$_1$-like receptor agonist. *British Journal of Pharmacology*, **96**, 379–87.

Curran, D. A., Hinterberger, H., and Lance, J. W. (1965). Total plasma serotonin aggregation responses in subjects with acute migraine headache. *Journal of Neurology, Neurosurgery and Psychiatry*, **35**, 505–9.

Curzon, G., Barrie, M., and Wilkinson, M. I. P. (1969). Relationships between headache and amine changes after administration of reserpine to migrainous patients. *Journal of Neurology, Neurosurgery and Psychiatry*, **32**, 555–61.

Doenicke, A., Brand, J., and Perrin, V. L. (1988). Possible benefit of GR 43175, a novel 5-HT$_1$-like receptor agaonist, for the acute treatment of severe migraine. *Lancet*, **i**, 1309–11.

Feinmann, C. (1985). Pain relief by antidepressants: possible modes of action. *Pain*, **23**, 1–8.

Fozard, J. (1990). 5-HT in migraine: evidence from 5-HT receptor antagonists for a neuronal aetiology. In *Migraine: a spectrum of ideas*, (ed. M. Sandler and G. Collins), pp. 128–46. Oxford University Press.

Garvey, M. J., Schaffer, C. B., and Tuason, V. B. (1983). Relationship of headaches to depression. *British Journal of Psychiatry*, **143**, 554–7.

Gawel, M., Burkitt, M., and Clifford Rose, F. (1979). The platelet release reaction during migraine attacks. *Headache*, **19**, 323–7.

Geaney, D. P., Rutterford, M. G., Elliott, J. M., Schachter, M., Peet, K. M. S., and Grahame-Smith, D. G. (1984). Decreased platelet [3H]imipramine binding sites in classical migraine. *Journal of Neurology, Neurosurgery and Psychiatry*, **47**, 720–3.

Glover, V., Peatfield, R., Zammit-Pace, R., Littlewood, J., Gawel, M., Clifford Rose, F., and Sandler, M. (1981). Platelet monoamine oxidase activity and headache. *Journal of Neurology, Neurosurgery and Psychiatry*, **44**, 786–90.

Glover, V. and Sandler, M. (1989). Can the vascular and neurogenic theories of migraine finally be reconciled? *Trends in Pharmacological Science*, **10**, 1–3.

Hale, A. S., Walker, P. L., Bridges, P. K., and Sandler, M. (1986). Tyramine conjugation deficit as a trait marker in endogenous depressive illness. *Journal of Psychiatric Research*, **20**, 251–61.

Hale, A. S., Sandler, M., Hannah, P., and Bridges, P. K. (1989). Tyramine conjugation for prediction of treatment response in depressed patients. *Lancet*, **i**, 234–6.

Hilton, B. P. and Cumings J. N. (1972). 5-Hydroxytryptamine levels and platelet aggregation responses in subjects with acute migraine headaches. *Journal of Neurology, Neurosurgery and Psychiatry*, **35**, 505–9.

Humphrey, P. P. A., Feniuk, W., and Perren, M. J. (1990). 5-HT in migraine: evidence from 5-HT$_1$-like receptor agonists for a vascular aetiology. In *Migraine: a spectrum of ideas*, (ed. M. Sandler and G. Collins), pp. 147–72. Oxford University Press.

Jarman, J., Fernandez, M., Davies, P. T. G., Glover, V., Steiner, T. J., Thompson, C., *et al.* (1990). High incidence of endogenous depression in migraine: confirmation by tyramine test. *Journal of Neurology, Neurosurgery and Psychiatry*, **55**, 573–5.

Kanof, P. D., Coccaro, E. F., Johns, C. A., Siever, L. J., and Davis, K. L. (1987). Platelet (^{3}H)-imipramine binding in psychiatric disorders. *Biological Psychiatry*, **22**, 278–86.

Littlewood, J. T., Gibb, C., Glover, V., Sandler, M., Davies, P. T. G., and Clifford Rose, F. (1988). Red wine as a cause of migraine. *Lancet*, **i**, 558–9.

Melzack, R. and Wall, P. (1988). *The challenge of pain*. Penguin, London.

Merikangas, K. R., Risch, N. J., Merikangas, J. R., Weissman, M. M., and Kidd, K. K. (1988). Migraine and depression: association and familial transmission. *Journal of Psychiatric Research*, **22**, 119–29.

Paul, S. M., Rehavi, M., Skolnick, P., Ballenger, J. C., and Goodwin, F. K. (1981). Depressed patients have decreased binding of tritiated imipramine to platelet serotonin transporter. *Archives of General Psychiatry*, **38**, 1315–17.

Peroutka, S. J. (1988*a*). 5-Hydroxytryptamine receptor subtypes. *Annual Review of Neuroscience*, **11**, 45–60.

Peroutka, S. J. (1988*b*). Antimigraine drug interactions with serotonin receptor subtypes in human brain. *Annals of Neurology*, **23**, 500–4.

Peroutka, S. J., Switzer, J. A., and Hamik, A. (1989). Identification of 5-hydroxytryptamine$_{1D}$ binding sites in human brain membranes. *Synapse*, **3**, 61–6.

Rolf, L. H., Wiele, G., and Brune, G. G. (1981). 5-Hydroxytryptamine in platelets of patients with muscle contraction headache. *Headache*, **21**, 10–11.

Sandler, M., Youdim, M. B. H., Southgate, J., and Hanington, E. (1970). The role of tyramine in migraine: some possible biochemical mechanisms. In *Background to migraine, 3rd Migraine Symposium*, (ed. A. L. Cochrane), pp. 104–15. Heinemann, London.

Sicuteri, F. (1972). 5-Hydroxytryptophan in the prophylaxis of migraine. *Pharmacological Research Communications*, **4**, 213–18.

Titus, F., Davalos, A., Alom, J., and Codina, A. (1986). 5-Hydroxytryptophan versus methysergide in the prophylaxis of migraine. *European Neurology*, **25**, 327–9.

Youdim, M. B. H., Bonham Carter, S., Sandler, M., Hanington, E., and Wilkinson, M. (1971). Conjugation defect in tyramine-sensitive migraine. *Nature*, **230**, 127–8.

Discussion

LÓPEZ-IBOR: Many years ago I did the opposite experiment, which was to look at somatic symptoms in patients with depression, studying so-called 'masked' depressions (López-Ibor 1979). A group of patients in this study had a history of migraine but they were never simultaneously depressed and afflicted with migraine. When the migraine attacks were relieved, depression returned and vice versa. It was described as a syndrome shift from one disorder to the other (Groen *et al.* 1957).

GLOVER: Garvey *et al.* (1983) studied depressed people during periods of depression and recovery. The patients suffered more migraine when they were depressed.

COPPEN: The study at the Migraine Clinic probably does not involve a random sample of migraine patients.

GLOVER: That is a problem. But population studies (Merikangas *et al.* 1988) suggest that there is a substantial overlap in the occurrence of migraine and depression.

COPPEN: We used the standardized migraine questionnaire to study depressed patients stabilized long-term on lithium. The prevalence of migraine was quite low, whereas patients with acute depression often have a history of migraine or headache. We have often wondered whether lithium has an effect on migraine.

GLOVER: It is generally believed not to.

YOUDIM: I am glad that you have confirmed the altered tyramine metabolism in patients with migraine. In an earlier paper (Youdim *et al.* 1971) we discussed the role of migraine in depression, because a number of depressed patients had the 'cheese effect' while on monoamine oxidase inhibitors. They developed migraine headache after eating certain foods.

GLOVER: There was no difference in the tyramine test results for those who said they were cheese-sensitive and those who were not. Your work began these studies, Professor Youdim, but I think the explanation will be different and will depend on a link with depression rather than on dietary triggers.

MENDLEWICZ: Depression is a very common disorder and overlaps have been reported between depression and several somatic disorders, such as low back pain, Crohn's disease, and cerebrovascular disorders. How can we discover which are relevant correlations?

SANDLER: Here, we have an objective marker, the tyramine test (see Hale *et al.* 1986).

GLOVER: The high degree of overlap between depression and several somatic disorders does make it difficult to find the relevant biochemical correlations. It is important to know which condition is really associated with a particular marker. We postulate a low 5-HT syndrome in migraine, pain, and depression, and there must be some way in which the 5-HT system and other systems are disturbed, partly in similar ways and partly in different ways, in these disorders.

References

Garvey, M. J., Schaffer, C. B., and Tuason, V. B. (1983). Relationship of headaches to depression. *British Journal of Psychiatry*, **143**, 323–7.

Groen, J., Bastiaans, J., and van der Valk, J. M. (1957). Psychosomatic aspects of syndrome shift and syndrome suppression. In: *Psychosomatics*, (ed. J. Booij). Elsevier, Amsterdam.

Hale, A. S., Walker, P. L., Bridges, P. K., and Sandler, M. (1986). Tyramine-conjugation deficit as a trait-marker in endogenous depressive illness. *Journal of Psychiatric Research*, **20**, 251–61.

López-Ibor Jr., J. J. (1979). Why do depressions become masked? In *Biological psychiatry today*, (ed. J. Obiols *et al.*). Elsevier, Amsterdam.

Merikangas, K. R., Risch, N. J., Merikangas, J. R., Weissman, M. M., and Kidd, K. K. (1988). Migraine and depression: association and familial transmission. *Journal of Psychiatric Research*, **22**, 119–29.

Youdim, M. B. H., Carter, S. B., Hanington, E., Sandler, M., and Wilkinson, M. (1971). Conjugation defect in tyramine-sensitive migraine. *Nature*, **230**, 128–8.

8. The acute effect of monoamine oxidase inhibitors on serotonin conversion to melatonin

Gregory F. Oxenkrug

Monoamine oxidase (MAO) inhibitors were introduced as antidepressants about 30 years ago (Crane 1957; Loomer *et al.* 1957). The pharmacological mechanism of their antidepressant effect was related to the inhibition of MAO activity and limitation of the catabolism of the monoamines, serotonin (5-hydroxytryptamine, 5-HT) and noradrenaline (NA)(Pare and Sandler 1959). Both monoamines play an important role in the regulation of melatonin biosynthesis from serotonin. This process involves the *N*-acetylation of serotonin to form *N*-acetylserotonin (NAS), which is catalysed by *N*-acetyltransferase (NAT). The synthesis of NAS is triggered by noradrenaline stimulation of the pinealocyte adrenoceptors (mainly β_1 receptors). The next step is methylation of NAS to form melatonin, which is catalysed by hydroxyindole-*O*-methyltransferase (HIOMT) (see Lewy 1983).

The inhibition of MAO by MAO inhibitors is acute: it occurs within hours of the administration of a single dose (Simpson *et al.* 1985; Oxenkrug *et al.* 1986*a*). Both tricyclic (Franey *et al.* 1986) and heterocyclic (Demisch *et al.* 1986) antidepressants increase the levels of melatonin in human plasma after administration of a single dose. A single electroconvulsive shock almost doubled rat pineal *N*-acetyltransferase activity (Nowak *et al.* 1988) and the concentrations of melatonin and serotonin (Oxenkrug *et al.*, this volume). This paper concentrates on our studies of the acute effect of MAO inhibitors on melatonin biosynthesis.

Animal Studies

The acute effect of the selective MAO-A and MAO-B inhibitors on rat pineal biosynthesis of melatonin

MAO inhibitors stimulated rat pineal biosynthesis of melatonin *in vitro* (Axelrod *et al.* 1969; Klein and Rowe, 1970) and *in vivo* (Deguchi and Axelrod 1972; Illnerova 1974; Bade *et al.* 1977; Heydorn *et al.* 1982). King *et al.* (1982) observed no difference between the effects of harmine (a selective MAO-A inhibitor) and pargyline (a relatively selective MAO-B inhibitor) on rat pineal NAT activity and melatonin content (measured by radioimmunoassay). However, at high doses pargyline inhibits both MAO-A and MAO-B (see McCauley 1981), and the dose of pargyline used by King *et al.* (1982) was rather high (20 mg kg^{-1}). They made no evaluation of the MAO-A and B activities. Therefore, we decided to re-evaluate the data.

Clorgyline, even at the rather high dose of 2.5 mg kg^{-1}, did not change the MAO-B activity, whereas a low dose of deprenyl (10 mg kg^{-1}) inhibited only MAO-B, but a higher dose (25 mg kg^{-1}) inhibited both A and B forms of MAO (Oxenkrug *et al.* 1984, 1985).

Accordingly, clorgyline increased the content of NAS and melatonin in the rat pineal 90 min after subcutaneous injection. A low dose of deprenyl (selective for MAO-B inhibition) did not affect melatonin synthesis, whereas a higher dose (non-selective MAO inhibition) stimulated melatonin biosynthesis (Oxenkrug *et al.* 1984, 1985).

Similar results were obtained in the *in vitro* experiments (Oxenkrug *et al.* 1988*b*). Clorgyline had a dose-dependent effect on melatonin synthesis, as did the other selective MAO-A inhibitors, brofaromine and moclobemide, and non-selective inhibitors, tranylcypromine, phenelzine, and pargyline, while the selective MAO-B inhibitor, Ro 19-6327, did not affect melatonin biosynthesis (Oxenkrug *et al.* 1986*b*, 1990, and unpublished). This suggests that *selective MAO-A (but not MAO-B) inhibitors stimulate the biosynthesis of melatonin in rat pineal.*

Mechanism(s) of the stimulation of melatonin biosynthesis induced by the selective MAO-A inhibitors

Although MAO inhibition after a single dose of the MAO inhibitors lasted for at least several days, the melatonin levels peaked after about 2 h and returned to baseline values after about 6 h (Oxenkrug *et al.* 1986*a,b*; Bieck *et al.* 1988). Also, melatonin contains no amino groups; therefore oxidative deamination cannot be directly involved in melatonin metabolism. Thus, the stimulation of melatonin biosynthesis induced by the MAO-A inhibitors is not the direct result of inhibition of the enzyme activity. Rather, the effect might be mediated by the changes induced by MAO inhibitors in the availability of serotonin and NA, in the activity of NAT and HIOMT, and/or in sensitivity of adrenoceptors.

Because MAO-A inhibitors prevent the degradation of both NA and 5-HT, we were specifically interested in determining which neurotransmitter was more important for the stimulation of melatonin biosynthesis.

Serotonin availability Wurtman and Ozaki (1978) proposed that the availability of serotonin is the main factor regulating melatonin biosynthesis. Bade *et al.* (1977) suggested that increased 5-HT availability mediated pargyline (20 mg kg^{-1}) induced stimulation of melatonin synthesis, because rat pineal NAT activation was observed in association with the elevation of serotonin (but not NA) content. Similarly, attenuation of clorgyline-induced stimulation of melatonin biosynthesis in rats subjected to superior cervical ganglionectomy (SCGX) (McIntyre *et al.* 1985) might be related to the 50 per cent reduction of pineal 5-HT content caused by this procedure.

However, in *in vitro* experiments clorgyline increased the rat pineal NAS and melatonin contents without affecting the tryptophan and 5-HT contents of both pineal gland and media (Oxenkrug *et al.* 1988*b*).

Noradrenaline availability In *in vitro* experiments an increase in the period of preincubation from 6 to 72 h resulted in a drastic decrease of pineal NA (but not 5-HT) content and almost complete prevention of clorgyline-induced stimulation of pineal melatonin biosynthesis (Oxenkrug *et al.* 1988*b*).

Thus, the prevention of NA degradation seems to be a major mechanism by which MAO-A inhibitors stimulate melatonin synthesis. There is, however, a certain level of 5-HT below which stimulation of melatonin synthesis by MAO-A inhibitors is not permitted.

NAT activity Experimental data suggest that MAO inhibitors affect the rate-limiting enzymic reaction of melatonin biosynthesis, *N*-acetylation of serotonin; pargyline (Deguchi and Axelrod 1972) and clorgyline (Oxenkrug *et al.* 1988*b*) enhanced NAT activity, and harmine stimulated 5-HT conversion to NAS *in vitro* (Klein and Rowe 1970). Clorgyline increased rat pineal NAS (and melatonin) contents *in vivo* and *in vitro* (Oxenkrug *et al.* 1984, 1985, 1988*b*). However, Bade *et al.* (1977) found no effect of pargyline on liver NAT activity. These authors argued that the NAT activation observed *in vivo* does not result from a direct stimulatory effect of pargyline on the NAT activity but occurs because of an enhanced concentration of 5-HT, the substrate for NAT.

β Receptor sensitivity The possibility of direct stimulation of pineal *β* receptors by MAO inhibitors has been suggested by Deguchi and Axelrod (1972). Our observation that surgical and chemical sympathectomy resulted in attenuation, but not prevention, of the clorgyline-induced stimulation of melatonin synthesis (McIntyre *et al.* 1985; Reuss and Oxenkrug 1989) might be at least partly explained by direct stimulation of pineal adrenoceptors by clorgyline. Although there is no clear evidence for the direct stimulation of pineal adrenoceptors by MAO inhibitors, up/down-regulation of the pineal $β_1$ receptors might be responsible for the circadian variations of the melatonin synthesis in response to pargyline (Illnerova 1974; Bade *et al.* 1977) and for the higher absolute increase of pineal NAS and melatonin contents in response to clorgyline in rats treated with 6-hydroxydopamine than in intact animals (Reuss and Oxenkrug 1989). The ability of a *β*-adrenoceptor blocker, propranolol, to prevent the pargyline-induced NAT stimulation *in vitro*

(Deguchi and Axelrod 1972) and *in vivo* (Heydorn *et al.* 1982) provides additional evidence for the involvement of the β_1 receptors in the mediation of the MAO inhibitor-induced stimulation of melatonin synthesis. Similarly, propranolol prevented the clorgyline-induced increases of pineal NAS and melatonin contents *in vivo* and *in vitro* (Oxenkrug *et al.* 1988*b*). Up-regulation of the pineal β receptors caused by continuous exposure to light for 24 h (Greenberg and Weiss 1978) significantly potentiated the increase of pineal NAS and melatonin caused by clorgyline. The lack of such potentiation in aged rats (Oxenkrug *et al.*, unpublished) might be attributed to an age-associated subsensitivity of the pineal β receptors to the up-regulative effect of light (Greenberg and Weiss 1978).

HIOMT activity   We have found only one study dedicated to this issue; harmine had no effect on rat pineal HIOMT activity *in vitro* (Klein and Rowe 1970).

Melatonin catabolism   See section on human studies: MAO inhibition and melatonin metabolites in urine.

Physiological and pathological activation of melatonin biosynthesis and the clorgyline-induced stimulation of melatonin biosynthesis

Sympathetic fibres from the superior cervical ganglion (SCG) are not the only source of NA able to stimulate pineal adrenoceptors. Because of its location outside the blood–brain barrier, the pineal gland might be affected by the blood NA produced in other parts of the sympathetic system. One of the most probable sources of blood NA is the adrenal medulla. Under physiological conditions, NA of non-SCG (superior cervical ganglion) origin does not affect the pineal melatonin biosynthesis because post-SCG sympathetic nerves are able to take up NA of non-SCG–pineal origin from the blood stream (Parfitt and Klein 1976). This protective mechanism might be compromised by stress (Lynch *et al.* 1977; Oxenkrug and McIntyre 1985).

Adrenal demedullation prevented stress-induced (Lynch *et al.* 1977), but not clorgyline-induced, stimulation of rat pineal melatonin biosynthesis, whereas SCGX did not affect the stimulation induced by stress but attenuated that induced by clorgyline (Oxenkrug and McCauley 1988). This suggests that *clorgyline stimulates melatonin biosynthesis by activation of the physiological pathways:* clorgyline increases the availability of NA released within the SCG–pineal complex.

The protective mechanism of the post-SCG sympathetic nerves might be compromised, as well as by stress, by surgical (McIntyre *et al.* 1985) or chemical (Reuss and Oxenkrug 1989) destruction of the SCG and by administration of desipramine (DMI), an inhibitor of NA uptake (Parfitt and

Klein 1976). Because both surgical and chemical SCGX did not affect adrenals, NA produced in the adrenal medulla might stimulate pineal melatonin synthesis in the absence of the protective mechanism. This might explain why surgical and chemical SCGX attenuated, but did not prevent, clorgyline-induced stimulation of melatonin biosynthesis.

In conclusion, MAO-A inhibitor-induced acute stimulation of melatonin biosynthesis represents the activation of physiological pathways of melatonin biosynthesis (that is, serotonin conversion to NAS) and probably depends on the preservation of the NA released from the post-SCG sympathetic nerve-endings. The amount of serotonin conversion to NAS is modulated mainly by the availability of the 5-HT as a substrate, and by the sensitivity of the pineal adrenoceptors.

Modulation of clorgyline- and stress-induced stimulation of melatonin biosynthesis by benzodiazepines

Because benzodiazepines (BZs) inhibit NA release (Lowenstein *et al.* 1985), we were interested to discover whether they affect the stimulation of melatonin biosynthesis induced by MAO-A inhibitors. Lorazepam and diazepam attenuated the clorgyline-induced increase of NAS and melatonin content in rat pineal (Oxenkrug and Harris 1988). Because both lorazepam and diazepam are mixed central/peripheral BZ agonists, we investigated whether the observed attentuation is a central or peripheral effect. Rat pineal contains only peripheral BZ receptors (Quirion 1984); therefore we expected only the peripheral BZ agonist to attentuate clorgyline-induced stimulation of melatonin biosynthesis. However, the central BZ agonist, clonazepam, (but not the peripheral BZ agonist, Ro 5-4864) attentuated the clorgyline-induced elevation of the rat pineal NAS and melatonin content (Oxenkrug and Requintina 1990). Our results suggest that BZ modulation of the effect of MAO-A inhibitors on melatonin synthesis depends on the inhibition of NA release (probably from the post-SCG sympathetic nerve endings) but not on direct BZ interaction with the pineal BZ receptors. This suggestion is in line with the observation that lorazepam attenuated the stress-induced stimulation of melatonin synthesis as well (Oxenkrug and McIntyre 1985). It is note-worthy that central, but not peripheral, types of BZ receptors were found on chromaffin cell membrane in the adrenal medulla (Kataoka *et al.* 1984).

Pharmacological versus physiological rhythm

The ability of clorgyline to stimulate melatonin biosynthesis at the beginning of the light phase of the light/dark cycle, i.e., at the time of the lowest pineal activity (Oxenkrug *et al.* 1990*b*), suggests that a single dose of MAO-A inhibitor may act as auxillary exogenous *Zeitgebers* (time cues). The suprachiasmatic nucleus (SCN) is considered the main regulator of circadian rhythms (CR) because its destruction resulted in the loss of the endogenous CR of melatonin synthesis, plasma corticosterone, feeding, drinking, heart rate, sleep-wake cycles, etc. (Moore 1974). In our study, SCN destruction did not affect clorgyline-induced stimulation of melatonin synthesis in rats kept under a 12:12 h light/dark schedule, although it abolished the additional stimulation of melatonin biosynthesis in rats exposed to 24 h of constant light (unpublished).

These results suggest that *administration of the MAO-A inhibitors might allow the substitution of an SCN-dependent, physiological melatonin rhythm, which is disturbed in depression, by a pharmacological one.* The parameters of the pharmacological rhythm might be designed according to clinical indications and the pharmacokinetics of the MAO-A inhibitors.

The endogenous MAO inhibitor and melatonin biosynthesis

The endogenous MAO inhibitor of indole origin (tribulin) was described by Sandler (1982). Cold-immobilization stress, known to stimulate urine tribulin excretion (Glover *et al.* 1981) and brain tribulin content (Bhattacharya *et al.* 1988), increases rat pineal NAS and melatonin content (Oxenkrug and McIntyre 1985; Bhattacharya *et al.* 1988).

It is unclear, however, whether the stress effect on melatonin is mediated by tribulin, which is not only an MAO inhibitor but also a BZ ligand. Therefore, the stimulation of melatonin synthesis caused by the MAO-inhibiting properties of tribulin may be balanced by the opposing effect of the BZ-like properties.

Human studies

The acute effect of the selective MAO-A and MAO-B inhibitors on the levels of melatonin in human plasma

The observation that a single dose of MAO-A, but not MAO-B, inhibitor stimulated rat pineal melatonin biosynthesis might be of clinical significance in view of the finding that only MAO-A (and not MAO-B) inhibitors have clinical antidepressant activity (Murphy *et al.* 1983). However, when we reported the stimulation of the rat pineal melatonin synthesis by the selective MAO-A inhibitor (Oxenkrug *et al.* 1984) it was not known whether MAO inhibitors might stimulate melatonin synthesis in humans and (if so) whether this effect was also related only to MAO-A inhibitors. We found that a single dose of tranylcypromine (non-selective MAO inhibitor available in the USA) transiently elevated human plasma melatonin levels (Oxenkrug *et al.* 1986*a*). Because the pineal gland is the only source of plasma melatonin in humans (Neuwelt and Lewy 1983), the observed increase of plasma melatonin after MAO inhibition is thought to reflect the stimulation of pineal melatonin synthesis. A single dose of the selective MAO-A inhibitor, brofaromine, but not of the relatively selective MAO-B inhibitor, pargyline (low dose; 5 mg kg^{-1}) increased plasma melatonin levels in healthy human volunteers (Bieck *et al.* 1988). A single dose of moclobemide increased night-time (P. R. Bieck, personal communication), but not daytime, human plasma melatonin levels (Scheinin *et al.* 1990). The clinical significance of the *acute* increase in daytime plasma melatonin levels induced by MAO inhibitors is emphasized by the fact that these levels were comparable with the night-time levels.

The elevation of plasma melatonin (Murphy *et al.* 1986) and urine 6-hydroxymelatonin levels (Golden *et al.* 1988) in depressed patients, and of CSF melatonin levels in rhesus monkeys (Murphy *et al.* 1985), have also been demonstrated after *chronic* administration of MAO-A, but not MAO-B, inhibitors.

MAO inhibitor-induced versus night-time elevation of human plasma melatonin   As in animals, the stimulation of melatonin synthesis in humans was observed in the daytime when melatonin synthesis activity is normally very low. Comparison of the daytime tranylcypromine-induced increase with the night-time peak (around 2.00 or 3.00) in the same human volunteers revealed a strong negative correlation between the peak plasma level of melatonin in the day and the night-time peak. Thus, the more active the melatonin synthesis is during the night, the more difficult it is to achieve the daytime stimulation (Oxenkrug *et al.* 1988a). This could arise from exhaustion of the substrate (5-HT) and/or down-regulation of the adrenergic receptors. Daytime response to MAO inhibition might be used for the assessment of the night-time melatonin synthesis.

MAO inhibition and melatonin metabolites in urine   Melatonin produced by the pineal is almost immediately released into the blood stream. Catabolism of the blood melatonin involves hydroxylation and conjugation with sulphuric or glucuronic acids (see Lewy 1983). 6-Sulphatoxymelatonin (6-SM) is the main melatonin metabolite and is excreted in urine (Arendt *et al.* 1985). Under conditions in which it increased plasma melatonin levels (Oxenkrug *et al.* 1986a), tranylcypromine did not change 6-SM urine excretion (Oxenkrug *et al.* 1988). A possible explanation for this is that MAO inhibitors inhibit not only MAO but also some other enzymes, including liver microsomal enzymes (hydroxylases) involved in melatonin hydroxylation (Belanger and Atitse-Gbeassor 1982). Thus, the elevation of blood melatonin levels induced by the action of MAO inhibitors on the pineal melatonin biosynthesis might be sustained because of the MAO inhibitor-induced suppression of melatonin transformation into 6-hydroxymelatonin. The effect of MAO inhibitors on melatonin hydroxylation might be of clinical significance because the changes in blood melatonin levels are apparently more important for regulation of the CR than changes in the pineal melatonin content.

In conclusion, the human data by and large confirmed the results from animal studies and, in addition, revealed a new aspect of the effect of MAO inhibitors on melatonin synthesis: *MAO inhibitors may be directly involved in melatonin catabolism although not through inhibition of MAO per se.*

Stimulation of melatonin synthesis and mechanism of antidepressant action of MAO inhibitors

In the past decade evidence accumulated that at least a subgroup of depressive disorders might be caused by the dysregulation in circadian rhythms (Kripke 1983) and that synchronization of the CR might be one mechanism for the antidepressant effect (Wehr and Wirz-Justice 1982). The literature and our own data reviewed here suggest that stimulation of melatonin biosynthesis is the *acute* pharmacological effect of MAO-A inhibitors. Melatonin seems to have an important role in the regulation of circadian rhythms: melatonin administration normalizes the rest–activity cycle in rodents (Armstrong *et al.* 1986) and the CR of exogenous melatonin in sighted (Arendt *et al.* 1985) and blind humans (Sack *et al.* 1987).

The results reviewed suggest that the clinical antidepressant effect of MAO inhibitors is mediated by the acute stimulation of melatonin synthesis and consequent normalization of the disturbed CR in depression. According to this hypothesis, the time-lag between the administration of MAO inhibitors and the clinical antidepressant effect depends upon the relative resistance of the endogenous CR of melatonin to the changes induced by MAO-A inhibitors. Normalization of the endogenous CR of melatonin requires the repetition of stimulation of melatonin synthesis by MAO-A inhibitors during several consecutive 24 h cycles. This view is at variance with the hypothesis that relates the clinical antidepressant effect with the adaptive changes (for example, β receptor down-regulation) induced by chronic antidepressant administration. If chronic administration of MAO inhibitors does down-regulate pineal β receptors (some antidepressants, such as fluoxetine, iprindole, and mianserin do not; Cowen *et al.* 1983), no further stimulation of the melatonin synthesis would be possible, and this would mark the end, not the beginning, of the clinical antidepressant effect. The proposed pharmacological mechanism for the clinical antidepressant action of MAO inhibitors might be used as a working hypothesis for further investigation of the involvement of melatonin in the antidepressant effect.

Acknowledgement

The support of the Lady Davis Fund is very much appreciated.

References

Arendt, J., Bojkowski, C., Folkard, S., Franey, C., Marks, V., Moniors, D., Waterhouse, J., *et al.* (1985). Some effects of melatonin and the control of its secretion in humans. In *Photoperiodism, melatonin and pineal*, Ciba Foundation Symposium 117, (ed. D. Evered and S. Clark), pp. 266–79. Pitman, London.

Armstrong, S. M., Cassone, V. M., Chesworth, M. J., Redman, J. R., and Short, V. (1986). Synchronization of mammalian circadian rhythms by melatonin. *Journal of Neural Transmission*, **S21**, 373–96.

Axelrod J., Shein X., and Wurtman, R. J. (1969). Stimulation of 14-C melatonin synthesis from 14-C-tryptophan by noradrenaline in rat pineal organ culture. *Proceedings of the National Academy of Sciences USA*, **62**, 544–9.

Bade, P., Rommerspacher, H., and Strauss, S. (1977). N-acetyltransferase activity in pineal gland of rats treated with pargyline. *Archives of Pharmacology*, **297**, 143–7.

Belanger, P-M. and Atitse-Gbeassor, A. (1982). The inhibitory effect of tranylcypromine on hepatic drug metabolism in the rat. *Biochemical Pharmacology*, **31**, 2679–83.

Bieck. P. R., Antonin, K. H., Balon, R., and Oxenkrug, G. F. (1988). Brofaromine and pargyline effect on human plasma melatonin. *Progress in Neuro-Psychopharmacology and Biological Psychiatry*, **12**, 93–101.

Bhattacharya, S. K., Glover, V., McIntyre, I. M., Oxenkrug, G. F., and Sandler M. (1988). Stress causes an increase in endogenous monoamine oxidase inhibitor (tribulin) in rat brain. *Neuroscience Letters*, **92**, 218–21.

Cowen, P. J., Frazer, S., Grahame-Smith, D. G., Green, A. R., and Stanford, C., (1983). The effect of chronic antidepressant administration on β-adrenoceptor function of the rat pineal. *British Journal of Pharmacology*, **78**, 89–96.

Crane, G., (1957). Iproniazid (Marsilid) phosphate, therapeutic agent for mental disorders and debilitating diseases. *Psychiatry Research Reports*, **8**, 142–52.

Deguchi, T. and Axelrod, J. (1972). Induction and superinduction of serotonin N-acetyltransferase by adrenergic drugs and denervation of rat pineal organ. *Proceedings of the National Academy of Sciences USA*, **69**, 2208–11.

Demisch, K., Demisch, L., Bochnik, H. J., Nickelsen, T., Althoff, P. H., Schoffling, K., and Rieth R. (1986). Melatonin and cortisol increase after fluvoxamine. *British Journal of Clinical Pharmacology*, **22**, 620–1.

Franey, C., Aldhous, M., Burton, S., Checkley, S., and Arendt, J. (1986). Acute treatment with desipramine stimulates melatonin and 6-sulphatoxy melatonin production in man. *British Journal of Clinical Pharmacology*, **22**, 73–9.

Glover, V., Bhattacharya, S. K., Sandler, M., and File, S. M. (1981). Benzodiazepines reduce stress-augmented increase in rat urine monoamine oxidase inhibitor. *Nature*, **292**, 347–9.

Golden, R. N., Markey, S. P., Risby, E. D., Rudorfer, M. V., Cowdry, R. W., and Potter, W. Z. (1988). Antidepressants reduce whole-body norepinephrine turnover while enhancing 6-hydroxymelatonin output. *Archives of General Psychiatry*, **45**, 150–4.

Greenberg, L. H. and Weiss, B. (1978). Beta-adrenergic receptors in aged rat brain reduced number and capacity of pineal gland to develop supersensitivity. *Science*, **201**, 62–3.

Heydorn, W. E., Brunswick, D. J., and Frazer, A. (1982). Effect of treatment of rats with antidepressants on melatonin concentrations in the pineal gland and serum. *Journal of Pharmacology and Experimental Therapeutics*, **222**, 534–43.

Illnerova, H. (1974). The effect of darkness and pargyline on the activity of serotonin N-acetyltransferase in the rat epiphysis. *Neuroendocrinology*, **16**, 202–11.

Kataoka, Y., Gutman, Y., Guidotti, A., Panula, P., Wroblewski, J., Cosenza-

Murphy, D., *et al.* (1984). Intrinsic GABAergic system of adrenal chromaffin cells. *Proceedings of the National Academy of Sciences USA*, **81**, 3218–22.

King, T. S., Richardson, B., and Reiter, R. J., (1982). Regulation of rat pineal melatonin synthesis: effect of monoamine oxidase inhibition. *Molecular and Cell Endocrinology*, **25**, 327–8.

Klein, D. and Rowe, J. (1970). Pineal gland in organ culture. I. Inhibition by harmine of serotonin-14-C oxidation accompanied by stimulation of melatonin 14-C production. *Molecular Pharmacology*, **6**, 164–71.

Kripke, D. (1983). Phase-advanced theories for affective disorders. In *Circadian rhythms in psychiatry*, (ed. T. Wehr and F. Goodwin), Vol. 2, pp. 41–69. Boxwood Press, California.

Lewy, A. (1983). Biochemistry and regulation of mammalian melatonin production. In *The pineal gland*, (ed. R. Relkin), pp. 77–128. Elsevier, New York.

Loomer, H., Saunders, J., and Kline, N. (1957). Clinical and pharmacodynamic evaluation of iproniazid as psychic energizer. *Psychiatry Research Reports*, **8**, 129–41.

Lowenstein, P., Solveyra, C., Sarmiento, M., and Cardinali, D. (1985). Benzodiazepines decreased norepinephrine release from rat pineal nerves by acting on peripheral type binding sites. *Acta Physiologica et Pharmacologica Latinoamericana*, **35**, 441–9.

Lynch, H. J., Ho, M., and Wurtman, R. J. (1977). The adrenal medulla may mediate the increase in pineal melatonin synthesis induced by stress, but not that caused by exposure to darkness. *Journal of Neural Transmission*, **40**, 87–97.

McCauley, R. B. (1981). Monoamine oxidases and the pharmacology of monoamine oxidase inhibitors. In *Neuropharmacology of central nervous system and behavioral disorders*, pp. 93–109. Academic Press, New York.

McIntyre, I. M., McCauley, R., Murphy, S., Goldman, H., and Oxenkrug, G. F. (1985). The effect of superior cervical ganglionectomy on melatonin stimulation by MAO-A inhibitor. *Biochemical Pharmacology*, **34**, 3394–5.

Moore, R. Y. (1974). Central nervous control of circadian rhythms. In *Frontiers in neuroendocrinology*, Vol. 5, (ed. W. F. Ganong,), pp. 185–205. Raven Press, New York.

Murphy, D., Cohen, R., Siever, L., Ray, B., Karoum, F., Wyatt, R., *et al.* (1983). Clinical and laboratory studies with selective monoamine-oxidase-inhibitory drugs. In *Problems in pharmacopsychiatry*, Vol 19, pp. 287–303. Karger, Basel.

Murphy, D. L., Garrick, N. A., Tamarkin, L., Taylor, P. L., and Markey, S.P. (1985). Effect of antidepressant and other psychotropic drugs on melatonin release and pineal gland function. In *Melatonin in humans*, (ed. R. J. Wurtman and F. Waldhauser), pp. 261–77. Center for Brain Sciences and Metabolism Charitable Trust, Cambridge, Massachussetts.

Murphy, D. L., Tamarkin, L., Sunderland, T., Garrick, N. A., and Cohen, R. (1986). Human plasma melatonin is elevated during treatment with the monoamine oxidase inhibitors clorgyline and tranylcypromine but not deprenyl. *Psychiatry Research*, **17**, 119–27.

Nowak, J. Z., Przybysz, M., and Zurawska, E. (1988). The melatonin generating system in the rat retina and pineal gland: effect of single and repeated electroconvulsive shock (ECS). *Polish Journal of Pharmacology*, **40**, 573–84.

Neuwelt, E. and Lewy, A. (1983). Disappearance of plasma melatonin after removal of a neoplastic pineal gland. *New England Journal of Medicine*, **308**, 1132–5.

Oxenkrug, G. F., and McIntyre, I. M. (1985). Stress-induced synthesis of melatonin:

possible involvement of the endogenous monoamine oxidase inhibitor (Tribulin). *Life Sciences*, **37**, 1743–6.

Oxenkrug, G. F., and McCauley, R. B. (1987). The effect of MAO inhibitors on melatonin synthesis: mechanism and clinical implication. *Pharmacology and Toxicology*, **60**, Suppl. 1, 36.

Oxenkrug, G. F. and Harris P. (1988). Benzodiazepines attenuate clorgyline-induced stimulation of melatonin synthesis. *Pharmacology Research Communication*, **20**, Suppl. 4, 139–40.

Oxenkrug, G. F. and Requintina, P. J. (1990). Central but not peripheral benzodiazepine agonists attenuate clorgyline effect on melatonin synthesis. *Biological Psychiatry*, **27**, 68A.

Oxenkrug, G., McCauley, R., McIntyre, I., and Filipowicz, C. (1984). Effect of clorgyline and deprenyl on rat pineal melatonin. *Journal of Pharmacy and Pharmacology*, **36**, 55W.

Oxenkrug, G., McIntyre, I., McCauley, R., and Filipowicz, C. (1985). Selective inhibition of MAO-A but not MAO-B activity increases rat pineal melatonin. *Journal of Neural Transmission*, **61**, 265–70.

Oxenkrug, G. F., Balon, R., Jain, A. K., McIntyre, I. M., and Appel, D. (1986a). Single dose of tranylcypromine increases human plasma melatonin. *Biological Psychiatry*, **21**, 1085–9.

Oxenkrug, G. F., McCauley, R. B., Fontana, D. J., McIntyre, I. M., and Commissaris, R. I. (1986b). Possible melatonin involvement in the hypotensive effect of MAO inhibitors. *Journal of Neural Transmission*, **66**, 271–80.

Oxenkrug, G. F., Balon, R., Jain, A. K., and McIntyre, I. M.(1988a). Melatonin plasma response to MAO inhibitor—an index of pineal activity? *Acta Psychiatrica Scandinavica*, **77**, 160–2.

Oxenkrug, G., McIntyre, I., McCauley, R., and Yuwiler, A. (1988b). The effect of selective MAO inhibitors on rat pineal melatonin synthesis in vitro. *Journal of Pineal Research*, **5**, 99–109.

Oxenkrug, G. F., Balon, R., Kroessler, D., Yeragani, V., Beardsley, G., and Lewy, A. (1989). Single dose administration of tranylcypromine does not change human 6-sulphatoxymelatonin urine excretion. *Biological Psychiatry*, **25** (7A), 53A.

Oxenkrug, G. F., Requintina, P. J., and Yuwiler, A. (1990a). Does moclobemide stimulate melatonin synthesis as the other selective MAO-A inhibitors do? *Journal of Neural Transmission*, **32**, in press.

Oxenkrug, G. F., Anderson, G., Dragovic, L., Blaivas, M., and Riederer, P. (1990b). Circadian rhythm of human plasma melatonin, related indoles and beta receptors: post-mortem evaluation. *Journal of Pineal Research*, in press.

Oxenkrug, G. F., Requintina, P., McIntyre, I. M., and Davis R. (1991). Stimulation of rat pineal melatonin synthesis by a single electroconvulsive shock: chronobiological effect of antidepressant therapy? In *5-Hydroxytryptamine in psychiatry: a spectrum of ideas*, (ed. M. Sandler, A. Coppen, and S. Harnett), pp. 110–15. Oxford University Press.

Pare, C. and Sandler, M. (1959). A clinical and biochemical study of a trial of iproniazid in the treatment of depression. *Journal of Neurology, Neurosurgery and Psychiatry*, **22**, 247–51.

Parfitt, A. G. and Klein, D. C. (1976). Sympathetic nerve terminals in pineal gland protect against acute stress induced increases in N-acetyltransferase activity. *Endocrinology*, **99**, 840–51.

Quirion, R. (1984). High density of Ro 5-4864 'peripheral' benzodiazepine binding sites in the rat pineal gland. *European Journal of Pharmacology*, **102**, 559–60.

Reuss, S., and Oxenkrug, G. F. (1989). Chemical sympathectomy and clorgyline-induced stimulation of rat pineal melatonin synthesis. *Journal of Neural Transmission*, **78**, 167–72.

Sack, R. L., Lewy, A. J., and Hoban, T. M. (1987). Free-running melatonin rhythms in blind people: phase shifts with melatonin and triazolam administration. In *Temporal disorders in human oscillatory systems*, (ed. L. Rensing, U. an der Heiden, and M. C. Mackey), pp. 219–24. Springer-Verlag, Heidelberg.

Sandler, M. (1982). The emergence of tribulin. *Trends in Pharmacological Sciences*, **3**, 471–2.

Scheinin, M., Koulu, M., Vakkuri, O., Vuorinen, J., and Zimmer, H. (1990). Moclobemide, an inhibitor of MAO-A, does not increase daytime melatonin levels in normal humans. *Progress in Neuro-Psychopharmacology and Biological Psychiatry*, **14**, 73–82.

Simpson, G. S., Frederickson, E., Palmer, R., Edmond, P., Bruce Sloan R., and White, K. (1985). Platelet monoamine oxidase inhibition by deprenyl and tranylcypromine: implications for clinical use. *Biological Psychiatry*, **20**, 680–4.

Wehr, T. and Wirz-Justice, A. (1982). Circadian rhythm mechanisms in affective illness and in antidepressant drug action. *Pharmacopsychiatria*, **15**, 31–9.

Wurtman, R. J. and Ozaki, Y. (1978). Physiological control of melatonin synthesis and secretion mechanisms generating rhythms in melatonin, methoxytryptophol and arginin vasotocin levels. *Journal of Neural Transmission*, **13**, Suppl., 59–70.

9. Stimulation of rat pineal melatonin synthesis by a single electroconvulsive shock: chronobiological effect of antidepressant therapy?

Gregory F. Oxenkrug, Pura J. Requintina, Iain M. McIntyre, and Rosseta Davis

Introduction

Electroconvulsive therapy is considered to be the most effective treatment for endogenous depression (Kendall 1981), but despite vigorous research there is no consensus on the mechanism of the antidepressant effect. One attempt to explain the mechanism uses a neuroendocrine hypothesis (Fink 1987). Because it is generally accepted that the therapeutic effect of electro-convulsive shock (ECS) (and of antidepressant drugs) occurs after chronic (but not single) administration, most researchers have studied the biological changes associated with chronic application (Gleiter and Nutt 1989). In the past decade, evidence accumulated that depression might result from desyn-chronization (mainly phase advance) of circadian rhythms (Kripke *et al.* 1978). Thus normalization of the circadian rhythm might be one mechanism of the antidepressant effect. Such normalization is achieved simply by a single administration of the pineal gland hormone melatonin in rats (Armstrong *et al.* 1986). Also, administration of a single dose of melatonin has been reported to change circadian rhythms in humans (R. L. Sack, A. J. Lewy, and J. M. Latham, unpublished paper, 28th American College of Neurophar-macologists Meeting, Hawaii, 1989). Elevation of human plasma melatonin levels was observed after a single dose of the heterocyclic antidepressants, desipramine (Franey *et al.* 1986) and fluvoxamine (Demisch *et al.* 1986), and of monoamine oxidase (MAO) inhibitors (Oxenkrug *et al.* 1986*a*, 1988; Bieck *et al.* 1988). If the stimulation of melatonin synthesis with consequent normalization of disrupted circadian rhythms is, indeed, the common denom-inator of the antidepressant effect, it is interesting to study the effect of ECS (especially a single application) on melatonin synthesis.

We have found only three reports (including our own) on the effect of

ECS on melatonin synthesis. Chronic administration of ECS had no effect on: rat pineal melatonin content (Cowen *et al.* 1983); rat pineal contents of serotonin (5-hydroxytryptamine, substrate of melatonin synthesis), *N*-acetyl-serotonin (NAS, the intermediate product of melatonin synthesis) and melatonin (McIntyre and Oxenkrug 1984); and the activities of both the enzymes of melatonin biosynthesis, *N*-acetyltransferase (NAT) and hydroxy-indole-*O*-methyltransferase (HIOMT) (Nowak *et al.* 1988). In contrast, acute administration of ECS nearly doubled the isoproterenol-induced stimulation of NAT in the rat pineal 2 h after ECS (Nowak *et al.* 1988). In a previous study, we failed to observe the acute effect of ECS on rat pineal melatonin biosynthesis, apparently because of the inopportune timing of our evalua-tions—12 h after ECS administration (McIntyre and Oxenkrug 1984).

We re-evaluated the effect of a single ECS on rat pineal melatonin biosynthesis by measuring the amount of rat pineal melatonin and related indoles 90 min after ECS administration. This choice of time-lag was influenced by the data of Nowak *et al.* (1988) and by our previous observa-tions of stimulation of the biosynthesis 90 min after a single dose of the selective MAO-A inhibitor, clorgyline (Oxenkrug *et al.* 1984, 1985) and after 2 h of cold-immobilization stress (Oxenkrug and McIntyre 1985), the con-dition associated with increased production of the endogenous MAO inhibi-tor (EMAOI) of indole origin, tribulin, in urine (Glover *et al.* 1981) and brain (Bhattacharya *et al.* 1988). Increased production of tribulin (Bhatta-charya *et al.*, unpublished) and an EMAOI of protein origin (Becker and Giambalvo 1982) was reported after a single ECS (Isaak *et al.* 1986).

Methods

Male Sprague-Dawley rats (150–200 g) were housed at a constant temperature (22 °C) and in diurnal lighting conditions (lights on from 06.00 to 18.00) for at least two weeks before use. Water and Purina Lab Chow were freely available.

An electroconvulsive shock was administered via ear clip electrodes at 10.00. Shocks (130 V; 0.75 s) were delivered from a Medcraft apparatus, and tonic-clonic seizures lasting 20–25 s were induced. Control animals had electrodes applied with no current passed (sham ECS). The rats were decapitated 90 min after treatment. The brains were removed rapidly, and pineals were dissected and frozen at −80 °C until the time of analysis.

The concentrations of melatonin and related indoles were determined by high-pressure liquid chromatography with a fluorimetric detector (Oxenkrug *et al.* 1986*b*). The results obtained were statistically treated (Student's *t*-test).

Results

The level of melatonin in the pineal was doubled 90 min after a single ECS. The amounts of serotonin increased by 50 per cent and those of its

TABLE 9.1.   *The effect of a single electroconvulsive shock on the rat pineal concentrations (ng per pineal) of melatonin and related indoles*

	N	Melatonin	Serotonin	5-HIAA	5-HIAA/ serotonin
Sham-treated	4	0.12 ± 0.03*	62.08 ± 10.78	4.22 ± 0.74	0.07 ± 0.02
ECS-treated	5	0.19 ± 0.05	90.08 ± 23.65	7.62 ± 2.47	0.08 ± 0.02
Student's *t*-test		$t=2.38, p <0.02$	$t=1.93, p <0.05$	$t=2.34, p <0.02$	

5-HIAA, 5-hydroxyindoleacetic acid.
* means ± S.D.

metabolite, 5-hydroxyindoleacetic acid (5-HIAA), increased by 80 per cent (Table 9.1). The concentrations of NAS were below the detectability level in both ECS- and sham-treated animals (data not shown). There were no differences between the 5-HIAA/serotonin ratios in both groups of animals (Table 9.1).

Discussion

These results are the first indication that a single ECS increases the daytime pineal concentrations of melatonin, serotonin, and 5-HIAA in otherwise un-treated rats. Our data are in line with the observation that a single ECS doubled the NAT activation induced by the β receptor agonist, isoproterenol (Nowak *et al.* 1988). The results of both studies are pertinent to the mechanism(s) of the changes in melatonin biosynthesis induced by a single ECS and to the possible role of these changes in the clinical effect of ECS.

The increase in pineal melatonin concentrations probably reflects a stimu-lation of the pineal melatonin biosynthesis by ECS. The simultaneous elevation of the pineal serotonin levels suggests the increased availability of this substrate as the most probable mechanism of the stimulation of melatonin biosynthesis (Wurtman and Ozaki 1978). Given that a single ECS enhanced the isoproterenol-induced NAT activation (Nowak *et al.* 1988), the ECS-induced elevation of the pineal melatonin levels might also result from NAT activation. Such an activation is expected to increase the pineal NAS content, which has not been noticed in our experiments. However, this does not rule out the possibility of ECS-induced NAT stimulation because HIOMT, the enzyme that converts NAS into melatonin, is unsaturated under physiological conditions; therefore, newly synthesized NAS might be rapidly converted into melatonin before it can be detected. We found, from the effect of different doses of the selective MAO-A inhibitor, clorgyline, on the concen-trations in rat pineal of melatonin and related indoles, that at least a fourfold increase in melatonin content must be reached before we can detect an

increase in NAS concentration. Therefore, the observed doubling of melatonin content would not be accompanied by a detectable elevation of NAS,
as measured by our method. Further experiments must include evaluations
of the NAT and HIOMT activities.

NAT activation might arise from ECS-induced elevation of the EMAOI of
protein origin (Isaak *et al.* 1986), because stimulation of melatonin synthesis
was observed after a single dose of non-selective MAO inhibitors (Deguchi
and Axelrod 1972) and selective MAO-A inhibitors (Oxenkrug *et al.* 1984,
1985, 1986*a*; Bieck *et al.* 1988). Stimulation of melatonin biosynthesis was
also observed in association with an increased production of the EMAOI of
indole origin, tribulin (Bhattacharya *et al.* 1988; Oxenkrug and McIntyre
1985), and ECS has been found to increase the brain tribulin content
(Bhattacharya *et al.*, unpublished). However, the absence of change in the 5-
HIAA/serotonin ratio after ECS speaks against the involvement of EMAOI
in the observed elevation of the pineal melatonin content (Table 9.1).

As to the possible role of the single ECS-induced changes of melatonin
biosynthesis in the clinical effect of ECS, it is noteworthy that ECS elevates
melatonin content during the day, when no significant melatonin biosynthetic
activity occurs under physiological conditions. A single administration of
melatonin at the correct time during the day was shown to resynchronize
disrupted circadian rhythms in humans (Sack *et al.* 1989) and rats (Armstrong
1986). We do not know whether the observed doubling of pineal melatonin
levels in ECS-treated rats is enough to affect the circadian rhythm—about a
fivefold increase of the rat pineal melatonin content might be observed during
the night (Pang and Yip 1988). It is possible that melatonin elevation reaches
its peak at times other than 90 min after ECS or that a consecutive ECS
might produce a greater increase of melatonin. These questions must be
answered in future studies. Nevertheless, it is tempting to speculate that the
antidepressive actions of ECS therapy might be mediated by the chronobiological effect of the ECS, that is stimulation of the melatonin synthesis with
consequent normalization of disrupted circadian rhythms (Kripke *et al.* 1978).
The endogenous circadian rhythms responded to a shift in environmental
24 h light/dark cycle with a slight change in the next 24 h cycle and only
gradually (in about a week) became synchronized with the new schedule
(Lewy *et al.* 1985). Thus, the requirement for repeated application before the
therapeutic effect of ECS is achieved might be explained by this necessity for
repeated (every 24 h cycle), exogenously induced alterations of the melatonin
rhythm before the endogenous circadian rhythms are changed. A similar
explanation—acute and repeated daytime elevations of plasma melatonin
levels—has been proposed for the antidepressant effect of MAO inhibitors
(Oxenkrug *et al.* 1986*a*).

This possibility of a chronobiological effect of ECS suggests a reinvestiga-
tion of the previously reported data on the effect of ECS on melatonin and
EMAOIs. We did not find changes in rat pineal melatonin after single and

repeated ECS because we only looked at one time at night (McIntyre and Oxenkrug 1984). The observation of the ECS-induced EMAOI activity in cats and rats (Isaak *et al.* 1986) was not confirmed in humans, apparently because EMAOI activity was measured on the day after ECS treatment, and not immediately after the application (Moriearty *et al.* 1987).

Further studies are necessary to investigate whether ECS-induced stimulation of melatonin synthesis is essential for the ECS antidepressive action or merely reflects ECS-induced changes in the metabolism of the monoamines (serotonin and noradrenaline) involved in melatonin synthesis (Gleiter and Nutt 1989).

References

Armstrong, S. M., Cassone, V. M., Chesworth, M. J., Redman, J. R., and Short, V. (1986). Synchronization of mammalian circadian rhythms by melatonin. *Journal of Neural Transmission*, **S21**, 373–96.

Becker, R. E. and Giambalvo, C. T. (1982). Endogenous modulation of monoamine oxidase in schizophrenic and normal humans. *American Journal of Psychiatry*, **139**, 1567–70.

Bieck, P. R., Antonin, K. H., Balon, R., and Oxenkrug, G. F. (1988). Brofaromine and pargyline effect on human plasma melatonin. *Progress in Neuro-Psychopharmacology and Biological Psychiatry*, **12**, 93–101.

Bhattacharya, S. K., Glover, V., McIntyre, I. M., Oxenkrug, G. F., and Sandler, M. (1988). Stress causes an increase in endogenous monoamine oxidase inhibitor (tribulin) in rat brain. *Neuroscience Letters*, **92**, 218–21.

Cowen, P. J., Frazer, S., Grahame-Smith, D. G., Green, A. R., and Stanford, C. (1983). The effect of chronic antidepressant administration on β-adrenoceptor function of the rat pineal. *British Journal of Pharmacology*, **78**, 89–96.

Deguchi, T. and Axelrod, J. (1972). Induction and superinduction of serotonin N-acetyltransferase by adrenergic drugs and denervation of rat pineal organ. *Proceedings of the National Academy of Sciences USA*, **69**, 2208–11.

Demisch, K., Demisch, L., Bochnick, H. J., Nickelsen, T., Althoff, P. H., Schoffling, K., and Rieth, R. (1986). Melatonin and cortisol increase after fluvoxamine. *British Journal of Clinical Pharmacology*, **22**, 620–1.

Franey, C., Aldhous, M., Burton, S., Checkley, S., and Arendt, J. (1986). Acute treatment with desipramine stimulates melatonin and 6-sulphatoxy melatonin production in man. *British Journal of Clinical Pharmacology*, **22**, 73–9.

Fink, M. (1987). Neuroendocrine aspects of convulsive thereapy: review of recent developments. In *Handbook of clinical psychoneuroendocrinology*, (ed. C. B. Nemeroff and P. T. Loosen), pp. 255–65. Guilford Press, New York.

Gleiter, C. H. and Nutt, D. J. (1989). Chronic electroconvulsive shock and neurotransmitter receptors: an update. *Life Sciences*, **44**, 985–1006.

Glover, V., Bhattacharya, S. K., Sandler, M., and File S. M. (1981). Benzodiazepines reduce stress-augmented increase in rat urine monoamine oxidase inhibitor. *Nature*, **292**, 347–9.

Isaak, L., Schoenbeck, R., Bacher, J., Skolnick, P., and Paul, S. M. (1986). Electroconvulsive shock increases endogenous monoamine oxidase inhibitor activity in brain and cerebrospinal fluid. *Neuroscience Letters*, **66**, 257–62.

Kendall, R. (1981). The present status of electroconvulsive therapy. *British Journal of Psychiatry*, **189**, 265–83.

Kripke, D. F., Mullaney, D. J., Atkinson, M., and Wolf, S. (1978). Circadian rhythm disorders in manic-depressives. *Biological Psychiatry*, **123**, 335–51.

Lewy, A. L., Sack, R. L., and Singer, C. M. (1985). Treating phase typed chronobiological sleep and mood disorders using approximately timed bright artificial light. *Psychopharmacology Bulletin*, **21**, 368–72.

McIntyre, I. M. and Oxenkrug, G. F. (1984). Electroconvulsive shock effect on pineal and hypothalamic indoles. *Journal of Pineal Research*, **1**, 273–9.

Moriearty, P. L., Herrick, C., Shafey, M., Bornstein, P., and Becker, R. E. (1987). Platelet MAO-B and endogenous MAO-A inhibitory activity in depressed patients: stability with electroconvulsive treatment. *Biological Psychiatry*, **22**, 1155–7.

Nowak, J. Z., Przybysz, M., and Zurawska, E. (1988). The melatonin generating system in the rat retina and pineal gland: effect of single and repeated electroconvulsive shock (ECS). *Polish Journal of Pharmacology*, **40**, 573–84.

Oxenkrug, G. F. and McIntyre, I. M. (1985). Stress-induced synthesis of melatonin: possible involvement of the endogenous monoamine oxidase inhibitor (Tribulin). *Life Sciences*, **37**, 1743–6.

Oxenkrug, G. F., McCauley, R. B., McIntyre, I. M., and Filipowicz, . (1984). Effect of clorgyline and deprenyl on rat pineal melatonin. *Journal of Pharmacy and Pharmacology*, **36**, 55W.

Oxenkrug, G. F., McIntyre, I., McCauley, R., and Filipowicz, C. (1985). Selective inhibition of MAO-A but not MAO-B activity increases rat pineal melatonin. *Journal of Neural Transmission*, **61**, 165–70.

Oxenkrug, G. F., Balon, R., Jain, A. K., McIntyre, I. M., Appel, D. (1986a). Single dose of tranylcypromine increases human plasma melatonin. *Biological Psychiatry*, **21**, 1085–9.

Oxenkrug, G. F., McCauley, R. B., Fontana, D. J., McIntyre, I. M., and Commissaris, R. L. (1986b). Possible melatonin involvement in the hypotensive effect of MAO inhibitors. *Journal of Neural Transmission*, **66**, 271–80.

Oxenkrug G. F., Balon, R., Jain, A. K., McIntyre, I. M. (1988). Melatonin plasma response to MAO inhibitor—an index of pineal activity? *Acta Psychiatrica Scandinavica*, **77**, 160–2.

Pang, S. F. and Yip, P. C. Y. (1988). Secretory patterns on pineal melatonin in the rat. *Journal of Neural Transmission*, **5**, 279–92.

Wurtman, R. J., and Ozaki, Y. (1978). Physiological control of melatonin synthesis and secretion mechanisms generating rhythms in melatonin, methoxytryptophol and arginin vasotocin levels. *Journal of Neural Transmission*, Suppl., **13**, 59–70.

10. cAMP-dependent binding proteins and endogenous phosphorylation after antidepressant treatment

G. Racagni, D. Tinelli, E. Bianchi, N. Brunello, and J. Perez

Introduction

The main antidepressants in clinical use elicit an increase in the synaptic availability of noradrenaline (NA) and serotonin (5-hydroxytryptamine, 5-HT), either by blocking NA and 5-HT re-uptake processes or by reducing the catabolism of the neurotransmitters through MAO inhibition (Racagni *et al*. 1982). However, whereas these effects occur after acute administration of antidepressants, the therapeutic effects of these drugs become evident only after about two weeks of treatment. Among the most significant changes induced in monoaminergic neurones by chronic antidepressant treatment are: reduction in tyrosine hydroxylase activity (Segal *et al*. 1974); decrease in the ability of NA to stimulate the activity of adenylate cyclase (Vetulani and Sulser 1975); and reduction in the concentration of noradrenergic (Banerjee *et al*. 1977; Brunello *et al*. 1988) and serotonergic receptors (Peroutka and Snyder 1980; Brunello *et al*. 1988). Many synaptic and trans-synaptic mechanisms may participate in the desensitization of neurotransmitter receptors after chronic treatment with antidepressants (Racagni and Brunello 1984). However, the intracellular events related to chronic antidepressant administration are still unclear. The most commonly described effector mechanism beyond the second messengers depends on protein phosphorylation mediated by activation of specific protein serine-threonine kinases (Edelman *et al*. 1987; Greengard 1987). Components of the protein phosphorylation system are associated with the cytoskeleton (Sloboda *et al*. 1975; Vallee 1980; Theurkauf and Vallee 1982; De Camilli *et al*. 1986; Goldenring *et al*. 1986), which suggests that cell surface receptors linked to second messengers could regulate cytoskeleton function. Therefore, it is a reasonable hypothesis that drugs capable of affecting synaptic transmission, such as antidepressants, could affect cytoskeleton function by changes in the components of the associated protein phosphorylation system. In this chapter we investigate whether the cAMP-dependent phosphorylation system associated with micro-tubules, which are constituents of neuronal cytoskeleton, could be an intracellular target for antidepressants acting on NA and 5-HT neurones.

Materials and methods

Male Sprague-Dawley rats were housed under standard laboratory conditions with water and food *ad libitum* and 14 h light-dark cycles (06.00–20.00). Animals received intraperitoneal injections of saline, desipramine (10 mg kg^{-1}), fluoxetine (10 mg kg^{-1}) or (+)-oxaprotiline (10 mg kg^{-1}) twice daily for 10 days and were killed 1 h after the last injection.

Preparation of microtubules

Microtubule fractions were obtained from rat cerebral cortex, as previously described (Shelanski *et al.* 1973). The tissues were homogenized (1 g ml^{-1}) in buffer containing 100 mM PIPES (pH 6.8), 1 mM MgCl$_2$, 1 mM EGTA, 1 mM 2-β-mercaptoethanol, 2 μg ml^{-1} pepstatin, 50 U ml^{-1} aprotinin, 1 mM phenylmethylsulphonyl fluoride (PMSF). The homogenate was centrifuged at 100 000 *g* for 1 h at 4 °C. The supernatant was incubated at 37 °C for 30 min with an equal volume of glycerol (8 M) and centrifuged at 100 000 *g* for 1 h at 37 °C. The translucent pellet, corresponding to the crude microtubule fraction, was resuspended in polymerization buffer (1/3 of initial volume), incubated at 0 °C for 30 min to depolymerize the microtubules, and centri-fuged at 100 000 *g* for 30 min at 4 °C. The supernatant was incubated at 37 °C with an equal volume of glycerol (8 M) and centrifuged as described above. This procedure was repeated and microtubules were obtained after two cycles of polymerization-depolymerization.

Photoaffinity labelling with 8-N$_3$-[^{32}P]cAMP

Assays were performed as described by Walter *et al.* (1978). Microtubule fractions obtained from rat cerebral cortex were resuspended in buffer containing 50 mM MES (pH 6.1), 10 mM MgCl$_2$, 1 mM 3-isobutyl-1-methylxanthine (IBMX), and 0.5 mM 2-β-mercaptoethanol. Aliquots of 50 μl (2 mg protein ml^{-1}) were incubated with 1 μM 8-N$_3$-[^{32}P]cAMP for 60 min in the dark at 4 °C. Non-specific binding was performed with 100 μM unlabelled cAMP. The samples were irradiated for 10 min at 254 nm with an ultraviolet lamp (Spectroline, model ENF/24F). The reaction was blocked by the addition of 50 μl of stop solution. The samples were mixed, boiled for 2 min, and subjected to sodium dodecyl sulphate-polyacrylamide gel electro-phoresis (SDS-PAGE), as described by Laemmli (1970). The gels were stained, destained, dried, and subjected to autoradiography.

Phosphorylation in vitro

Endogenous phosphorylation was performed as previously described (Sloboda *et al.* 1975). Crude microtubule fractions obtained from rat cerebral cortex were resuspended in buffer containing 50 mM PIPES (pH 6.8), 0.1 mM $MgCl_2$, 0.1 mM 2-β-mercaptoethanol, 50 U ml^{-1} aprotinin, 2 mg ml^{-1} pepstatin, and 0.1 mM PMSF. Aliquots of 50 μl (2 mg protein ml^{-1}) were preincubated at 30 °C for 90 s with or without 5 μM cAMP plus IBMX (1 mM). The reaction was initiated by addition of 2 μM [γ-^{32}P]ATP and was terminated after 1 min by addition of 100 μl of stop solution. The samples were mixed, boiled for 2 min, and subjected to SDS-PAGE (Laemmli 1970). The gels were stained, destained, dried, and subjected to autoradiography. Radioactive bands were localized by autoradiography and cut out from the dried gel. The ^{32}P content was quantified by liquid scintillation counting.

Protein assay

Protein concentrations were determined by the method of Bradford (1976).

Results and discussion

The effects of the second messenger cAMP on cell function are mediated through its binding to the regulatory subunits of protein kinases (Edelman *et al.* 1987). cAMP-dependent protein kinase type II is associated with microtubules and cAMP is implicated in the regulation of microtubule function (Vallee *et al.* 1981; Theurkauf and Vallee 1982). We evaluated the binding of cAMP to proteins of the microtubule fraction by measuring the photoaffinity labelling with 8-N$_3$-[^{32}P]cAMP. Partial characterization of the cerebrocortical microtubule fraction was obtained by Western blotting, as described by Perez *et al.* (1989). The major protein component of microtubules is tubulin, which is a heterodimer composed of α- and β-subunits of about 50 kDa molecular mass. In addition, a rich variety of polypeptides, known as the microtubule-associated proteins (MAPs), co-purify with tubulin through cycles of *in vitro* assembly-disassembly (Matus 1988). Prolonged administration of antidepressants with different mechanisms of action affected the photoactivated incorporation of 8-N$_3$[^{32}P]cAMP into a protein band with apparent molecular mass of 52 kDa. Lane 1 of Fig. 10.1 shows the photoactivated incorporation into the microtubule fraction of control animals. Chronic treatment with desipramine (DMI), a tricyclic antidepressant, induced an increase in the photoactivated incorporation into a protein band of apparent molecular mass 52 kDa (Fig. 10.1, lane 3). The bands labelled were shown to be specific because their labelling was prevented by the presence of excess unlabelled cAMP (Fig. 10.1, lanes 2 and 4). Figure 10.2 shows the data obtained after administration of antidepressants that specifically inhibit 5-HT or NA uptake, fluoxetine and (+)-oxaprotiline

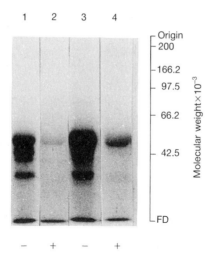

FIG. 10.1. Photoaffinity labelling with 8-N₃-[³²P]cAMP of cerebrocortical crude microtubule fraction after 10 days of treatment with desipramine (DMI). Autoradiography showing the covalent binding of 8-N₃-[³²P]cAMP into a 52 kDa protein band from saline- (lanes 1 and 2) and DMI- (lanes 3 and 4) treated rats. +, with 100μM unlabelled cAMP; −, in absence of unlabelled cAMP.

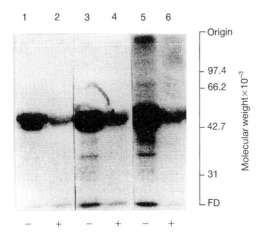

FIG. 10.2. Photoaffinity labelling with 8-N₃-[³²P]cAMP of cerebrocortical crude microtubule fraction after 10 days of treatment with fluoxetine and (+)-oxaprotiline. Autoradiography showing the covalent binding of 8-N₃-[³²P]cAMP into 52 kDa protein band from saline- (lanes 1 and 2), fluoxetine- (lanes 3 and 4), and (+)-oxaprotiline- (lanes 5 and 6) treated rats. +, with 100 μM unlabelled cAMP; −, in absence of unlabelled cAMP.

respectively. Given for 10 days, these drugs enhanced covalent binding into the 52 kDa protein band (Fig. 10.2, lanes 3 and 5) when compared to the control (lane 1). Non-specific binding was obtained by addition of unlabelled cAMP (Fig. 10.2, lanes 2, 4, and 6). To demonstrate that the increase in the photoactivated incorporation into the 52 kDA protein after prolonged DMI treatment was tightly associated with the microtubule, we did photoaffinity labelling after two cycles of microtubule polymerization-depolymerization. Under these conditions, the 8-N_3-[^{32}P]cAMP binding was clearly increased after chronic DMI treatment (Fig. 10.3, lane 3) when compared to the control (lane 1). Non-specific binding was obtained by addition of unlabelled cAMP (Fig. 10.2, lanes 2, 4, and 6).

cAMP-dependent endogenous phosphorylation was studied in the microtubule fraction of rat cerebral cortex. It has been shown that a protein band of high molecular mass, designated MAP$_2$, incorporated radioactive phosphate in the presence of cAMP (Sloboda *et al.* 1975). In our experiments repeated administration of DMI modified the cAMP-dependent endogenous phosphorylation of a protein band which had an apparent molecular mass of 280 kDa (Fig. 10.4) and was immunologically recognized as MAP$_2$ (Perez *et al.* 1989).

In this study we investigated the effect of prolonged treatment with different antidepressant drugs on effector mechanisms mediated by activation of specific cAMP-dependent protein kinases associated with microtubule fractions. We observed that in the microtubule fraction the 8-N_3-[^{32}P]cAMP binding to the 52 kDa protein band was increased after chronic treatment with DMI, fluoxetine, and (+)-oxaprotiline when compared to controls. Because the regulatory subunit of protein kinase is the only well-characterized receptor for cAMP, our data indicate that antidepressants might affect the regulatory subunit of protein kinase type II associated with the microtubule fraction. Accordingly, in the same fraction, chronic DMI treatment induced specific changes in the cAMP-dependent endogenous phosphorylation of MAP$_2$, which is a substrate protein for protein kinase type II (Lohmann *et al.* 1980).

In conclusion, our studies suggest that, besides the modifications elicited at the receptor level, antidepressants might affect neuronal signal transduction processes beyond the receptor. Among the different intracellular mechanisms, cAMP-binding proteins and the cAMP-dependent phosphorylation system in the microtubule fraction could be considered as neurochemical targets in the action of antidepressant drugs.

References

Banerjee, S. P., Kung, L. S., Riggi, S. S., and Chanda, S. K. (1977). Development of beta adrenergic receptor subsensitivity by antidepressants. *Nature*, **268**, 455–6.

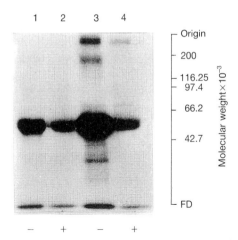

FIG. 10.3.   Photoaffinity labelling with 8-N$_3$-[^{32}P]cAMP of cerebrocortical microtubule fraction after 10 days of treatment with desipramine (DMI). Microtubules were obtained after two cycles of polymerization-depolymerization as described in text. Autoradiography showing the covalent binding of 8-N$_3$-[^{32}P]cAMP from saline- (lanes 1 and 2) and DMI- (lanes 3 and 4) treated rats. +, with 100 μM unlabelled cAMP; −, in absence of unlabelled cAMP.

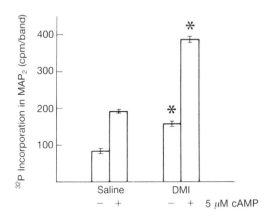

FIG. 10.4. ^{32}P incorporation in 280 kDa protein band after cAMP-dependent endogenous phosphorylation of a cerebrocortical crude microtubule fraction after chronic desipramine treatment. The radioactive bands localized by autoradiography were cut out from the dried gel and counted by liquid scintillation, as described in text. The values are the means of three experiments. *, $p < 0.001$ versus saline (Student's t-test).

Bradford, M. (1976). A rapid and sensitive method for the quantitation of microgram quantities of protein utilizing the principle of protein-dye binding. *Analytical Biochemistry*. **72**, 255–60.

Brunello, N., Riva, M., Rovescalli, A. C., Galimberti, R., and Racagni, G. (1988). Age related changes in rat serotoninergic and adrenergic systems and in receptor responsiveness to subchronic desipramine treatment. *Pharmacology and Toxicology*, **63**, 150–5.

De Camilli, P., Moretti, M., Denis-Donini, S., Walter, V., and Lohmann, S. M. (1986). Heterogenous distribution of cAMP receptor protein RII in the nervous system: evidence for its intracellular accumulation in microtubules, microtubule-organizing centers, and in the area of the Golgi Complex. *Journal of Cell Biology*, **103**, 189–203.

Edelman, A. M., Blumenthal, D. K., and Krebs, E. G. (1987). Protein serine/threonine kinases. *Annual Review of Biochemistry*, **56**, 567–613.

Goldenring, J. R., Vallano, M. L., Lasher, R. S., Ueda, T., and DeLorenzo, R. J. (1986). Association of calmodulin-dependent kinase II and its substrate protein with neuronal cytoskeleton. *Progress in Brain Research*, **69**, 341–54.

Greengard, P. (1987). Neuronal phosphoproteins. Mediators of signal transduction. *Molecular Neurobiology*, **1**, 81–119.

Laemmli, U. K. (1970). Cleavage of structural proteins during the assembly of the head of the bacteriophaghe T_4. *Nature*, **227**, 680–5.

Lohmann, S. M., Walter, U., and Greengard, P. (1980). Identification of endogenous substrate protein for cAMP-dependent protein kinase in bovine brain. *Journal of Biological Chemistry*, **256**, 9985–92.

Matus, A. (1988). Microtubule-associated proteins: their potential role in determining neuronal morphology. *Annual Review of Neuroscience*, **11**, 29–44.

Perez, J., Tinelli, D., Brunello, N., and Racagni, G. (1989). cAMP-dependent phosphorylation of soluble and crude microtubule fractions of rat cerebral cortex after prolonged desmethylimipramine treatment. *European Journal of Pharmacology*, **172**, 305–16.

Peroutka, S. J. and Snyder, S. H. (1980). Long term antidepressant treatment decreases spiroperidol labelled serotonin receptor binding. *Science*, **210**, 88–90.

Racagni, G. and Brunello, N. (1984). Transsynaptic mechanisms in the action of antidepressant drugs. *Trends in Pharmacological Sciences*, **5**, 527–31.

Racagni, G., Mocchetti, I., Renna, G., and Cuomo, V. (1982). In vivo studies on central noradrenergic synaptic mechanisms after acute and chronic antidepressant drug treatment: biochemical and behavioral comparison. *Journal of Pharmacology and Experimental Therapeutics*, **223**, 227–34.

Segal, D. S., Kuckzenski, R., and Mandell, A. J. (1974). Theoretical implication of drug-induced adaptive regulation for biogenic-amine hypothesis of affective disorders. *Biological Psychiatry*, **9**, 135–47.

Shelanski, M. L., Gaskin, F., and Cantor, C. R. (1973). Microtubule assembly in the absence of added nucleotides. *Proceedings of the National Academy of Sciences USA*, **70**, 765–8.

Sloboda, R. D., Rudolph, S. A., Rosenbaum, J. L., and Greengard, P. (1975). Cyclic AMP-dependent endogenous phosphorylation of a microtubule associated protein. *Proceedings of the National Academy of Sciences USA*, **72**, 177–81.

Theurkauf, W. E. and Vallee, R. B. (1982). Molecular characterization of the cAMP-dependent protein kinase bound to microtubule associated protein 2. *Journal of Biological Chemistry*, **257**, 3284–90.

Vallee, R. B. (1980). Structure and phosphorylation of microtubule-associated protein 2 (MAP 2). *Proceedings of the National Academy of Sciences USA*, **77**, 3206–10.

Vallee, R. B., Dibartolomeis, M. J., and Theurkauf, W. E. (1981). A protein kinase bound to the projection portion of MAP₂ (microtubule-associated protein 2). *Journal of Cell Biology*, **90**, 568–76.

Vetulani, J. and Sulser, F. (1975). Action of various antidepressant treatments reduces reactivity of noradrenergic cyclic AMP generating system in limbic forebrain. *Nature*, **297**, 479–96.

Walter, U., Kanof, P., Schulman, H., and Greengard, P. (1978). Adenosine 3′-5′-monophosphate receptor proteins in mammalian brain. *Journal of Biological Chemistry*, **253**, 6275–80.

11. Abnormal 5-HT neuroendocrine function in depression: association or artefact?

P. J. Cowen and I. M. Anderson

Introduction

The indoleamine hypothesis of depression was formulated over 20 years ago, but consistent evidence for abnormal brain 5-hydroxytryptamine (5-HT, serotonin) function in depressed patients is still lacking (Cowen 1988). Part of the reason for this is the difficulty of investigating the biochemistry of the human brain *in vivo*. While post-mortem investigations allow a direct examination of brain 5-HT metabolism in patients with an ante-mortem diagnosis of depression, results from such investigations are still extremely conflicting (Cooper *et al.* 1986).

Neuroendocrine challenge tests

It is well established that the secretion of anterior pituitary hormones is partly controlled by brain monoamine pathways (Checkley 1980; Tuomisto and Mannisto 1985). Stimulation of a particular monoamine pathway by a specific drug leads to a characteristic hormonal response that can be detected in plasma. In principle, therefore, neuroendocrine challenge tests offer a dynamic means of assessing brain monoamine function in the living human brain.

The methodological difficulties inherent in neuroendocrine tests have been described by Checkley (1980). Scrupulous control for age, sex, and psychotropic drug exposure is required. In addition, three other methodological conundrums are apparent in the following discussion. First, how specific are drug challenges of 5-HT pathways? Second, what is the role of weight loss in the abnormal 5-HT neuroendocrine responses seen in depressed patients? Third, where a 5-HT-mediated endocrine response is abnormal in depression, is it possible to distinguish between a defect in 5-HT neurotransmission and a primary impairment in the secretion of the hormone concerned?

5-HT neuroendocrine challenges

Increasing brain 5-HT function in humans leads to an elevation in plasma concentration of prolactin (PRL), growth hormone (GH), adrenocortico-

TABLE 11.1.   *5-HT neuroendocrine challenges in humans*

Drug	Mechanism	Hormone response
Tryptophan	5-HT precursor	PRL, GH
5-HTP	5-HT precursor	CORT, PRL, GH
Fenfluramine	5-HT releaser	PRL, CORT
Clomipramine	5-HT uptake inhibitor	PRL, CORT
Buspirone	5-HT$_{1A}$ agonist	PRL, GH, CORT
Gepirone	5-HT$_{1A}$ agonist	PRL, GH, CORT
Ipsapirone	5-HT$_{1A}$ agonist	CORT
m-CPP	5-HT$_{1C}$ agonist	PRL, CORT
MK 212	5-HT$_{1C}$ agonist	PRL, CORT

PRL, prolactin; GH, growth hormone; 5-HTP, 5-hydroxytryptophan; CORT, cortisol, *m*-CPP, *m*-chlorophenylpiperazine; MK 212, 6-chloro-2-(1-piperazinyl)-pyrazine.

tropic hormone (ACTH), and cortisol. Changes in thyroid-stimulating hormone and luteinising-releasing hormone may also occur but are less well characterized (Tuomisto and Mannisto 1985; Anderson and Cowen 1986; Meltzer and Nash 1988). A major difficulty in 5-HT neuroendocrine challenge tests is that increasing brain 5-HT function may lead to feelings of nausea and dizziness which can themselves increase the secretion of anterior pituitary hormones through 'stress' effects. A further problem is the lack of specificity of some of the agents employed to probe 5-HT function (Table 11.1), as is discussed below.

5-HT precursors

Tryptophan   Administration of tryptophan (TRP), the amino acid precursor of 5-HT, increases brain 5-HT synthesis in humans, because tryptophan hydroxylase, the rate-limiting step in the synthesis of 5-HT, is not saturated with TRP under physiological conditions (Fernstrom and Wurtman 1971). Whereas oral TRP is generally ineffective in elevating plasma hormone concentrations, administration of intravenous TRP in doses of 5 g or greater increases plasma PRL and, usually, plasma GH (MacIndoe and Turkington 1973; Charney *et al.* 1982; Cowen *et al.* 1985; Cowen and Anderson 1986). However, some have argued that the increase in hormone concentrations produced by intravenous TRP may not be mediated by an enhancement of brain 5-HT function, but rather by an effect of TRP on brain tyrosine concentrations, or through the formation of an active metabolite, such as tryptamine (van Praag *et al.* 1986).

We have carried out some pharmacological studies in normal subjects to establish how TRP increases plasma PRL and GH. Both endocrine responses were enhanced by pretreatment with the 5-HT uptake inhibitor, clomipramine, suggesting the involvement of 5-HT pathways (Anderson and Cowen 1986). The PRL response to TRP was attenuated by the non-selective 5-HT receptor antagonist, metergoline (McCance *et al.* 1987), but not by the 5-$HT_{2/1C}$ antagonist, ritanserin (Charig *et al.* 1987), or the 5-HT_3 antagonist, BRL 43694 (Anderson *et al.* 1988). We therefore tentatively concluded that the PRL response to TRP was mediated by post-synaptic 5-HT_1 receptors, perhaps of the 5-HT_{1A} subtype (McCance *et al.* 1987). To test this proposal we are studying the effect of pindolol, which has a high affinity for brain 5-HT_{1A} receptors (Hoyer 1988) and antagonizes some 5-HT_{1A}-mediated neuroendocrine responses in animals (Gilbert *et al.* 1988).

The GH response to TRP was not antagonized by metergoline (McCance *et al.* 1987), ritanserin (Charig *et al.* 1987) or BRL 43694 (Anderson *et al.* 1988): accordingly the 5-HT receptor subtype mediating this response is not yet clear. Further studies with more selective antagonists are required.

5-Hydroxytryptophan Intravenous administration of 5-hydroxytryptophan (5-HTP) increases plasma concentrations of PRL, GH, and cortisol, but this route of administration may cause severe side-effects (MacIndoe and Turkington 1973). Oral DL-5-HTP, in acceptable doses, is unreliable in increasing plasma hormone concentrations in normal subjects, but the L-isomer of 5-HTP may be more efficacious (Meltzer and Nash 1988). 5-HTP is a less specific stimulus of brain 5-HT function than TRP because it may also displace catecholamines from nerve terminals (see Meltzer and Nash 1988).

Meltzer (1990) has presented evidence that PRL and cortisol responses to L-5-HTP are attenuated by ritanserin and therefore may be mediated by 5-$HT_{2/1C}$ receptors. However, Facchinetti *et al.* (1987) found that the cortisol response to DL-5-HTP was not reduced by pretreatment with ritanserin; further studies seem necessary. It may be thought unlikely that the endocrine responses to TRP and 5-HTP could be mediated by different receptor subtypes; however, both animal and human data suggest that 5-HT_{1A} and 5-HT_{1C} agonists are capable of producing similar endocrine responses (Cowen 1990), and it is therefore conceivable that different 5-HT precursors could selectively activate different post-synaptic 5-HT receptor subtypes.

Fenfluramine

Fenfluramine is a 5-HT-releasing agent that at oral doses of 60 mg and greater increases plasma PRL and cortisol in humans (Quattrone *et al.* 1983; Meltzer and Nash 1988). Interestingly, plasma GH is not reliably altered. Fenfluramine, at the doses employed in humans, seems a relatively specific stimulus of brain 5-HT function, and this is particularly true of the more recently available d-fenfluramine (Meltzer and Nash 1988). The PRL response to d-fenfluramine was blocked by metergoline, suggesting mediation by post-synaptic 5-HT receptors (Quattrone *et al.* 1983), although the subtype involved has not been elucidated. The cortisol and ACTH responses to dl-fenfluramine were attenuated by cyproheptadine (Lewis and Sherman 1984) which could suggest involvement of $5-HT_{2/1C}$ receptors (Leysen *et al.* 1981).

The main problem with fenfluramine as a neuroendocrine challenge is that it is usually adminstered orally and the peak response tends to occur after four hours, which makes it rather a tedious investigation for subjects. Dysphoria can also occur. Finally, the uncertainties of oral absorption complicate the interpretation of the results.

Clomipramine

Intravenous administration of the tricyclic antidepressant, clomipramine, increases plasma PRL and cortisol, probably through 5-HT mechanisms (Laakmann *et al.* 1984*a,b*). Clomipramine itself is a highly selective inhibitor of 5-HT uptake and while its metabolite, desmethylclomipramine, is a potent inhibitor of noradrenaline uptake, we have not been able to detect this latter compound in the first hour after intravenous clomipramine administration (I. M. Anderson and P. J. Cowen, unpublished observations). Laakmann (1983) has reported that the PRL response to intravenous clomipramine is abolished by the non-selective 5-HT receptor antagonist, methysergide, suggesting that post-synaptic 5-HT receptors are involved in this response.

The main problem with intravenous clomipramine in neuroendocrine challenge tests is its tendency to cause nausea and vomiting even at quite low doses. While some authors have suggested that a dose of 10 mg intravenously increases plasma PRL without causing significant side-effects (Rudorfer *et al.* 1986), our own experience is that doses that cause minimal adverse effects (6–8 mg) produce very modest PRL responses.

5-HT receptor agonists

Non-selective 5-HT receptor agonists have been available for some years but because of their propensity to cause psychotomimetic side-effects have been employed only rarely in neuroendocrine studies. More recently the development of more selective 5-HT receptor agonists that lack such side-effects has allowed the study of the neuroendocrine responses to post-synaptic 5-HT receptor challenge.

m-*Chlorophenylpiperazine*   This trazodone metabolite is a non-selective agonist at $5-HT_1$ receptors (Hoyer 1988; Hamik and Peroutka 1989). Oral *m*-chlorophenylpiperazine (*m*-CPP) increases plasma PRL and cortisol and these effects are antagonized by metergoline (Mueller *et al.* 1986). Behavioural (Kennett and Curzon 1988) and ligand-binding (Hoyer 1988) studies in animals suggest that *m*-CPP may be a preferential agonist at $5-HT_{1C}$ receptors. These receptors might also therefore mediate the cortisol and prolactin responses (Cowen 1990). Side-effects of *m*-CPP, which include nausea, flushing, headache, and anxiety, are more pronounced after intravenous administration (Murphy *et al.* 1989). Intravenous *m*-CPP also elevates plasma GH (Charney *et al.* 1987), an effect not seen after oral treatment (Mueller *et al.* 1986).

6-Chloro-2-(1-piperazinyl)-pyrazine (MK 212)   Like *m*-CPP, the 5-HT receptor agonist, MK 212, increases plasma PRL and cortisol (Lowy and Meltzer 1988). MK 212 is also a non-selective 5-HT receptor agonist, but animal studies seem to indicate that 5-HT$_{1C}$ receptors may be involved in its ability to increase plasma cortisol (Koenig *et al.* 1987). The side-effects of MK 212 are similar to those of *m*-CPP (Lowy and Meltzer 1988).

Pyrimidinylpiperazine derivatives   This group of drugs includes compounds such as buspirone, gepirone, and ipsapirone which have a high and selective affinity for 5-HT$_{1A}$ receptors (Traber and Glaser 1987). In humans, buspirone, ipsapirone, and gepirone all increase plasma cortisol (Meltzer and Nash 1988; Lesch *et al.* 1989; Anderson *et al.* 1990) and there is good evidence from animal studies that this effect is mediated by post-synaptic 5-HT$_{1A}$ receptors (Gilbert *et al.* 1988). Buspirone and gepirone also elevate plasma concentrations of PRL and GH in humans (Meltzer *et al.* 1983; Anderson *et al.* 1990). While these effects could be produced by 5-HT$_{1A}$ receptor activation, it is also possible that actions on dopamine pathways are involved (Meltzer *et al.* 1982; Nash and Meltzer 1989). We found that the PRL but not the GH response to buspirone was antagonized by metergoline (Gregory *et al.* 1990), and we are also assessing the effect of pindolol on these endocrine responses.

5-HT$_{1A}$ agonists tend to cause light-headedness and dizziness which can complicate interpretation of neuroendocrine tests. In addition, they are generally administered orally which may lead to inconsistent responses.

5-HT neuroendocrine function in depression

From the above it is apparent that a number of drugs can be used to produce a variety of 5-HT-mediated neuroendocrine responses. The following discussion explores the patterns of response of different hormones to 5-HT challenge in depressed patients.

ACTH and cortisol

Studies using 5-HTP   Two studies have reported that the cortisol response to 5-HTP may be enhanced in depressed patients (Table 11.2), but in one of these investigations the abnormality was seen only in females (Maes *et al.* 1987). Meltzer *et al.* (1984*a,b*) found that the enhanced cortisol response to 5-HTP correlated with the extent of depression, suicidal behaviour, and weight loss. These authors proposed that the enhanced cortisol responses to

TABLE 11.2. *5-HT-mediated cortisol release in depression*

Study	Drug	Cortisol response
Meltzer *et al.* (1984*a*)	5-HTP	↑
Maes *et al.* (1987)	5-HTP	↑ (females)
Weizman *et al.* (1988)	FEN	↓
Asnis *et al.* (1988)	FEN	NC
López-Ibor *et al.* (1989)	FEN	NC
Mitchell and Smythe (1990)	FEN	NC
Kahn *et al.* (1988)	*m*-CPP	NC

5-HTP, 5-hydroxytryptophan; NC, no change; FEN, fenfluramine; *m*-CPP, *m*-chlorophenylpiperazine.

5-HTP might reflect a 'supersensitivity' of post-synaptic 5-HT receptors, arising from decreased 5-HT release. However, Kahn *et al.* (1988) found that the cortisol response to *m*-CPP was unchanged in depression (Table 11.2), although enhanced in panic disorder.

Studies using fenfluramine Three studies have reported that the cortisol response to fenfluramine is unaltered in depression (Asnis *et al.* 1988; López-Ibor *et al.* 1989; Mitchell and Smythe 1990) (Table 11.2). Weizman *et al.* (1988) found a reduced cortisol response to fenfluramine, but the baseline cortisol was elevated in the depressed patients, making interpretation of this effect difficult.

Abnormal hypothalamo-pituitary-adrenal function in depression
A major problem in assessing 5-HT-mediated cortisol responses in depression is that many depressed patients have pre-existing abnormalities in hypothalamo-pituitary-adrenal function (see Charlton and Ferrier 1989). For example, administration of corticotropin-releasing hormone to depressed patients provokes a smaller increase in plasma ACTH than in controls, but a similar output of cortisol (Gold *et al.* 1984; Holsboer *et al.* 1986). Interpretation of neurotransmitter effects in such a dysregulated neuroendocrine system poses formidable difficulties.

Growth hormone
An early study by Takahashi *et al.* (1973) reported that the GH response to 5-HTP was blunted in depressed patients. More recently, three studies (Koyama and Meltzer 1986; Cowen and Charig 1987; Deakin *et al.* 1990) have found blunted GH responses to intravenous TRP in depression, an impressive consensus (Table 11.3). Deakin *et al.* (1990) reported that the blunted GH response to TRP was correlated with the presence of endogenous depression; however, this was not apparent in the study of Cowen and Charig

TABLE 11.3. *5-HT-mediated growth hormone (GH) release in depression*

Study	Drug	GH response
Takahashi *et al.* (1973)	5-HTP	↓
Koyama and Meltzer (1986)	TRP	↓
Cowen and Charig (1987)	TRP	↓
Deakin *et al.* (1989)	TRP	↓

5-HTP, 5-hydroxytryptophan; TRP, tryptophan

(1987) where a confounding effect of weight loss in the endogenously depressed patients may have obscured this relationship (see below).

A major obstacle in interpreting this intriguing abnormality is that the mechanism of the GH response to TRP has not been clarified (see above). If it does indeed reflect a 5-HT-mediated neuroendocrine response the results obtained would be consistent with an abnormality of brain 5-HT function in depression. In this case, studies using post-synaptic receptor agonists would be of great interest.

Growth hormone release in depression   In view of the blunted GH response to TRP in depression it is worthwhile asking whether this phenomenon reflects a primary abnormality in GH secretion. It is well established that the GH response to clonidine is blunted in depressed patients (Checkley *et al.* 1986), but, with one exception (Ansseau *et al.* 1988), GH responses to apomorphine have been reported as normal (Caspar *et al.* 1977; Jimerson *et al.* 1986). It has become possible to test pituitary GH secretion directly by administering growth hormone-releasing hormone. However, the results in depressed patients have been conflicting, with some studies finding a blunted GH response (Lesch *et al.* 1987), and others normal or even enhanced GH secretion (Eriksson *et al.* 1988; Krishnan *et al.* 1988; Thomas *et al.* 1989). Taken together, these data do not suggest that the blunted GH response to TRP in depression stems from a primary abnormality in GH secretion.

Prolactin

Studies with intravenous tryptophan   Heninger *et al.* (1984) first reported that the PRL responses to intravenous TRP were blunted in patients with major depression. This has been confirmed by three other groups (Koyama and Meltzer 1986; Cowen and Charig 1987; Deakin *et al.* 1990) (Table 11.4), but there are some caveats. Koyama and Meltzer (1986) found that the TRP concentrations following intravenous infusion were significantly lower in depressed patients and this may have accounted for the blunted PRL responses. Deakin *et al.* (1990) also found reduced TRP levels in their patients post-infusion; however, the reduction did not correlate with the blunted PRL responses. Finally, in the study of Cowen and Charig (1987)

TABLE 11.4. *5-HT-mediated prolactin (PRL) release in depression*

Study	Drug	PRL response
Heninger *et al.* (1984)	TRP	↓
Koyama and Meltzer (1986)	TRP	↓
Cowen and Charig (1987)	TRP	↓ *
Deakin *et al.* (1990)	TRP	↓ *
Siever *et al.* (1984)	FEN	↓
Asnis *et al.* (1988)	FEN	NC
Weizman *et al.* (1988)	FEN	? ↓
López-Ibor *et al.* (1989)	FEN	↓
Mitchell and Smythe (1990)	FEN	↓
Coccaro *et al.* (1989)	FEN	↓ †
Anderson and Cowen (1990)	CLO	↓
Golden *et al.* (1990)	CLO	↓

TRP, tryptophan; FEN, fenfluramine; CLO, clomipramine; NC, no change.
* In patients without severe weight loss.
† In patients with suicidal behaviour.

TRP levels following intravenous TRP were the same in patients and controls.

Effect of weight loss In the studies of Cowen and Charig (1987) and Deakin *et al.* (1990) blunted PRL responses to TRP were apparent only in depressed patients without significant recent weight loss (Fig. 11.1). There is a rationale for the separate examination of this subcategory of patients, because Goodwin *et al.* (1987) demonstrated that weight reduction by dieting in normal female volunteers markedly enhances the PRL and GH responses to TRP. The mechanism of this enhancement may involve dieting-induced lowering of plasma TRP (Anderson *et al.* 1989); a TRP-deficient diet in animals does lead to reduced brain 5-HT turnover and enhanced neuroendocrine responses to challenge with TRP (Gil-Ad *et al.* 1976) and 5-HTP (Clemens *et al.* 1980). The mechanism of these enhanced responses is uncertain but may represent a supersensitivity effect, perhaps of post-synaptic 5-HT receptors. Intriguingly, a recent report suggests that reduced dietary intake of TRP increases the PRL responses to TRP in normal volunteers (Delgado *et al.* 1989).

These findings indicate the importance of weight loss in studies of 5-HT neuroendocrine function in depressed patients. In fact, Cowen and Charig (1987) showed that depressed women with severe weight loss had significantly greater PRL responses to TRP than either depressed women without weight loss or normal female controls. Thus enhanced neuroendocrine responses to 5-HT precursors in depressed patients may arise from a primary effect of weight loss rather than depression.

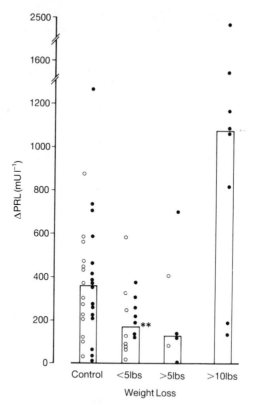

FIG. 11.1. Peak ($\triangle$) PRL responses to tryptophan (100 mg kg⁻¹) in control subjects and depressed patients categorized by weight loss on Beck Scale. ○, men; ●, women; histograms, median values. Significant difference exists between groups ($p < 0.005$, Kruskal-Wallis test): **, significantly less than control and 10 lb weight loss groups ($p < 0.01$); ††, significantly greater than controls ($p < 0.02$, Mann–Whitney U test).

Other correlates of abnormal TRP-mediated PRL responses in depression Deakin *et al.* (1990) found that, in contrast to blunted GH responses to TRP which correlated with endogenicity (see above), reduced PRL responses in depression were associated with chronic psychosocial difficulties and raised basal plasma cortisol. However, Cowen and Charig (1987) found that dexamethasone non-suppression was correlated with greater PRL responses to TRP, although weight loss may have played a confounding role. Further studies are needed to resolve this issue.

Other 5-HT challenges of PRL release There have been a number of studies of PRL responses to fenfluramine in depressed patients (Table 11.4). Siever *et al.* (1984), Mitchell and Smythe (1990), and López-Ibor *et al.* (1989) have reported blunted PRL responses, but Asnis *et al.* (1988) found no change. However, the latter study involved outpatients and in general a reduced PRL response to fenfluramine is associated with more severe depression (López-Ibor *et al.* 1989). The data of Weizman *et al.* (1988) are difficult to interpret; a statistically insignificant reduction in PRL responses to fenfluramine was noted in depressed patients, but the small number of subjects and high baseline PRL make it difficult to draw firm conclusions.

Coccaro *et al.* (1989) examined the PRL response to fenfluramine in a group of patients with major depression and personality disorder. A blunted PRL response to fenfluramine was observed in the depressed patients, but the reduction was correlated with a history of suicidal behaviour rather than the presence of major depression. This study is consistent with suggestions from a number of workers that reduced brain 5-HT function in depressed patients is associated with self-harm rather than depression *per se* (see van Praag 1986).

We also studied intravenous clomipramine in major depression. The PRL responses were significantly less in depressed patients than healthy controls (Cowen and Anderson 1990). A similar finding has been reported by Golden *et al.* (1990) (Table 11.4).

Taken together, these studies provide considerable evidence that 5-HT-mediated PRL release is blunted in depression. The drugs discussed above all increase brain 5-HT function by an action on pre-synaptic 5-HT neurones (Table 11.1) and it would be interesting to study the PRL release produced by a direct post-synaptic receptor agonist in depressed patients. Published studies of the effects of these compounds are few; Heninger *et al.* (1990) reported that the PRL response to *m*-CPP was not altered in depressed patients. Combined study of pre- and post-synaptic 5-HT neuroendocrine challenges could help to localize the abnormality in 5-HT-mediated PRL release to a pre- or post-synaptic site.

PRL release in depression As with the blunted TRP-mediated GH responses described above, it is important to ask whether the apparent reduction in 5-HT-mediated PRL release in depression is caused by a generalized abnormality of pituitary PRL secretion. Thyrotropin-releasing hormone (TRH) stimulates PRL release by a direct action on the pituitary (Diefenbach *et al.* 1976), although there is also some evidence that 5-HT may modulate this response (Sartani *et al.* 1984; Apfelbaum 1987). Studies on the PRL response to TRH in depression have been extremely contradictory with normal, reduced, and increased responses being reported (Linnoila *et al.* 1979; Witschy *et al.* 1984; Zis *et al.* 1985; Rubin *et al.* 1989).

Previous investigations of TRH-mediated PRL release in depression have used doses of TRH that produce a maximal response in PRL output from the pituitary. We decided to use a submaximal TRH dose (Jacobs *et al.* 1973) to explore a possible shift in the TRH/PRL dose-response relationship. This investigation was combined with the clomipramine study mentioned above,

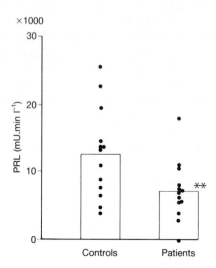

FIG. 11.2. Prolactin (PRL) response to thyrotropin-releasing hormone (TRH, 6.25 μg), in depressed patients and matched controls. Values are area under the curve of PRL secretion. Histograms give mean values. **, significantly less than controls (*p* < 0.02, Mann–Whitney U test).

so that TRH (6.25 μg) was administered intravenously to depressed patients and controls 90 min after the clomipramine infusion, when PRL levels had returned to baseline. We found that the PRL response to TRH was blunted in the depressed patients (Fig. 11.2) and the PRL responses to TRH and clomipramine in the patients were significantly correlated (r = 0.63; *p* < 0.02).

This finding raises the possibility that the blunted PRL response of depressed patients to drugs increasing brain 5-HT function is due to a reduction in the pituitary release of PRL, rather than an impairment of brain 5-HT function. However, as mentioned above, 5-HT may modulate the PRL response to TRH (Sartani *et al.* 1984; Apfelbaum 1987) and in support of this view we found that pretreatment with oral clomipramine enhanced the PRL response to 6.25 μg of TRH in normal volunteers (I. M. Anderson, unpublished). Therefore it is possible that the blunted PRL response to TRH seen in our study may still reflect impaired brain 5-HT function. However, we have not excluded a primary pituitary abnormality.

To help resolve this issue we are studying the PRL response to the dopamine antagonist metoclopramide. Thus far there does not appear to be a reduced response in depressed patients (Fig. 11.3). Therefore it is possible that the PRL response to dopamine receptor blockade may not be altered in depression.

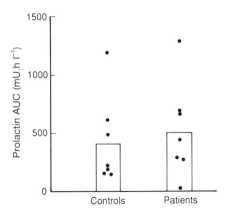

FIG. 11.3. Prolactin (PRL) response to metoclopramide (0.3 mg) in depressed patients and matched controls. Values are area under the curve of PRL secretion. Histograms give mean values.

Conclusions

There is strong evidence tht 5-HT neuroendocrine responses are abnormal in depression. We believe that the enhanced endocrine responses to 5-HT precursors seen in some depressed patients are probably due to weight loss; however, this factor does not seem a likely explanation for the more common finding of blunted 5-HT neuroendocrine responses.

While the evidence suggests that 5-HT-mediated PRL release is reduced in depression, it is not yet established whether this abnormality reflects a specific impairment of 5-HT neurotransmission or a more general neuroendocrine abnormality, perhaps at pituitary level. If it is established that 5-HT neurotransmission is impaired, further studies with selective 5-HT receptor agonists will be required to identify more precisely the nature of the abnormality. Finally, larger scale clinical investigations will be needed to determine the relationship of abnormal brain 5-HT function to the syndrome of depressive illness and its implications for treatment with drugs that alter brain 5-HT function.

Acknowledgements

The authors thank Professors D. G. Grahame-Smith and M. G. Gelder for advice and encouragement. The studies of the authors were supported by the Medical Research Council. IMA is an MRC Training Fellow. L-tryptophan was kindly supplied by E. Merck.

References

Anderson, I. M. and Cowen, P. J. (1986). Clomipramine enhances prolactin and growth hormone responses to L-tryptophan. *Psychopharmacology*, **89**, 131–3.

Anderson, I. M., Cowen, P. J., and Grahame-Smith, D. G. (1988). The effect of BRL 43694 on the neuroendocrine responses to L-tryptophan infusion. *Journal of Psychopharmacology*, **2**, 2.

Anderson, I. M., Crook, W. S., Gartside, S. E., Parry-Billings, M., Newsholme, E. A., and Cowen, P. J. (1989). Effect of moderate weight loss on prolactin secretion in normal female volunteers. *Psychiatry Research*, **29**, 161–7.

Anderson, I. M., Cowen, P. J., and Grahame-Smith, D. G. (1990). Neuroendocrine and temperature responses to gepirone in humans. *Psychopharmacology*, **100**, 498–503.

Ansseau, M., von Krenckell, R., Cerfontaine, J. L., Papart, P., Franck, G., Timsit-Berthier, M., *et al.* (1988). Blunted response of growth hormone to clonidine and apomorphine in endogenous depression. *British Journal of Psychiatry*. **153**, 65–71.

Apfelbaum, M. E. (1987). Effect of serotonin on basal and TRH-induced release of prolactin from rat pituitary glands in vivo. *Acta Endocrinologica*, **114**, 556–71.

Asnis, G. M., Eisenberg, J., van Praag, H. M., Lemus, C. Z., Harkavy Friedman, J. M., and Miller, A. M. (1988). The neuroendocrine responses to fenfluramine in depressives and normal controls. *Biological Psychiatry*, **24**, 117–20.

Caspar, R. C., Davies, J. M., Pandey, G. N., Graver, D. L., and Dekirmenjion, H. (1977). Neuroendocrine and amine studies in affective illness. *Psychoneuroendocrinology*, **2**, 105–10.

Charlton, B. G. and Ferrier, I. N. (1989). Hypothalamo-pituitary-adrenal axis abnormalities in depression: a review and model. *Psychological Medicine*, **19**, 331–6.

Charig, E. M., Anderson, I. M., Robinson, J. M., Nutt, D. J., and Cowen, P.J. (1987). L-tryptophan and prolactin release: evidence for interaction between 5-HT$_1$ and 5-HT$_2$ receptors. *Human Psychopharmocology*, **1**, 91–7.

Charney, D. S., Heninger, G. R., Reinhard, J. F., Sternberg, D. E., and Hafstead, K. M. (1982). The effect of intravenous L-tryptophan on prolactin, growth hormone and mood in healthy subjects. *Psychopharmacology*, **77**, 217–22.

Charney, D. S., Woods, S. W., Goodman, W. K., and Heninger, G. R. (1987). Serotonin function in anxiety. II. Effects of the serotonin agonist mCPP in panic disorder patients and healthy subjects. *Psychopharmacology*, **92**, 14–24.

Checkley, S. A. (1980). Neuroendocrine tests of monoamine function. A review of basic theory and its application to the study of depressive illness. *Psychological Medicine*, **10**, 35–53.

Checkley, S. A., Corn, T. H., Glass, I. B., Burton, S. W., and Burke, C. A. (1986). The responsivity of central alpha$_2$ adrenoceptors in depression. In *The biology of depression*, (ed. J. F. W. Deakin), pp. 100–20. Gaskell, London.

Clemens, J. A., Bennet, D. R., and Fuller, R. W. (1980). The effect of a tryptophan-free diet on prolactin and corticosterone release by serotonergic stimuli. *Hormone and Metabolism Research*, **12**, 35–8.

Coccaro, E. F., Siever, L. J., Klar, H. M., Maurer, G., Cochrane, M., Cooper, T. B., *et al.* (1989). Serotonergic studies in patients with affective and personality disorders. *Archives of General Psychiatry*, **46**, 587–99.

Cooper, S. J., Owen, F., Chambers, D. R., Crow, T. J., Johnson, J., and Poulter, M. (1986). Post-mortem neurochemical findings in suicide and depression: a study of the serotenergic system and imipramine binding in suicide victims. In *The biology of depression*, (ed. J. F. W. Deakin), pp. 53–70. Gaskell, London.

Cowen, P. J. (1988). Recent views on the role of 5-hydroxytryptamine in depression. *Current Opinion in Psychiatry*, **1**, 56–9.

Cowen, P. J. (1990). Endocrinological responses to 5-HT. *Annals of the New York Academy of Sciences*, in press.

Cowen, P. J. and Anderson, I. M. (1986). 5-HT neuroendocrinology: changes during depressive illness and antidepressant drug treatment. In *The biology of depression*, (ed. J. F. W. Deakin), pp. 71–89. Gaskell, London.

Cowen, P. J. and Charig, E. M. (1987). Neuroendocrine responses to intravenous tryptophan in major depression. *Archives of General Psychiatry*, **44**, 958–66.

Cowen, P. J. and Anderson, I. M. (1990). Investigations of 5-HT neuroendocrine function in depression. In *Serotonin: from cell biology to pharmacology and therapeutics*, pp. 493–7. Kluwer, Amsterdam.

Cowen, P. J., Gadhvi, H., Gosden, B., and Kolakowska, T. (1985). Responses of prolactin and growth hormone to L-tryptophan infusion: effects in normal subjects and schizophrenic patients receiving neuroleptics. *Psychopharmacology*, **86**, 164–9.

Deakin, J. F. W., Pennell, I., Upadhyaya, A. J., and Lofthouse, R. (1990). A neuroendocrine study of 5-HT function in depression: evidence for biological mechanisms of endogenous and psychosocial causation. *Psychopharmacology*, **101**, 85–92.

Delgado, P. L., Charney, D. S., Price, L. H., Landis, H., and Heninger, G. R. (1989). Neuroendocrine and behavioural effects of dietary tryptophan restriction in healthy subjects. *Life Sciences*, **45**, 2323–32.

Diefenbach, W. P., Carme, P. W., Frantz, A. G., and Ferin, M. (1976). Suppression of prolactin secretion by L-dopa in the stalk-sectioned Rhesus monkey. *Journal of Clinical Endocrinology and Metabolism*, **43**, 638–42.

Eriksson, E., Balldin, J., Lindstedt, G., and Modigh, K. (1988). Growth hormone responses to the alpha$_2$-adrenoceptor agonist, guanfacine and to growth hormone releasing hormone in depressed patients and controls. *Psychiatry Research*, **26**, 59–67.

Fachinetti, F., Martignoni, E., Nappi, G., Petraglia, F., Sandrini, G., and Genazzani, A.R. (1987). Ritanserin, a serotonin-S$_2$ receptor antagonist does not prevent 5-hydroxytryptophan-induced β-EP, β-LPH and cortisol secretion. *Hormone Research*, **27**, 42–6.

Fernstrom, J. D. and Wurtman, R.J. (1971). Brain serotonin content: physiological dependence on plasma tryptophan levels. *Science*, **173**, 149–52.

Gil-Ad, I., Zambotti, F., Carruba, M., Vicenti, L., and Muller, E. E. (1976). Stimulatory role for brain serotonergic system on prolactin secretion in the male rat. *Proceedings of the Society for Experimental Biology and Medicine*, **151**, 512–18.

Gilbert, F. M., Brazell, C., Tricklebank, M. D., and Stahl, S. M. (1988). Activation of the 5-HT$_{1A}$ receptor subtype increases rat ACTH concentration. *European Journal of Pharmacology*, **147**, 431–9.

Gold, P. W., Crousos, G. P., Kellner, C., Post, R., Roy, A., Augerinos, P., *et al.* (1984). Psychiatric implications of basic and clinical studies with corticotropin-releasing factor. *American Journal of Psychiatry*, **141**, 619–27.

Golden, R. N., Hsiao, J. K., Lane, E., Eckstrom, D., Rogers, S., Hicks, R., and Potter, W. Z. (1990). Abnormal neuroendocrine responsivity to acute clomipramine challenge in depressed patients. *Psychiatry Research*, **31**, 39–47.

Goodwin, G. M., Fairburn, C. G., and Cowen, P. J. (1987). The effects of dieting and weight loss on neuroendocrine responses to tryptophan, apomorphine and clonidine in normal volunteers: important implications for neuroendocrine investigations in depression. *Archives of General Psychiatry*, **44**, 952–7.

Gregory, C. A., Anderson, I. M., and Cowen, P. J. (1990). Metergoline abolishes the prolactin response to buspirone. *Psychopharmacology*, **100**, 283–4.

Hamik, A. and Peroutka, S. J. (1989). 1-(m-chlorophenyl)piperazine (mCPP) interactions with neurotransmitter receptors in the human brain. *Biological Psychiatry*, **25**, 569–75.

Heninger, G. R., Charney, D. S., and Sternberg, D. E. (1984). Serotonergic function in depression: prolactin response to intravenous tryptophan in depressed patients and healthy controls. *Archives of General Psychiatry*, **41**, 398–402.

Heninger, G. R., Charney, D. S., Price, L., Delgado, P., Woods, S., and Goodman, W. (1990). Neuroendocrine effects of serotonin agonists in rhesus monkeys, healthy humans and patients with depression or anxiety disorders: effects of antidepressant treatment. In *Serotonin: from cell biology to pharmacology and therapeutics*, pp. 559–63. Kluwer, Amsterdam.

Holsboer, F., Gerken, A., Von Bradelbeau, U., Grimm., M., Beyer, H., Muller, O. A., and Stalla, G. K. (1986). Human corticotropin-releasing hormone in depression: correlation with thyrotropin secretion following thyrotropin-releasing hormone. *Biological Psychiatry*, **21**, 601–11.

Hoyer, D. (1988). Functional correlates of serotonin 5-HT$_1$ recognition sites. *Journal of Receptor Research*, **8**, 59–81.

Jacobs, L. S., Snyder, P. J., Utiger, R. D., and Daughaday, W. H. (1973). Prolactin response to thyrotropin-releasing hormone in normal subjects. *Journal of Clinical Endocrinology and Metabolism*, **36**, 1069–73.

Jimerson, D. C., Cutler, N. R., Post, R. M., Dey, A., Gold, P. W., Brown, G. M., and Bunney, W. E. (1986). Neuroendocrine responses to apomorphine in depressed patients and healthy control subjects. *Psychiatry Research*, **13**, 1–12.

Kahn, R. S., Asnis, G. M., Wetzler, S., and van Praag, H. M. (1988). Neuroendocrine evidence for serotonin receptor hypersensitivity in panic disorder. *Psychopharmacology*, **96**, 360–4.

Kennett, G. A. and Curzon, G. (1988). Evidence that hypophagia induced by mCPP and TFMPP requires 5-HT$_{1C}$ and 5-HT$_{1B}$ receptors: hypophagia induced by RU 24969 only requires 5-HT$_{1B}$ receptors. *Psychopharmacology*, **96**, 93–100.

Koenig, J. I., Gudelsky, G. A., and Meltzer, H. Y. (1987). Stimulation of corticosterone and β-endorphin secretion in the rat by selective 5-HT receptor activation. *European Journal of Pharmacology*, **137**, 1–8.

Koyama, T. and Meltzer, H. Y. (1986). A biochemical and neuroendocrine study of the serotonergic system in depression. In *New results of depression research*, (ed. H. Hippius), pp. 169–88. Springer-Verlag, Berlin.

Krishnan, K. R. R., Manepalli, A. N., Ritchie, J. C., Rayasam, K., Melville, M. L., Daughtry, G., *et al.* (1988). Growth hormone-releasing factor stimulation test in depression. *American Journal of Psychiatry*, **145**, 90–2.

Laakmann, G., Chuang, I., Gugath, M., Ortner, M., Schmauss, M., and Wittemann, M. (1983). Prolactin and antidepressants. In *Prolactin and prolactinomas*, (ed. G. Tolis, C. Stefanis, T. Mountokalakis, and F. Labrie). Raven Press, New York.

Laakmann, G., Gugath, M., Kuss, H-J., and Zygan, K. (1984a). Comparison of growth hormone and prolactin stimulation induced by chlorimipramine and desipramine in man in connection with chlorimipramine metabolism. *Psychopharmacology*, **82**, 62–7.

Laakmann, G., Wittmann, M., Gugath, M., Mueller, O. A., Treusch, T. J. Wahlster, U., and Stalla, G. K. (1984*b*). Effects of psychotropic drugs (desipramine, chlorimipramine, sulpiride and diazepam) on the human HPA axis. *Psychopharmacology*, **84**, 66–70.

Lesch, K. P., Laux, G., Erb, A., Pfuller, H., and Beckmann, H. (1987). Growth hormone (GH) responses to GH releasing hormone in depression: correlation with GH release following clonidine. *Psychiatry Research*, **25**, 301–10.

Lesch, K. P., Rupprecht, R., Poten, B., Muller, U., Sohnle, K., Fritze, J., and Schulte, H. M. (1989). Endocrine responses to 5-HT-1A receptor activation by isapirone in humans. *Biological Psychiatry*, **26**, 203–5.

Leysen, J. E., Awouters, F., Kennis, L., Laduron, P. M., Vandenberg, J., and Janssen, P. A. J. (1981). Receptor binding profile of R41468, a novel antagonist at 5-HT$_2$ receptors. *Life Sciences*, **28**, 1115–22.

Lewis, D. A. and Sherman, B. M. (1984). Serotonergic stimulation of adrenocorticotropin secretion in man. *Journal of Clinical Endocrinology and Metabolism*, **58**, 458–62.

Linnoila, M., Lamberg, B. A., Rosberg, G., Karonen, S. L., and Melin, S. G. (1979). Thyroid hormones and TSH, prolactin and LH responses to repeated TRH and LRH injections in depressed patients. *Acta Psychiatrica Scandinavica*, **59**, 536–44.

López-Ibor, J. J., Sáiz-Ruiz, J., and Moral Iglesias, L. (1989). Neuroendocrine challenges in the diagnosis of depressive disorders. *British Journal of Psychiatry*, **154**, Suppl. 4, 73–6.

Lowy, M. T. and Meltzer, H. Y. (1988). Stimulation of serum cortisol and prolactin secretion in humans by MK-212, a centrally active serotonin agonist. *Biological Psychiatry*, **23**, 818–28.

McCance, S. L., Cowen, P. J., Waller, H., and Grahame-Smith, D. G. (1987). The effect of metergoline on endocrine responses to L-tryptophan. *Journal of Psychopharmacology*, **2**, 90–4.

MacIndoe, J. H. and Turkington, R. W. (1973). Stimulation of human prolactin secretion by intravenous L-tryptophan. *Journal of Clinical Investigation*, **52**, 1972–8.

Maes, M., De Ruyter, M., Claes, R., Bosma, G., and Suy E. (1987). The cortisol responses to 5-hydroxytryptophan, orally, in depressive inpatients. *Journal of Affective Disorders*, **13**, 23–30.

Meltzer, H. Y. (1990). Serotonin in depression. *Annals of the New York Academy of Science*, in press.

Meltzer, H. Y. and Nash, J. F. (1988). Serotonin and mood: neuroendocrine aspects. In *Current topics in neuroendocrinology*, (ed. D. Ganten and D. Pfaff), Vol. 8, pp. 183–210. Springer-Verlag, Berlin.

Meltzer, H. Y., Simonovic, M., Fang, V. S., and Gudelsky, G. A. (1982). Effect of buspirone on rat plasma prolactin levels and striatal dopamine turnover. *Psychopharmacology*, **78**, 49–53.

Meltzer, H. Y., Flemming, R., and Robertson, A. (1983). The effect of buspirone on prolactin and growth hormone secretion in man. *Archives of General Psychiatry*, **40**, 1099–102.

Meltzer, H. Y., Perline, R., Tricou, B. J., Lowy, M., and Robertson, A. (1984*a*). Effect of 5-hydroxytryptophan on serum cortisol levels in major affective disorders: I. Enhanced responses in depression and mania. *Archives of General Psychiatry*, **41**, 366–74.

Meltzer, H. Y., Perline, R., Tricou, B. J., Lowy, M., and Robertson, A. (1984*b*). Effect of 5-hydroxytryptophan on serum cortisol levels in major affective disorders. II. Relation to suicide, psychosis and depressive symptoms. *Archives of General Psychiatry*, **41**, 379–87.

Mitchell, P. and Smythe, G. (1990). Hormonal responses to fenfluramine in depressed and control subjects. *Journal of Affective Disorders*, **19**, 43–51.

Mueller, E. A., Murphy, D. L., and Sunderland, T. (1986). Further studies of the putative serotonin agonist, m-chlorophenylpiperazine: evidence for a serotonin receptor-mediated mechanism of action in humans. *Psychopharmacology*, **89**, 388–91.

Murphy, D. L., Mueller, E. A., Hill, J. L., Tolliver, T. J., and Jacobsen, F. M. (1989). Comparative anxiogenic, neuroendocrine and other physiologic effects of m-chlorophenylpiperazine given intravenously or orally to healthy volunteers. *Psychopharmacology*, **98**, 275–82.

Nash, J. F. and Meltzer, H. Y. (1989). The effect of gepirone and ipsapirone on the stimulated and unstimulated secretion of prolactin in the rat. *Journal of Pharmacology and Experimental Therapeutics*, **249**, 236–41.

Quattrone, A., Tedeschi, A., Aguglia, U., Scopacasa, F., Direnzo, G. F., and Annunziato, L. (1983). Prolactin secretion in man: a useful tool with which to evaluate the activity of drugs on central 5-hydroxytryptamine neurones: studies with fenfluramine. *British Journal of Clinical Pharmacology*, **16**, 471–5.

Rubin, R. T., Poland, R. E., Lesser, I. M., and Martin, D. J. (1989). Neuroendocrine aspects of primary endogenous depression. V. Serum prolactin measures in patients and matched control subjects. *Biological Psychiatry*, **25**, 4–21.

Rudorfer, M. V., Golden, R. N., Sherer, M. A., Lesieur, P., and Potter, W. Z. (1986). Antidepressant challenge tests in man. In *Proceedings of the world congress of biological psychiatry*, (ed. C. Shagass), pp. 789–91. Elsevier, Amsterdam.

Sartani, A., de Pasqua, A., Cesati, R., Farina, L., and Pontiroli, A. E. (1984). Effect of metergoline on prolactin, follicle stimulating hormone, luteinising hormone and thyroid stimulating hormone response to TRH and LRH in normal men and women. *Hormone and Metabolism Research*, **16**, 535–8.

Siever, L. J., Murphy, D. L., Slater, S., De la Vega, E., and Lippen, S. (1984). Plasma prolactin following fenfluramine in depressed patients compared to controls: an evaluation of central serotonin responsivity in depression. *Life Sciences*, **34**, 1029–39.

Takahashi, S., Kondo, H., Yoshimura, M., Ochi, Y., and Yoshimi, T. (1973). Growth hormone response to administration of L-5-hydroxytryptophan (L-5-HTP) in manic depressive psychoses. *Japanese Journal of Psychiatry and Neurology*, **27**, 197–206.

Thomas, R., Beer, R., Harris, B., John, R., and Scanlon, M. (1989). GH responses to growth hormone releasing factor in depression. *Journal of Affective Disorders*, **16**, 133–7.

Traber, J. and Glaser, T. (1987). 5-HT$_{1A}$ receptor anxiolytics. *Trends in Pharmacological Sciences*, **8**, 432–7.

Tuomisto, J. and Mannisto, P. (1985). Neurotransmitter regulation of anterior pituitary hormones. *Pharmacological Reviews*, **37**, 249–332.

van Praag, H. M. (1986). Biological suicide research: outcome and limitations. *Biological Psychiatry*, **21**, 1305–23.

van Praag, H. M., Lemus, C., and Kahn, R. (1986). The pitfalls of serotonin precursors as challengers in hormonal probes of central serotonin activity. *Psychopharmacology Bulletin*, **22**, 565–70.

Weizman, A., Mark, M., Gil-Ad, I., Tyano, S., and Laron, Z. (1988). Plasma cortisol, growth hormone and immunoreactive β-endorphin response to fenfluramine challenge in depressed patients. *Clinical Neuropharmacology*, **11**, 250–6.

Witschy, J. K., Schlessen, M. A., Fulton, C. L., Orsukak, P. J., Giles, D. E., Fairchild, C., *et al.* (1984). TRH-induced prolactin release is blunted in females with endogenous unipolar major depression. *Psychiatry Research*, **12**, 321–31.

Zis, A. P., Albala, A. A., Haskett, R., Carroll, B. J., and Lohr, N. E. (1985). Prolactin response to TRH in depression. *Journal of Psychiatry Research*, **20**, 77–82.

Discussion

CURZON: I was fascinated by your results on the effect of dieting on prolactin release in healthy females. In females, plasma tryptophan decreased by about 20 per cent; in males it decreased by about 10 per cent. I cannot believe that such a profound effect on the hormonal response can be caused by such a small change of tryptophan availability to the brain. Surely the effect on prolactin must occur through a different mechanism? If you repeated your experiment but gave the females a small tryptophan supplement to make their plasma tryptophan levels the same as that in the males, I would predict that the dietary effect on prolactin response in the females would still occur.

COWEN: We are doing that study now. If we are correct, when we feed people enough tryptophan to normalize the plasma tryptophan levels, we should lose the enhanced prolactin responses. I wonder if small decreases in plasma tryptophan might not be functionally important. It seems quite hard to increase brain 5-hydroxytryptamine (5-HT, serotonin) function; you have to give large doses of tryptophan. However, the system may be more vulnerable to decreased tryptophan availability. There might be some functional sense in that,

MURPHY: Is another possible mechanism a competitive action of large neutral amino acids on tryptophan transport? What happens during fasting? Could there be protein breakdown and increased amounts of large neutral amino acids that compete with tryptophan?

COWEN: We measured the amounts of branched chain amino acids during dieting; they were unchanged. Thus the ratio of tryptophan to branched chain amino acids was lowered. Some people would feel that this ratio is the important determinant of tryptophan availability for brain 5-HT synthesis.

CURZON: But the ratio was only lowered by 20 per cent in the females and 10 per cent in the males. It is a very small sex difference.

MELTZER: Does pindolol block the prolactin response to tryptophan or just the growth hormone response?

COWEN: We don't know the answer to that yet. The data for the growth hormone response are fairly convincing. The prolactin response may be blocked, but it is not as striking an effect.

MELTZER: Did propranolol also block the growth hormone response?

DEAKIN: Enough propranolol to reduce the heart rate by about 10 beats per minute— a β-blocking dose—did not block the growth hormone or the prolactin response. However, propranolol is not as good a 5-HT antagonist as pindolol.

COWEN: There are other explanations for that result and we would like to use the more selective 5-HT$_{1A}$ blockers that are becoming available to study the receptor subtypes mediating the endocrine responses to tryptophan.

12. Experimental tests of the 5-HT receptor imbalance theory of affective disturbance

J. F. W. Deakin, F. S. Guimaraes, M. Wang, and R. Hensman

Introduction

Contradiction and synthesis

Symptoms of anxiety and depression usually coexist (Goldberg *et al.* 1987). Scores on anxiety rating scales strongly predict scores on depression rating scales. Symptoms of anxiety predict symptoms of depression. Symptoms of anxiety may ante-date and outlast depressive symptoms, and depression may be a higher level of affective disturbance than anxiety (Foulds and Bedford 1975). However, there is no antithesis between the two sets of symptoms. The same treatments are effective in both and the most effective is treatment with 5-hydroxytryptamine (5-HT, serotonin) re-uptake-blocking antidepressants. It is therefore a very considerable paradox that excessive 5-HT neurotransmission has been associated with symptoms of anxiety (Briley and Chopin, this volume) whereas deficient 5-HT function has been associated with depressive illness. How can symptoms which occur together and which have the same treatment have an opposed pathogenesis?

I have suggested that 5-HT systems have a unitary function in mediating adaptive responses to aversive events (Table 12.1), but that different anatomical and pharmacological 5-HT subsystems have different roles (Deakin 1983, 1989; Deakin and Pennell 1986). According to this formulation, aversive events release 5-HT. The 5-HT$_2$ receptor family mediates the short-term consequence—anxiety. Anxiety is a normal protective response which terminates contact with aversive stimuli by avoidance behaviour. Bolles and Fanselow (1980) pointed out that fear inhibits pain. Fear also inhibits aggression, eating, sleeping, sexual behaviour, and impulsiveness—hence the release of such behaviours in 5-HT-depleted animals and their association with low concentrations of 5-hydroxyindoleacetic acid (5-HIAA) in human cerebrospinal fluid (Linnoila and Virkkunen, this volume). Suppression of these behaviours may involve 5-HT$_1$ and 5-HT$_2$ receptor families (Table 12.1). The continuing presence of aversive stimuli triggers long-term protective

TABLE 12.1. *Differential involvement of 5-HT subsystems in the mediation of normal and pathological responses to aversive events*

	Responses to aversive events	
	Short-term	Long-term
Uncoditioned responses *(pain, defence)*		
Behaviours	Panic: flight/fight Non-opioid-5-HT analgesia	Opioid-5-HT analgesia
Anatomy	PAG	PAG-raphe magnus
Conditioned responses		
Behaviours	Anxiety Behavioural inhibition Analgesia Autonomic defence	Resilience Slow-wave sleep? Self-esteem?
	Inhibition fight/flight Inhibition panic?	
Anatomy	Fronto-temporal cortex Amygdala–hypothalamus– PAG Basal ganglia	Hippocampus
5-HT system	Dorsal raphe	Median raphe
Receptors	$5\text{-HT}_{2/1C}$, 5-HT_3	5-HT_{1A}
Affective illness		
Symptom	Anxiety	Depression, helplessness, panic
Functional change	↑ $5\text{-HT}_2/5\text{-HT}_{1C}$, ↑ 5-HT_3	↓ 5-HT_1
Antidepressants	↓ 5-HT_2	↑ 5-HT_1

PAG, periacqueductal grey matter

mechanisms (e.g., stress-induced analgesia). 5-HT_1 receptors may mediate longer-term adaptation to aversive events (Table 12.1). Depression, it was suggested, is associated with a failure of the 5-HT_1 'resilience' system. This chapter describes some tests of this hypothesis and reports evidence supporting a mechanism by which chronic adversity results in impaired 5-HT_1 receptor function in humans.

The 5-HT$_2$ receptor family and anxiety

A clinical trial

The potency of some antidepressants as 5-HT$_2$ receptor antagonists (for example, amitriptyline, trazodone, clomipramine; Fluxe *et al.* 1977) and the shared ability of all antidepressants to induce a delayed down-regulation of 5-HT$_2$ receptor numbers (Peroutka and Snyder 1980) might be related to their efficacy as anxiolytics and only indirectly related to antidepressant actions (Deakin 1988). To test this theory we made a clinical trial of a 5-HT$_{2/1C}$ receptor antagonist, ritanserin, in neurotic outpatients (Deakin and Wang 1990). Fifty-six patients completed the trial. Patients with major depression were excluded. Patients entered the trial if significant symptoms of anxiety and/or depression were detected with the Goldberg Clinical Interview Schedule. Patients were stratified into anxious, mixed anxious/depressed, and depressed groups before being randomly assigned to ritanserin or placebo. After four weeks of treatment there were no significant differences in the interviewer ratings for ritanserin-treated and placebo-treated patients (Global Impression, Hamilton scales). Thus, the treatment effects were small, as in other trials in mixed neurotic patients. However, analysis of covariance of self-rating scales (Beck, Hopkins symptom check list [SCL90], Spielberger) revealed on every scale that ritanserin had significant anxiolytic effects. These were most marked in males and in those with mixed anxiety and depression. These results are compatible with the theory that morbid anxiety involves excessive 5-HT$_{2/1C}$ neurotransmission.

5-HT$_{2/1C}$ receptors and aversive conditioning

Classical conditioning has long been held to be an important mechanism by which anxiety occurs in innocuous circumstances. Neutral stimuli acquire the ability to elicit fear if they have predicted noxious events (the unconditioned stimulus). We have investigated the role of 5-HT mechanisms in aversive conditioning of skin conductance responses (SCRs). Normal subjects listened to a series of ten ramdomly presented neutral tones. Skin conductance responses rapidly habituated. If the eleventh tone was followed immediately by a loud, unpleasant, but brief, white noise, skin conductance responses were reinstated and did not habituate over a further ten presentations. If the eleventh tone was omitted and the white noise occurred in isolation, no enhancement of skin conductance responses to the subsequent tone presentations was seen. Thus, responses to the second series of ten tones were maintained by an associative mechanism.

In ten normal subjects pretreated with ritanserin, the skin conductance responses after the tone-noise pairing rapidly habituated (Fig. 12.1), which was not the case in ten subjects who had no pill and ten who received placebo. Ritanserin had no effect on habituation of responses to the first ten

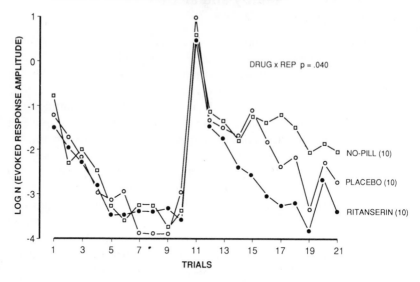

FIG. 12.1. Amplitude of skin conductance responses to a sequence of innocuous tones before (1–10) and after (12–21) tone 11 which was followed by a loud aversive white noise. Ten volunteers matched for age and sex for each treatment group.

tones. The results suggest that the 5-HT$_2$ receptor family has a specific involvement in aversive conditioning. The aversive white noise also increased the number of spontaneous fluctuations of skin conductance and this increase was almost completely blocked by pretreatment with ritanserin (Fig. 12.2).

Similar effects were seen in the neurotic patients during the ritanserin trial. After four weeks of ritanserin, previously acquired conditioned SCRs were absent, whereas they were maintained in placebo-treated patients. Thus, in patients with morbid anxiety, as well as in normal subjects, the 5-HT$_2$ receptor family appears to have a role in aversively conditioned skin conductance responses.

Panic

A difficulty with classical conditioning theories of anxiety is that the noxious (unconditioned stimulus) is almost never identifiable. According to Klein's (1964) formulation of agoraphobia, the conditioning event is a spontaneous panic attack. Contextual and other associated stimuli acquire the ability to elicit anticipatory fear. The two forms of anxiety may have different pharmacological mechanisms. A single, but decisive, trial in humans indicated that ritanserin had no effect on the number of panic attacks in patients with panic disorder, whereas fluvoxamine, a 5-HT re-uptake blocker, caused

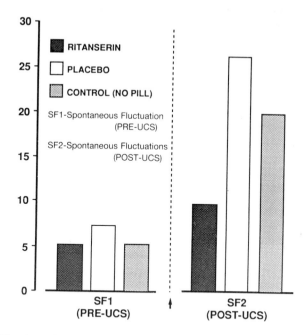

FIG. 12.2.   Number of spontaneous fluctuations in skin conductance before and after the unconditioned stimulus (UCS)—aversive white noise (indicated by arrow). Ten healthy subjects in each treatment group.

a highly significant reduction compared with placebo (Westenberg and Den Boer 1988).

In animals, anticipatory anxiety may be modelled by conditioning paradigms, such as the conflict test, and perhaps by the open-field, elevated plus-maze, and social interaction tests. These are all paradigms that would involve the 'behavioural inhibition system' proposed by Gray (1971) which we suggest involves the 5-HT$_2$ receptor family. Panic, in contrast, is unconditioned, unelicited, spontaneous, and probably arises from activation of the emergency flight/fight system, which runs from amygdala–hypothalamus–periacqueductal grey matter (PAG). Electrical stimulation of these structures in animals produces autonomic activation, flight, and attack behaviour (fight) if another animal is in the vicinity (Graeff 1990). As with panic disorder, 5-HT re-uptake blockers attenuate stimulation-induced flight or fight, and this may involve an enhancement of 5-HT$_1$ receptor function because 5-HT$_1$ receptor agonists that act directly are also effective (Broekkamp and Jenck 1989). According to this view, panic is a spontaneous activation of fight/flight pathways which, in contrast to conditioned fear/anxiety, is modulated rather than mediated by 5-HT systems.

The 5-HT$_1$ receptor family and depression

Cowen and Anderson (this volume) review the neuroendocrine evidence that depression involves reduced neurotransmission in systems which have 5-HT$_1$ receptors. There are various possible mechanisms for this.

Deakin (1989) pointed out a number of physiological and pharmacological functions where 5-HT$_1$ and 5-HT$_2$ receptor families exert opposed influences. Excessive function in 5-HT$_2$ systems would be one mechanism for attenuation of 5-HT$_1$ functions, including attenuation of prolactin responses to intravenous tryptophan infusions (Charig *et al.* 1987). Thus, it was suggested that depression could, in some cases, arise from pathological enhancement of 5-HT$_2$ receptor function, resulting in symptoms of anxiety, and secondary impairment of 5-HT$_1$ receptor function, resulting in symptoms of depression. In other types of depression, deficient 5-HT$_1$ mechanisms might be the primary defect with secondary enhancement of 5-HT$_{2/1C}$ functions.

We found evidence that hypercortisolaemia may reduce 5-HT$_1$ receptor function by a central mechanism. Prolactin responses to tryptophan infusion were attenuated in patients with major depression who had not lost weight (Fig. 12.3; Deakin and Upadhyaya 1990; Cowen and Anderson, this volume). We found strong negative correlations between basal cortisol concentrations and the magnitude of the prolactin response to tryptophan in controls, in depressives (Fig. 12.4b), in the total group (Fig. 12.4a), in females, and in those without weight loss.

Three groups have reported that prolactin responses to fenfluramine are blunted in those with raised cortisol secretion (Mitchell and Smythe 1989; López-Ibor *et al.* 1988; Bagdy *et al.* 1989). This suggests that cortisol may interact with central mechanisms involving 5-HT$_1$ receptors. Table 12.2 summarizes the animal experiments which suggest that chronic treatment with corticosteroids reduces 5-HT$_1$ receptor function. One study suggests that chronic corticosterone treatment enhances the 5-HT$_2$-mediated head-twitch responses to 5-hydroxytryptophan (Buckett and Luscombe 1984). Thus, several experiments in animals and humans strongly suggest that chronic hypercortisolaemia can cause precisely the imbalance in 5-HT$_2$/5-HT$_1$ receptor functioning which we have suggested as a cause of depression (Deakin and Pennell 1986; Deakin 1989).

We observed that basal cortisol concentrations were 30 per cent greater in patients with independently rated chronic psychosocial difficulties and with chronic symptoms than in those without (Deakin and Upadhyaya 1990). We suggested that chronic psychosocial difficulties might cause depression because hypercortisolaemia reduces function in 5-HT$_1$ receptor systems. If deficient 5-HT$_1$ function causes depression, and if antidepressants work by reversing the deficit, then blunted prolactin responses to tryptophan, a putative index of 5-HT$_1$ receptor function, should be associated with the depressed state and should be corrected with clinical recovery.

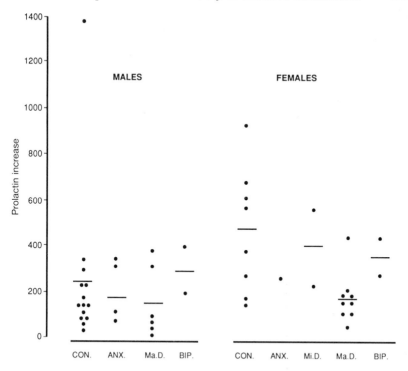

FIG. 12.3. Prolactin responses (peak–base) following infusion of L-tryptophan (100 mg kg^{-1},N.) in DSM-III diagnostic groups (Deakin and Upadhyaya 1990). CON, control; ANX, anxiety diagnoses; Ma.D, major depression; Mi.D, minor depression (dysthymia minus 2 year criterion); BIP, bipolar depression.

The Manchester and Oxford groups have retested ten depressives when free of drugs after full clinical recovery. In male depressives there was clear evidence of normalization of prolactin responses (Table 12.3). Only four females were retested and interpretation is confused by the effect of weight loss on prolactin responses. Growth hormone responses showed unequivocal recovery, but the involvement of 5-HT in this response is not clear (Cowen and Anderson, this volume).

These data suggest that reduced 5-HT$_1$ receptor function is not a vulnerability or trait marker for depression. We have proposed that 5-HT$_1$ receptor function has a close and causal relationship with the depressed state and its reversal by antidepressant drugs.

TABLE 12.2. *Evidence that chronic treatment with corticosteroids in experimental animals decreases 5-HT$_1$ receptor function and enhances 5-HT$_2$ receptor function*

(a)   5-HT$_1$ function
    ▼ 5-HTP myoclonus, guinea-pig (Nausieda *et al.* 1982)
    ▼ 5-MeO-DMT syndrome, rats (Dickinson *et al.* 1985)
    ▼ *m*-CPP effects on eating, locomotion, prolactin response (Bagdy *et al.* 1989)
    ▼ ³H-5-HT binding (De Kloet *et al.* 1986; Biegon *et al.* 1985)

(b)   5-HT$_2$ function
    ▲ 5-HTP head-twitching in mice (Buckett and Luscombe 1984)

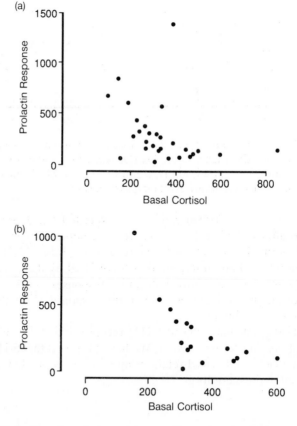

FIG. 12.4.   Raised basal cortisol secretion predicts reduced prolactin responses to L-tryptophan. (a) depressives and controls, r = −0.52, *p* = 0.001; (b) depressives, r = −0.66, *p* = 0.001.

TABLE 12.3. *Prolactin (mU l⁻¹) responses to L-tryptophan in depression and recovery*

Males		Females	
Depressed	Recovered	Depressed	Recovered
30	133	207	1824
60	436	274	137
86	106	640	576
247	365	833	143
292	564		
589	1081		

How does reduced 5-HT$_1$ receptor function cause depression?

5-HT$_1$ receptors and resilience

The experiments of Kennett *et al.* (1985 *a,b*; 1987) in rats suggest that 5-HT$_1$ receptors may have a role in adaptation to chronic aversive stimulation. They showed that two hours of immobilization stress resulted, 24 hours later, in reduced locomotion and increased defaecation in an open-field test. However, the acute effect of immobilization stress disappeared after seven daily immobilizations, and this was associated with an enhancement of 5-HT$_1$ receptor function. The acute effects of immobilization stress were reversed by immediate treatment with a single large dose of the 5-HT$_{1A}$ receptor agonist 8-hydroxy-*N,N*-dipropyl-2-aminotetralin (8-OH-DPAT) or if the animals had been treated with an antidepressant. Furthermore, Kennett *et al.* demonstrated that stress-induced glucocorticoid release retarded development of tolerance to repeated stress, and this could involve the steroid-induced down-regulation of 5-HT$_1$ receptor function described above.

5-HT$_1$ receptors show a striking localization to the hippocampus, which also contains a high concentration of glucocorticoid receptors; the influence of hypercortisolaemia on 5-HT$_1$ receptors might be mediated here. The hippocampus is selectively innervated by the median raphe nucleus and animal and human results are compatible with the suggestion that the median raphe–hippocampal 5-HT$_1$ system is concerned with long-term adaptive responses to chronic aversive stimulation—the median raphe 'resilience' system (Deakin 1989). Hypercortisolaemia caused by chronic psychosocial stress may be one way in which this system breaks down to cause depression. However, the mechanisms of resilience are ill-defined.

What is resilience?

Social scientists have identified psychosocial factors which predispose to depressive illness, including lack of social supports, early loss of a parent, and low self-esteem (Brown and Harris 1978). The obverse of these factors might be termed resilience factors—good social support, good early parenting experiences, and high self-esteem. Might such resilience factors involve neurochemical mechanisms?

In the tolerance to immobilization model, C. T. Dourish (unpublished) found that in rats acute immobilization stress had no effect on open-field behaviour 24 hours later if the intervening period was spent with other rats. In other words, group housing had the same effect as a single dose of the 5-HT$_{1A}$ agonist 8-OH-DPAT or as treatment with an antidepressant. Perhaps group housing in some way stabilizes or maintains 5-HT$_1$ receptor function. Nothing is known of how social signals are translated into neurochemical consequences. The neurochemical effects of group housing in rats are likely to involve tactile pathways (for example, grooming) and olfactory stimulation. In primates and humans, tactile stimuli might still be important (grooming, embracing, holding), but other modalities (for example, vision) and cognitive processes are likely to be important in mediating the protective effects of social supports.

The effects of social contact might also be related to dominance hierarchies. Tactile, olfactory, and visual signals are important in the maintenance of such hierarchies. Subordinate primates show hypercortisolaemia and reduced concentrations of circulating 5-HT (Raleigh *et al.* 1984). Low self-esteem in humans, a putative vulnerability factor for depression, could be an analogue of low position in a primate dominance hierarchy. Low self-esteem and social isolation could predispose to depression because 5-HT$_1$ resilience systems are not maintained by sufficient afferent social signals.

Much research effort has been expended on investigations of the social aetiology of depression. Social psychiatrists hold that most cases of depression have social origins. There now seems to be a need for a major effort to understand the biological mechanisms that mediate the social origins of depression.

References

Bagdy, G., Calogero, A. E., Aulakh, C. S., Szeeredi, K., and Murphy, D. L. (1989). Long-term cortisol treatment impairs behavioural and neuroendocrine responses to 5-HT$_1$ agonists in the rat. *Neuroendocrinology*, **50**, 241–7.

Biegon, A., Rainbow, T. C., and McEwan, B. S. (1985). Corticosterone modulation of neurotransmitter receptors in rat hippocampus: a quantitative autoradiographic study. *Brain Research*, **332**, 309–14.

Bolles, R. C. and Fanselow, M. S. (1980). A perceptual-defensive-recuperative model of fear and pain. *Behavioral and Brain Science*, **3**, 291–323.

Briley, M. and Chopin, P. (1991). Serotonin in anxiety: evidence from animal models. In *5-Hydroxytryptamine in psychiatry: a spectrum of ideas*, (ed. M. Sandler, A. Coppen, and S. Harnett), pp. 177–197, Oxford University Press.

Broekkamp, C. L. and Jenck, F. (1989). The relationship between various animal models of anxiety, fear-related psychiatric symptoms and responses to serotonergic drugs. In *Behavioural pharmacology of 5-HT*, (ed. P. Bevan, A. R. Cools, and T. Archer), pp. 321–36. Lawrence Erlbaum, New York.

Brown, G. W. and Harris, T. O. (1978). *Depression: a study of psychiatric disorder in women*. Tavistock, London.

Buckett, W. R. and Luscombe, G. P. (1984). Chronic hydrocortisone induces central serotonergic supersensitivity without affecting a behaviour paradigm for depression. *British Journal of Pharmacology*, **81**, 132.

Charig, E. M., Anderson, I. M., Robinson, J. M., Nutt, D. J., and Cowen, P. J. (1987). L-Tryptophan and prolactin release: evidence for interaction between 5-HT$_1$ and 5-HT$_2$ receptors. *Human Psychopharmacology*, **1**, 93–7.

Cowen, P. and Anderson, I. M. (1991). Abnormal 5-HT neuroendocrine function in depression: association or artefact? In *5-Hydroxytryptamine in psychiatry: a spectrum of ideas*, (ed. M. Sandler, A. Coppen, and S. Harnett), pp. 124–142. Oxford University Press.

De Kloet, E. R., Sybesma, H., and Reul, J. M. H. M. (1986). Selective control by corticosterone of serotonin receptor capacity in raphe–hippocampal system. *Neuroendocrinology*, **42**, 513–22.

Deakin, J. F. W. (1988). 5-HT$_2$ receptors, depression and anxiety. *Pharmacology Biochemistry and Behavior*, **29**, 819–20.

Deakin, J. F. W. (1989). 5-HT receptor subtypes in depression. In *Behavioural pharmacology of 5-HT*, (ed. P. Bevan, A. R. Cools, and T. Archer). Lawrence Erlbaum, New York.

Deakin, J. F. W. and Pennell, I. (1986). 5-HT receptor subtypes in depression. *Psychopharmacology*, **89**, 524.

Deakin, J. F. W. and Upadhyaya, A. K. (1990). Hormonal response to L-tryptophan infusion: effect of propranolol. *Psychopharmacology*, in press.

Deakin, J. F. W. and Wang, M. (1990). Role of 5-HT$_2$ receptors in anxiety and depression. In *Serotonin from cell biology to pharmacology and therapeutics*, (ed. P. Paulette and P. M. Vanhoutte). Kluwer, Dordrecht.

Dickinson, S. L., Kennett, G. A., and Curzon, G. (1985). Reduced 5-hydroxytryptamine dependent behaviour in rats following chronic corticosterone treatment. *Brain Research*, **345**, 10–18.

Foulds, G. A. and Bedford, A. (1975). Hierarchy of classes of personal illness. *Psychological Medicine*, **5**, 181–92.

Fluxe, K., Ogren, S., Agnati, L., Gustafsson, J. A., and Jonsson, G. (1977). On the mechanism of action of the antidepressant drugs amitriptyline and nortriptyline. Evidence of 5-hydroxytryptamine receptor blocking activity. *Neuroscience Letters*, **6**, 339–43.

Goldberg, D. P., Bridges K., Duncan-Jones, P. and Grayson, D. (1987). Dimensions of neuroses seen in primary care settings. *Psychological Medicine*, **17**, 461–70.

Graeff, F. G. (1990). Brain defence systems and anxiety. In *Handbook of anxiety*, Vol. 3., (ed. M. Roth, G. B. Burrows, and R. Noynes). Elsevier, Amsterdam, in press.

Gray, J. (1971). The psychology of fear and stress. Weidenfeld and Nicholson.

Kennett, G. A., Dickinson, S., and Curzon, G. (1985a). Enhancement of some 5-HT-dependent behavioural responses following repeated immobilization in rats. *Brain Research*, **330**, 253–63.

Kennett, G. A., Dickinson, S. L., and Curzon, G. (1985b). Central serotonergic responses and behavioural adaptation to repeated immobilisation: The effect of the corticosterone synthesis inhibitor metyrapone. *European Journal of Pharmacology*, **119**, 143–274.

Kennett, G. A., Dourish, C. T., and Curzon, G. (1987). Antidepressant-like action of 5-HT$_{1A}$ agonists and conventional antidepressants in an animal model of depression. *European Journal of Pharmacology*, **134**, 265–74.

Klein, D. F. (1964). Delineation of two drug-responsive anxiety syndromes. *Psychopharmacology*, **5**, 397–408.

Linnoila, M. and Virkkunen, M. (1991). Monoamines, glucose metabolism, and impulse control. In *5-Hydroxytryptamine in psychiatry: a spectrum of ideas*, (ed. M. Sandler, A. Coppen, and S. Harnett), pp. 258–78. Oxford University Press.

López-Ibor, J. J. Jr., Sáiz-Ruiz, J., and Iglesias, M. (1988). The fenfluramine challenge test in the affective spectrum: a possible marker of endogeneity and severity. *Pharmacopsychiatry*, **21**, 9–14.

Mitchell, P. and Smythe, G. (1990). Hormonal responses to fenfluramine in depressed and control subjects. *Journal of Affective Disorders*, **19**, 43–52.

Nausieda, P. A., Carvey, P. M., and Weiner, W. J. (1982). Modification of central serotonergic and dopaminergic behaviour in the course of chronic corticosteroid administration. *European Journal of Pharmacology*, **78**, 335–43.

Peroutka, S. J. and Snyder, S. H. (1980). Long-term antidepressant treatment decreases spiroperidol-labelled serotonin receptor binding. *Science*, **210**, 88–90.

Raleigh, M. J., Mcguire, M. T., Brammer, G. L., and Yuwiler, A. (1984). Social and environmental influence on blood serotonin concentrations in monkeys. *Archives of General Psychiatry*, **41**, 405–10.

Westenberg, H. G. M. and den Boer, J. A. (1988). Serotonin uptake inhibitors and agonists in the treatment of panic disorders. *Psychopharmacology*, **96**, Suppl., 56.

Discussion

COPPEN: The classification of depression arouses a heated debate. I like the Newcastle Scale because it has shown correlation with many pharmacological variants. What is the correlation between psychosocial disturbance and high scores on the Newcastle Scale?

DEAKIN: They cannot be correlated. The evidence is that psychosocial factors can trigger off all sorts of affective illnesses, including mania and psychotic depression; there is an increase in adverse life events before those conditions. Psychosocial stresses non-specifically activate a predisposition.

COPPEN: What about subsequent attacks? Are people with repeated endogenous illness those who are subjected to continuing psychosocial stress?

DEAKIN: Acute life events seem to be important in the timing of these illnesses, and not in who suffers them. It is an underlying biological vulnerability that determines whether a person suffers from endogenous depression or becomes manic or schizophrenic in response to a life event.

LINNOILA: In a fairly sizeable group of unipolar depressed patients that Dr Alec Roy and I studied, there was a striking correlation between those patients who had a large number of adverse life events in the year before their latest depressive episode and those who had relatively high concentrations of 5-hydroxyindoleacetic acid (5-HIAA) in cerebrospinal fluid (CSF). On the other hand, equally severely depressed individuals whose illness did not seem to be connected with negative life events had a lower concentration of CSF 5-HIAA.

PALFREYMAN: Dr Deakin suggested that $5-HT_{1A}$ receptors might be involved in increasing 'resilience' to stress. Both Tom Insel and John Kehne have developed a model in which a rat pup is separated from its mother. The rat pup signals with ultrasonic vocalization at a defined wavelength and as soon as it is returned to its mother the signalling stops. By treating the separated pups with buspirone or other $5-HT_{1A}$ agonists one can completely block the signalling response. This model might give interesting ideas on how to develop serotonin (5-HT) drugs that increase resilience to stress.

INSEL: In addition to concerns about the false positives in the endocrine responses to serotonergic challenge, there is a tremendous risk of false negatives. For example, we studied 3,4-methylene dioxymethamphetamine (MDMA, Ecstasy) as a neuro-toxin in the rhesus monkey. We were able to destroy 50 to 70 per cent of the serotonin terminals across all cortical fields and across all subcortical fields with the conspicuous exception of the hypothalamus, in which there was a total conservation of serotonin terminals (assessed by [³H]paroxetine-binding sites). There may be something special about hypothalamic 5-HT which can be preserved even in the face of a tremendous denervation of the rest of the brain.

LINNOILA: Price *et al.* (1989*a*) reported reduced prolactin responses to L-tryptophan in patients who had used Ecstasy.

INSEL: For the nine subjects in that study, the prolactin results were not significantly different between MDMA users and controls. We have done similar studies in monkeys. Both in acute studies and when we followed MDMA-lesioned monkeys for 15 weeks there did not seem to be a change in the plasma prolactin concentration. There was, however, a continued decrease in CSF 5-HIAA throughout that time, but no change in other metabolites or uptake sites in the brain.

COWEN: An absence of abnormal 5-HT neuroendocrine changes in obsessional neurosis would not be surprising, but there is so much evidence of disordered hypothalamic regulation in depressed patients that neuroendocrine challenge tests seem an appropriate means of assessing the integrity of the hypothalamic–limbic circuits.

INSEL: This approach has been described as a window into the brain. However, it may be a window into a very narrow room in the brain, and many other windows might be overlooked.

COWEN: That is true. My point is that in this room we know that something is definitely wrong.

MELTZER: I pointed out this sort of inverse relationship between cortisol and prolactin some years ago in the context of the effect of dexamethasone administration on plasma prolactin levels (Meltzer *et al.* 1982). In analysis of the prolactin response in depressed patients, it may be useful to co-vary out the basal cortisol levels, which should adjust for that effect. How would that influence the blunting of the prolactin response?

COWEN: We divided patients into dexamethasone suppressors and non-suppressors. The non-suppressors had the greater L-tryptophan prolactin responses. That was also found by Price *et al.* (1989*b*). Thus, if you take dexamethasone non-suppression as an index of cortisol hypersecretion, those two studies do not agree with Dr

Deakin's results. A problem with our investigation is that the patients who were non-suppressors had also lost a lot of weight; this might have confounded the effect of cortisol on prolactin responses. However, I don't think that the inverse relationship between cortisol and prolactin is very consistent across studies.

OXENKRUG: Exposure of the brain to elevated levels of cortisol specifically affects cognitive function. Corticosteroids might also stimulate the dopaminergic system. We should consider this when we discuss the effect of cortisol on prolactin responses.

DEAKIN: The hippocampus has a very high concentration of glucocorticoid receptors and 5-HT$_1$ receptors. The cognitive changes are said to be due to glucocorticoid-induced cell death in the hippocampus.

OXENKRUG: Dr Linnoila showed that alcoholics who go through withdrawal often have cognitive dysfunction.

LINNOILA: Even long-term abstinent alcoholics show a response compatible with adrenocortical hypertrophy when challenged with corticotropin-releasing hormone. If there is a kindling phenomenon in alcoholism, this may be its peripheral component. After repeated untreated withdrawals the adrenals probably begin to respond increasingly vigorously to adrenocorticotropic hormone stimulation. Furthermore, there is a strong reduction in the length of diurnal cortisol cycle during the first week after alcohol withdrawal, and there is an inverse correlation between the length of the cycle and the severity of withdrawal.

References

Meltzer, H. Y., Fang, V. S., Tricous, B. J., Robertson, A., and Piyaka, S. K. (1982). Effect of dexamethasone on plasma prolactin and cortisol levels in psychiatric patients. *American Journal of Psychiatry*, **139**, 763–8.

Price, L. H., Ricaurte, G. A., Krystal, J. H., and Heninger, G. R. (1989*a*). Neuroendocrine and mood responses to intravenous L-tryptophan in 3,4-methylene dioxymethamphetamine (MDMA) users. *Archives of General Psychiatry*, **46**, 20–2.

Price, L. H., Charney, D. S., Delgado, P. L., and Heninger, G. R., (1989*b*) Lithium treatment and serotoninergic function: the neuroendocrine and behavioural responses to intravenous tryptophan in affective disorder. *Archives of General Psychiatry*, **46**, 13–19.

13. Antidepressant efficacy of 5-HT$_{1A}$ partial agonist drugs

Donald S. Robinson

A clinical development programme for buspirone as an anti-anxiety drug was initiated following the fortuitous finding that it had a profoundly calming effect on aggressive rhesus monkeys (Tompkins *et al.* 1980). It was thought that buspirone might have useful anxiolytic properties which, along with its benign safety profile, could offer important therapeutic advantages over the benzodiazepine class of anti-anxiety drugs.

Buspirone's initial clinical development involved treatment of chronic anxiety in patients generally corresponding to the DSM-III *(Diagnostic and Statistical Manual*; American Psychiatric Association 1980) diagnostic category of generalized anxiety disorder. Its approval as a drug was based on demonstration of efficacy in a series of placebo-controlled trials involving over 700 patients. Results of three representative studies, each conducted in a different country and clinical setting, are shown in Figure 13.1. It was evident from studies such as these that buspirone and the benzodiazepine comparison drug exhibited generally comparable efficacy compared to placebo treatment, based on the extent of improvement in Hamilton Anxiety (Ham-A) scale scores. Buspirone has been widely available for clinical use as an anti-anxiety drug in several countries, including the USA, since 1987.

During buspirone's initial development the field of neuroscience was undergoing a period of rapid discovery and change. In the 1980s there emerged the ability to quantify the numbers of receptors and their affinities for drug ligands, the discovery and characterization of receptor subtypes, and the description of more discriminative behavioural models with improved predictive value.

Buspirone's unique pharmacology became better understood with the demonstration of its high affinity for the serotonin (5-hydroxytryptamine, 5-HT) type-1A (5-HT$_{1A}$) receptor. In parallel with knowledge of its receptor interactions, buspirone's behavioural pharmacology continued to be characterized more comprehensively. Preclinical studies yielded evidence that buspirone may have potential as an antidepressant drug (Table 13.1). It became apparent that buspirone, gepirone, and other drugs of the azapirone class produced down-regulation of serotonin type-2 (5-HT$_2$) receptors on chronic administration, a property shared by most antidepressant drugs.

D. S. Robinson

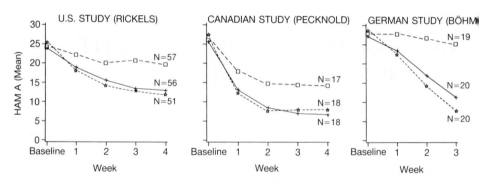

FIG. 13.1. Comparisons of buspirone, benzodiazepine, and placebo in the treatment of generalized anxiety disorder. Three representative efficacy trials conducted in different countries and clinical settings. Both active treatments were significantly better than placebo, based on mean inprovement in Hamilton Anxiety scale (HAM A) ratings. □, placebo; +, buspirone; ☆, benzodiazepine.

Buspirone was also found to be active in the learned helplessness and differential reinforcement at low rates of response tests, two behavioural models regarded as reliably predictive of antidepressant activity.

A preliminary uncontrolled study of buspirone in patients with major depression indicated that some depressed patients responded favourably to treatment (Schweizer *et al.* 1986). Based on the promising preclinical and clinical data, Bristol-Myers Squibb Company initiated a series of Phase II placebo-controlled trials of buspirone in major depression to assess whether it possessed clinically useful potential as an antidepressant as well as an anxiolytic drug. Three studies involving five sites were recently completed (Table 13.2). Four of the five investigators found buspirone to be superior to placebo, with only one of the multicentre sites yielding a negative result. The consistency of the favourable response pattern across these studies strongly supported the concept that 5-HT$_{1A}$ partial agonists have antidepressant activity clinically. Analyses of the composite database from all five study sites for the major efficacy outcome measures are summarized in Table 13.3. Significantly greater improvement was seen with buspirone treatment compared to placebo, based on the Hamilton Depression (Ham-D) scale total and subscale scores as well as on an assessment of global improvement, the CGI (Clinical Global Impressions) scale.

To establish intrinsic antidepressant efficacy for an anti-anxiety drug we require convincing evidence that it produces improvement in core depression symptoms and that more severely depressed patients benefit from treatment, to exclude the possibility that the drug might primarily be ameliorating non-specific anxiety symptoms. For this reason we conducted several additional analyses to establish buspirone's antidepressant properties (Robinson *et al.* 1989).

TABLE 13.1. *Azapirones: preclinical pharmacological profile predictive of antidepressant activity*

1. Agonist activity at serotonin type-1A (5-HT$_{1A}$) post-synaptic receptors

2. Induction of serotonin syndrome in rodents

3. Down-regulation of serotonin type-2 (5-HT$_2$) receptors

4. Active in learned helplessness behavioural models

5. Active in differential reinforcement at low rates of response behavioural model

6. Active in behavioural despair test

7. Desensitization of somatic autoreceptors with chronic administration leading to enhanced serotonergic neurotransmission at hippocampal 5-HT$_{1A}$ sites

TABLE 13.2. *Phase II placebo-controlled studies of buspirone in patients with DSM-IIIR major depression*

Investigator (site)	No. of patients	Efficacy outcome*
Rickels (Philadelphia)	153	Buspirone > placebo
Fabre (Houston)	122	Buspirone > placebo
Multicentre study	127	Buspirone > placebo
Feighner (San Diego)	41	
Branconnier (Boston)	38	
Hartford (Cincinnati)	38	

* Assessment based on outcomes ($p < 0.05$) on major efficacy scales (Hamilton Depression and Clinical Global Impressions-Improvement scales).

Those patients in the entire sample meeting criteria for DSM-IIIR major depression, melancholic subtype, were separately analysed. These patients responded significantly better to buspirone than to placebo treatment, as measured by mean improvement ratings in Ham-D scores. After only one week of treatment the benefit with buspirone was significantly greater than with placebo (Figure 13.2). Additional analyses were performed by stratifying patients based on their pretreatment Ham-D symptom severity scores. Buspirone treatment was significantly better than placebo treatment in the more severely depressed patients (pretreatment Ham-D scores above the median) as well as in the less ill patients (Ham-D scores below the median).

TABLE 13.3. *Comparison of buspirone and placebo treatment of patients with DSM-IIIR major depression: major efficacy scales**

Scale	Baseline score		Improvement		$P^\dagger$
	Buspirone	Placebo	Buspirone	Placebo	
Ham-D					
17-item total	23.5	22.8	−8.4	−5.3	< 0.001
25-item total	28.2	27.2	−10.6	−6.5	< 0.001
Retardation factor	7.7	7.4	−2.6	−1.6	< 0.001
Anxiety factor	7.9	8.0	−2.7	−1.7	< 0.001
CGI‡	4.5	4.4	101/183 (55%)	63/199 (32%)	< 0.001

* Mean pretreatment and change from baseline scores are shown.
† 2-Way Analysis of Variance (ANOVA) (except CGI).
‡ Based on Clinical Global Impressions ratings, mean severity score at baseline; responders are indicated based on improvement rating of much improved or very much improved at end of treatment. Probability test used for responder rate is Cochran–Mantel–Haenszel test.

TABLE 13.4. *Buspirone depression study treatment: response of major depression subtypes*

Depression type	No. of patients	Treatment group (responders)*		$P^\dagger$
		Buspirone ($n = 182$)	Placebo ($n = 200$)	
Melancholia	126	38 (60%)	22 (35%)	<0.005
Non-melancholia	256	63 (53%)	136 (30%)	<0.001

* Responder defined as Clinical Global Impresions rating of much improved or very much improved.
† Cochran–Mantel–Haenszel test.

These consistent findings, supporting the therapeutic usefulness of buspirone in major depression, including the melancholic subtype, and in more severely ill patients, prompted Bristol-Myers Squibb Company to initiate a clinical development programme for buspirone as an antidepressant drug. A full programme of studies is now in progress, including comparisons of buspirone with active treatments and with placebo controls.

Gepirone, an analogue of buspirone that binds specifically to 5-HT_{1A} receptors and is a more complete agonist than buspirone, is now in clinical investigation as an anxiolytic and an antidepressant drug. It shares the pharmacological profile of buspirone and, in addition, possesses certain desirable features including greater bioavailability and greater intrinsic

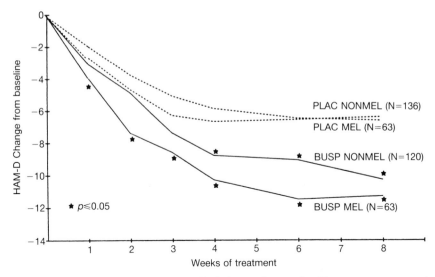

FIG. 13.2. Buspirone placebo-controlled depression study. Treatment response in DSM-IIIR major depression for those patients of the melancholic subtype (MEL) and those lacking symptoms of melancholia (NONMEL). Improvement in mean Hamilton Depression (HAM-D) ratings from pretreatment values are shown for each group. PLAC, placebo; BUSP, buspirone.

activity measured by the 5-HT$_{1A}$ adenylate cyclase assay. Gepirone falls between buspirone and the full 5-HT$_{1A}$ agonists, such as serotonin, in its activity in this *in vitro* system.

Figure 13.3 gives results of an initial phase II, placebo-controlled study of gepirone in major depression. In this double-blind trial, gepirone, titrated within two different dose ranges (one using a 5 mg capsule and the other a 10 mg capsule), was compared to placebo treatment using a random assignment, parallel group design. After a baseline wash-out period, patients meeting DSM-IIIR criteria for major depression were treated for eight weeks with the study medication. Both gepirone treatment groups exhibited significantly greater improvement in the principal efficacy measure, as indicated by Ham-D ratings (Figure 13.3). These preliminary results are consistent with the buspirone findings and support gepirone's clinical utility as an antidepressant drug.

Summary

Dysfunction of central serotonergic neuronal systems is implicated in mood disorders, and treatment of these disorders has recently been focused on this neurotransmitter. The 5-HT$_{1A}$ partial agonists possess a pharmacological

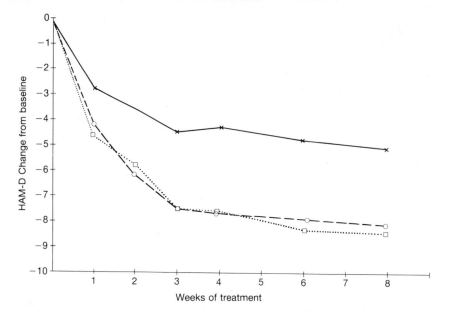

FIG. 13.3. Gepirone placebo-controlled depression study. Response of patients with DSM-III major depression receiving gepirone titrated between either 10–90 mg per day (□), or 5–45 mg per day (○), or placebo, 1–9 capsules per day (×). Improvement in mean Hamilton Depression (HAM-D) ratings from pretreatment values are shown for each group. Both gepirone treatment groups produced significantly greater improvement in HAM-D ratings than placebo treatment.

profile predictive of both antidepressant and anxiolytic activity. Placebo-controlled studies with buspirone and gepirone in depressive disorders have shown that these agents produce significant therapeutic benefit. Buspirone and gepirone treatment resulted in global improvement of depressed patients, and specifically benefited symptoms of depressed mood, work and activity, anergia, diurnal variation, and other cardinal symptoms of depression. The 5-HT$_{1A}$ partial agonists offer the prospect of significant therapeutic advance in the treatment of mood disorders because of their highly selective serotonergic effects.

Acknowledgement

The excellent secretarial assistance of Mary Ellen Doolittle is greatly appreciated.

References

American Psychiatric Association (1980). *Diagnostic and statistical manual of mental disorders*, (3rd edn). American Psychiatric Association, Washington DC.
Robinson, D. S., Alms, D. R., Shrotriya, R. C., Messina, M., and Wickramaratne,

P. (1989). Serotonergic anxiolytics and treatment of depression. *Psychopathology*, **22**, Suppl. 1, 27–36.

Schweizer, E. E., Amsterdam, J., Rickels, K., Kaplan, M., and Droba, M. (1986). Open trial of buspirone in the treatment of major depressive disorder. *Psychopharmacology Bulletin*, **22**, 183–5.

Tompkins, E. C., Clemento, A. J., Taylor, D. P., and Perhach, J. L. Jr. (1980). Inhibition of aggressive behaviour in rhesus monkeys by buspirone. *Research Communications in Psychology Psychiatry and Behavior*, **5**, 337–52.

Discussion

RACAGNI: Buspirone generates an active metabolite, 1-phenylpiperazine (1-PP), which is a potent serotonin (5-hydroxytryptamine, 5-HT) re-uptake blocker at micromolar concentrations. Could the antidepressant activity of buspirone be related to the action of this metabolite?

ROBINSON: The concentrations of 1-PP in human plasma are as high or higher than those of the parent drug, but are still in the nanomolar range. So that is possible, but I would think it unlikely. Buspirone does have a very short half-life.

BRILEY: 1-PP is also quite a potent α_2 antagonist. That fits with other hypotheses of antidepressant action. All these small activities may work together.

ROBINSON: That is certainly reasonable. With gepirone the 1-PP concentrations relative to those of the parent drug are lower, yet we still see robust antidepressant activity. We tend to discount the clinical effects of 1-PP.

CURZON: We need a hypothesis for how the same drug can be both anxiolytic and antidepressant. I can understand why many 5-HT$_{1A}$ agonists are anxiolytic; by their pre-synaptic effect they decrease release of 5-HT in the hippocampus, as do conventional anxiolytics. However, the antidepressant effects of 5-HT$_{1A}$ agonists generally have been ascribed to increased post-synaptic 5-HT function. Do the anxiolytic and antidepressant effects occur with different dose and time schedules?

ROBINSON: The average dose in the anxiety trials was about half that in the depression trials. So whether anxiolytic or antidepressant activity is expressed might be concentration sensitive at the receptor level.

CURZON: Does the anxiolytic response occur more rapidly than the antidepressant response?

ROBINSON: No; the onset of the anxiolysis is gradual, and is very reminiscent of what is seen with antidepressants. This is difficult to understand mechanistically because the acute shut-down of dorsal raphe activity with the first dose might be thought important in the expression of the anxiolytic activity; yet most patients do not experience any subjective effects of the initial dose of buspirone. It seems that the drug has to be given chronically for anxiolysis.

CURZON: Do conventional anxiolytics have an equally slow response?

ROBINSON: Patients given benzodiazepines are aware of effects at the first dose; they say that they are sedated and report other effects related to the non-specific pharmacology of the drugs. This is interpreted as a therapeutic effect. On the Hamilton Anxiety scale, parallel decreases are noted for benzodiazepines and buspirone. Perhaps the so-called anxiolytic effect represents both specific and non-specific effects of benzodiazepines.

CARLSSON: Could it be that we are dealing with one and the same action? *p*-Chlorophenylalanine elicits irritability and aggressiveness in animals. There could be a broad function controlling the threshold for lots of unpleasant experiences, including depressed mood and anxiety.

DEAKIN: Might this relate to the receptor imbalance? Chronic buspirone down-regulates 5-HT$_2$ receptors, as do the most clinically useful anxiolytic agents, including the tricyclic antidepressants which are re-uptake-blocking drugs. According to my scheme, 5-HT$_2$ receptors mediate the acute response to an aversive stimulus, anxiety. Buspirone does not work immediately because time is required for down-regulation of 5-HT$_2$ receptors. The antidepressant effect involves enhancement of 5-HT$_1$ receptor function.

LINNOILA: Dr Robinson's results on the timing of anxiolytic and antidepressant effects are contrary to those of large-scale studies comparing diazepam and amitriptyline (E. Johnstone and T. Crow) and imipramine and chlordiazepoxide (L. Covi and K. Rickels) in patients with depression, mixed anxiety/depression, and primarily generalized anxiety. There was a significant response to benzodiazepines within the first and second weeks, but after four to six weeks the tricyclics were more effective, if the patients were able to continue taking their medication.

Many animal studies still use only single doses of 5-HT$_{1A}$ agonists in various models of anxiety. For animal models to be relevant to the human disorders chronic treatment should be used.

Dr Deakin, given that there seems to be up-regulation of 5-HT$_2$ receptors after electroconvulsive therapy (ECT) in rodents, how do you fit ECT into the 5-HT$_2$, 5-HT$_{1A}$ model?

DEAKIN: ECT is really a treatment for psychotic depression, similar to neuroleptic drugs. There is evidence that if ECT is given to patients with neurotic symptoms, especially patients with anxiety, the anxiety is intensified. I would suggest that is because ECT enhances 5-HT$_2$ receptor function.

LINNOILA: I agree that ECT is not a good treatment for anxious depression, but it is effective in non-psychotic melancholia.

DEAKIN: At Northwick Park (London) simulated and real ECT groups were compared (Crow *et al.* 1984) The difference was only significant for those who suffered depressive delusions. All subjects had endogenous depression defined by the Newcastle criteria. A study at Leicester found the same results (Freeman *et al.* 1978).

MENDLEWICZ: What percentage improvement was seen in the melancholic subtype of patients?

ROBINSON: The melancholic patients were sicker and more symptomatic; their baseline Hamilton Depression scale (Ham-D) scores averaged about 26, higher than that for the whole sample. They had a greater drop in Ham-D on average from about 26 to 13. Global improvement ratings are also reliable indicators. About 65 per cent of all the patients receiving buspirone were rated as responders; a somewhat higher percentage of the melancholic patients responded.

SANDLER: I am sceptical about this use of 5-HT$_{1A}$ partial agonists as antidepressants. Much depends on how the drugs are marketed. The pharmaceutical company Duphar has a research programme centred on so-called 'serenics', which seem to be 5-HT$_{1A}$ agonists. Their reference compound at present, eltoprazine hydrochloride, seems to possess substantial anti-aggressive action but also suppresses sexual drive.

ROBINSON: How a drug is marketed depends heavily on the initial clinical findings, some of which are chance observations. If imipramine were discovered today, it might be marketed as an anxiolytic for the treatment of panic disorder, for example.

There is a patent, not held by Bristol-Myers, for buspirone to enhance sexual performance; there is a pharmacological rationale for this.

MELTZER: Low-dose thioridazine is an effective antidepressant, and dopamine (DA) agonists, such as bromocriptine, have also been reported to be effective antidepressants in man. Could the actions of buspirone and gepirone be related to their DA$_2$ effects? Buspirone shows significant DA$_2$ antagonism. We showed in the rat pituitary that gepirone directly inhibited prolactin release, an effect blocked by haloperidol (Nash and Meltzer 1989). Gepirone suppressed rat prolactin secretion *in vivo*. It behaved just like a straight DA$_2$ agonist, although we could not show in binding studies that it had a high affinity for the DA$_2$ receptor.

YOUDIM: We showed that buspirone behaved exactly the same way in the rat (Skolnick *et al.* 1986).

CURZON: But in the animal model that Dr Deakin mentioned the antidepressant-like effect of 5-HT$_{1A}$ agonists seemed to occur whether they interacted directly with dopaminergic systems or not.

References

Crow, T. J., Deakin, J. F. W., Johnstone, E. C., Joseph, M. H., and Lawler, P. D. (1984). The Northwick Park ECT trial: predictors of response to real and simulated ECT. *British Journal of Psychiatry*, **144**, 227–37.

Freeman, C. P. L., Basson, J. V., and Creighton, A. (1978). A double-blind controlled trial of electroconvulsive therapy (ECT) and simulated ECT in depressive illness. *Lancet*, **i**, 738–40.

Nash, J. F., and Meltzer, H. Y. (1989). Effect of gepirone and ipsapirone on the stimulated and unstimulated secretion of prolactin in the rat. *Journal of Pharmacology and Experimental Therapeutics*, **249**, 236–41.

Skolnick, P., Weissman, A., and Youdim, M. B. H. (1986). Monoaminergic involvement in the pharmacological action of buspirone. *British Journal of Pharmacology*, **86**, 637–46.

14. Neuroendocrine serotonergic challenges in clinical research

Juan J. López-Ibor Jr, Jerónimo Sáiz-Ruiz, Leticia Moral, Isabel Moreno, and Rosa Viñas

Biological research in psychiatry tries to correlate psychopathological and biological data in order to find mutual interactions. The methodological problems of this approach are immense because one has to look simultaneously at at least two very complex, interacting systems. Pitfalls are therefore the norm rather than the exception.

The investigation of the metabolism of serotonin (5-hydroxytryptamine, 5-HT) in psychiatry is based on several methodological approaches which study the concentrations of the neurotransmitter itself or its metabolites in post-mortem brain tissue, platelets, cerebrospinal fluid (CSF), or other body fluids. Often the activity of the 5-HT receptors in some of these samples is evaluated. Clinical trials designed to test the involvement of serotonin in a specific disorder have also been used in this endeavour.

CSF studies have been for some years the main route for this area of research, focusing on the measurement of the concentrations of 5-hydroxyindoleacetic acid (5-HIAA), the 5-HT metabolite, in both baseline conditions and after probenecid. But CSF studies have some drawbacks. They are often not feasible in a psychiatric unit, which reduces the availability of patients and also how representative the sample is. Moreover, metabolite concentration ratios in CSF obtained from the lumbar space may not be representative of events taking place in higher parts of the nervous system (Bulat 1984). Further difficulties include the cross-sectional nature of most CSF evaluations and the limited availability of controls.

The secretion of the hypothalamic factors that regulate the secretion of hypophyseal hormones is under the control of several neurotransmitters and peptides. It is therefore possible to get an idea of the functional status of a system, such as the 5-HT system, by manipulating the metabolism of the substance itself and evaluating the consequences for the secretion of different hormones by measuring the modifications of their concentrations in blood. Such a procedure allows one to gather information on the functional status of the hypothalamus, a much more selective approach than measurement of events in spinal lumbar fluid.

Serotonergic activity is involved in the control of the secretion of prolactin

TABLE 14.1.   *Proposed or possible serotonergic challenges*

Type of challenge	Agent	Reference
5-HT precursors	Tryptophan (i.v.)	Heninger *et al.* (1984)
	(p.o.)	Koyama and Meltzer (1986)
	5-HTP (p.o.)	Meltzer *et al.* (1982)
		Takahashi *et al.* (1983)
		Koyama and Meltzer (1986)
	5-HTP-ester (i.v.)	Lancranjan *et al.* (1976)
Direct agonists	Quipazine	Parati *et al.* (1987)
	m-Clorophenylpiperazine	Brewerton *et al.* (1986)
Synthesis blockers	*p*-Chlorophenylalanine	
Receptor blockers	Methysergide	
	Metergoline	
	Zimelidine	Holsboer *et al.* (1983)
Re-uptake blockers	Fluoxetine	
	Clovoxamine	
	Fluvoxamine	
	Clomipramine	Laakmann *et al.* (1984)
Monoamine oxidase inhibitors (type A)	Pirlindole	Demisch *et al.* (1986)
Indirect agonists (releasing agents)	Fenfluramine	Siever *et al.* (1984)

i.v., intravenously; p.o., orally.

(PRL), adrenocorticotropic hormone (ACTH), growth hormone (GH), and renin (Fuller 1981; Meltzer *et al.* 1982; Leong *et al.* 1983; Preziosi 1983). Some physiological or behavioural modifications induced by substances activating the serotonergic system have also been studied (for example, anxiety responses, body temperature). PRL secretion is controlled by 5-HT stimulation and dopamine inhibition (Horowski and Gräf 1976; Müller *et al.* 1983). Stress, hypoglycaemia, exercise, and sexual activity (in women) also increase its secretion. GH secretion is regulated by dopamine, noradrenaline, 5-HT, physical and emotional stress, and hypoglycaemia.

Several serotonergic challenges have been proposed (Table 14.1). Some act by promoting the synthesis or liberation of 5-HT, some by inhibiting its re-uptake, and others by influencing the activity of receptors. It is also possible to combine several of them with the aim of targeting the research on a specific kind of receptor. Unfortunately, none of the 5-HT probes has been accepted as a standard and all have been criticized, mainly because they are not 'clean' enough; none of the proposed substances acts exclusively on the 5-HT system (van Praag *et al.* 1987).

Despite all the difficulties we have obtained interesting results with two 5-HT probes, fenfluramine and clomipramine, using methodologies which are simple enough for use in normal clinical conditions. Consequently we have been able to study samples which are not as biased as the ones usually employed for CSF studies.

Fenfluramine challenge

dl-Fenfluramine induces release of 5-HT from its storage sites. It also has a re-uptake blocking effect and, unlike the l-enantiomer produces changes in other neurotransmitters, mainly dopamine (Garattini *et al.* 1975). The test, described by Siever *et al.* (1984), is done in the following way. Blood samples are taken 30 minutes and immediately before the oral administration of 60 mg of dl-fenfluramine in fasting conditions after a normal night rest and 60, 120, 180, and 240 minutes afterwards. After the intake of fenfluramine a light breakfast is permitted. PRL, cortisol (CORT), and GH are measured in every sample. The technique and the neuroendocrine foundations of the fenfluramine challenge test are described in López-Ibor *et al.* (1988a, 1989). Absolute and differential (maximum minus baseline) concentrations of the hormones are considered. The average of the two samples before the intake of fenfluramine is taken as the baseline value.

In our study of PRL secretion (Fig. 14.1), we were able to differentiate patients with major depression (with and without melancholia) from dysthymic patients (López-Ibor *et al.* 1988a, 1989), the former having a blunted response to the fenfluramine administration. In another sample (López-Ibor *et al.* 1990), a group of borderline suicidal patients who did not meet DSM-III criteria for any depressive disorders, showed, in comparison to an age and sex-matched control group, a very blunted response (Fig. 14.2), similar to the melancholics in the first study.

When cortisol secretion is studied, patients with major depression have a higher response than the dysthymic disorder group. The non-depressed borderline patients have significantly higher baseline CORT concentrations, but during the challenge they show a very modest increase in CORT concentration when compared with the controls (Fig. 14.3). We interpret this finding as suggesting a baseline highly stressed situation accompanied by a reduced ability to respond to new stressful events.

Clomipramine challenge

Fenfluramine has several drawbacks: it is administered orally and its intestinal absorption cannot be controlled; it is a 'dirty' drug; and the test requires

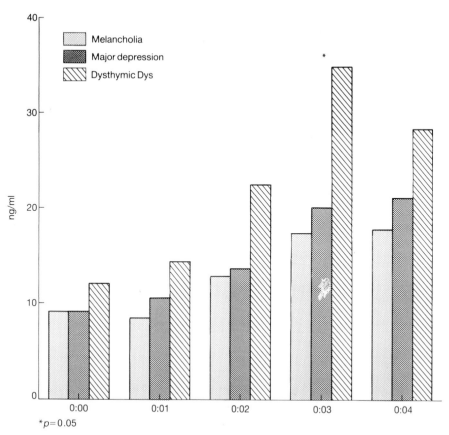

FIG. 14.1. Prolactin concentration after fenfluramine challenge. Patients suffering from major depression and major depression with melancholia show a blunted response to the serotonergic challenge when compared with patients suffering from dysthymic disorder, who show a response within the normal range.

several hours. Clomipramine lacks these drawbacks and the responses can be studied within two hours. Francis *et al.* (1976), Cole *et al.* (1976), Jones *et al.* (1977), and Murphy *et al.* (1986) described increased PRL concentrations after oral or intravenous administration of clomipramine in healthy subjects or depressed patients. Laakmann *et al.* (1984a, b) studied PRL and CORT secretion variations after the administration of clomipramine or desipramine in healthy subjects and also showed a response to the challenge. We perform the test using a similar methodology to the fenfluramine challenge. The patient remains lying down and after a venepuncture a saline infusion is administered, during which clomipramine (12.5 mg) is administered over 10 minutes. Samples are taken 30 minutes before, during and 30, 60, 90, and

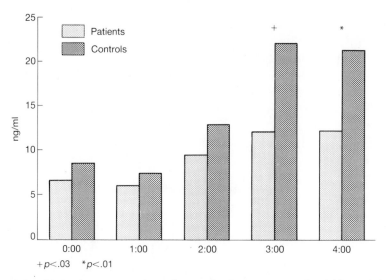

+*p*<.03   *p<.01

FIG. 14.2.   Prolactin response in patients who have attempted suicide and do not meet diagnostic criteria for any kind of depressive disorder is blunted compared with that in age and sex-matched controls.

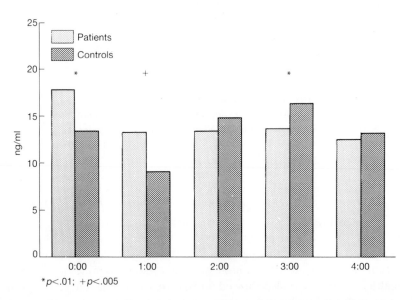

*p<.01; +*p*<.005

FIG. 14.3.   Cortisol concentrations in borderline suicidal patients tend to be higher at baseline and one hour after ingestion of fenfluramine, and do not show an increase in the following hours, whereas controls have lower concentrations at baseline and one hour after fenfluramine, and show a significant increase in the following hours.

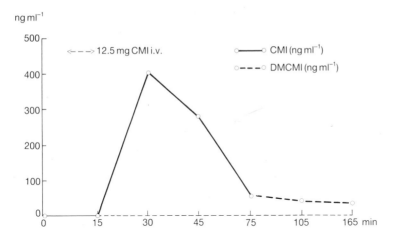

FIG. 14.4. Clomipramine (CMI) concentrations after 12.5 mg intravenously are shown. Desmethylclomipramine (DMCMI) is absent from all the samples because of the short duration of the test and the administration route, which avoids the first pass effect through the liver.

120 minutes after the infusion. PRL, CORT, GH, clomipramine and desmethylclomipramine are analysed in each sample. The concentrations of the latter two compounds show (Fig. 14.4) that, because of the short time elapsed and the avoidance of the first pass effect through the liver, no desmethylclomipramine is produced. Thus, the test is quite clean, because clomipramine is a selective 5-HT re-uptake blocker whereas its metabolite, desmethylclomipramine, has noradrenergic activity also.

With this probe we have also found a significant difference between PRL responses in major depressions and dysthymic disorders (López-Ibor *et al.* 1988*b*). The same blunted response is to be found in a group of patients suffering from a disorder characterized by a poor control of impulses, manifested by a gambling dependence, and selected by the absence of any kind of depressive disorders. We found the same pattern in the CORT secretion as with the impulsive borderlines, namely, high baseline concentration and a blunted response to the challenge (Moreno *et al.* 1990). A sample of drug addicts after naltrexone maintenance treatment shows a similar pattern (López-Ibor *et al.* 1990, Fig. 14.5).

Finally, in all the investigations, GH concentrations do not show significant differences among the groups studied, and their values show high dispersion, a finding which is in accordance with the great variations in the secretion of this hormone and how much this is influenced by external stresses.

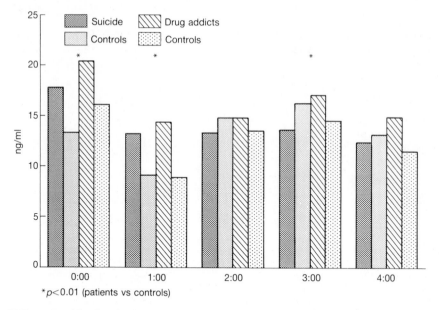

FIG. 14.5. The borderline suicidal patients and controls in Fig. 14.3 are compared with a sample of drug addicts after naltrexone maintenance treatment. Drug addicts have a similar pattern to borderline patients in their cortisol concentration modifications during the fenfluramine challenge test.

References

Brewerton, T., Mueller, E., and George, T. (1986). Blunted prolactin response to the serotonin agonist m-chlorophenylpiperazine (m-CPP) in bulimia. *Abstracts of the 15th congress of the CINP*. San Juan, Puerto Rico.

Bulat, M. (1984). Some criteria for the study of biochemical processes in CNS by analysis of the cerebrospinal fluid (CSF). *Clinical Neuropharmacology*, **7**, Suppl. 1, 286–7.

Cole, D. N., Groom, G. V., Link, J., *et al.* (1976). Plasma prolactin concentrations in patients on clomipramine. *Postgraduate Medical Journal*, **52**, 93–100.

Demisch, K., Demisch, L., Buchholz, G., Althiff, P., Rosak, C., and Magnet, W. (1986). Effect of Pirlindole on endocrine parameters in healthy man. In *Psychiatry. The state of the art*, (ed. P. Pichot, P. Berner, R. Wolf, and K. Thay), Vol. 3. Plenum, New York.

Fuller, R. W. (1981). Serotonergic stimulation of pituitary-adrenocortical function in rats. *Neuroendocrinology*, **32**, 118–27.

Francis, A. F., Williams, P., Williams, R., *et al.* (1976). The effect of clomipramine on prolactin levels—pilot studies. *Postgraduate Medical Journal*, **52**, 87–91.

Garattini, S., Buczko, W., Jori, A., and Samanin, R. (1975). The mechanism of action of fenfluramine. *Postgraduate Medical Journal*, **51**, Suppl. 1, 27–35.

Heninger, G. R., Charney, D. S., and Sternberg, D. E. (1984). Serotonergic function in depressed patients and healthy subjects. *Archives of General Psychiatry*, **41**, 398–402.

Holsboer, F., Muller, O. A., Winter, K., Doerr, H. G., and Sippell, W. G. (1983). Effect of serotonin uptake inhibition by Zimelidine on hypothalamic-pituitary-adrenal activity. *Psychopharmacology*, **80**, 85–7.

Horowski, R. and Gräf, K. J. (1976). Influence of dopaminergic agonist and antagonist on serum prolactin concentrations in the rat. *Neuroendocrinology*, **22**, 273–86.

Jones, R. B., Luscombe, D. K., and Groom, G. V. (1977). Plasma concentrations in normal subjects and depressive patients following oral clomipramine. *Postgraduate Medical Journal*, **53**, 166–71.

Koyama, T. and Meltzer, H.Y. (1986). A biochemical and neuroendocrine study of the serotonergic system in depression. In *New results in depression research*, (ed. H. Hippius *et al.*). Springer-Verlag, Berlin.

Laakmann, G., Gugath, M., Kuss, H. J., and Zygan, K. (1984*a*). Comparison of growth hormone and prolactin stimulation induced by chlorimipramine and desimipramine in man in connection with chlorimipramine metabolism. *Psychopharmacology*, **82**, 62–7.

Laakmann, G., Wittman, M., Gugath, M., Müller, O. A., Treusch, J., Wahlster, U., and Stalla, G. K. (1984*b*). Effects of psychotropic drugs (desimipramine, chlorimipramine, sulpiride and diazepam) on the human HPA axis. *Psychopharmacology*, **84**, 66–70.

Laakmann, G., Hinz, A., and Neulinger. E. (1986). Pharmacoendocrine studies in healthy subjects and depressed patients. In *New results in depression research*, (ed. H. Hippius *et al.*), pp. 250–60. Springer-Verlag, Berlin.

Lancranjan, I., Wirz-Justice, A., Puhringer, W., and Del Pozo, E. (1976). Effect of L-5-Hydroxytryptophan infusion on growth hormone and prolactin secretion. *Clinical Endocrinology and Metabolism*, **15**, 588–93.

Leong, D., Frawley, L. S., and Neill, J. D. (1983). Neuroendocrine control of prolactin secretion. *Annual Review of Physiology*, **45**, 109–27.

López-Ibor Jr., J. J., Sáiz-Ruiz, J., and Pérez de los Cobos, J. C. (1985). Biological correlations of suicide and aggressivity in major depressions (with melancholia): 5-hydroxyindoleacetic acid and cortisol in cerebral spinal fluid, dexamethasone suppression test and therapeutic response to 5-hydroxytryptophan. *Neuropsychobiology*, **14**, 67–74.

López-Ibor Jr., J. J., Sáiz-Ruiz, J., and Moral-Iglesias, L. (1988*a*). The fenfluramine challenge test in the affective spectrum: A possible marker of endogeneity and severity. *Pharmacopsychiatry*, **21**, 9–14.

López-Ibor Jr., J. J., Sáiz-Ruiz, J., and González-Pinto, A. (1988*b*). The clomipramine challenge test. *Abstracts of the CINP Congress*, Munich.

López-Ibor Jr., J. J. (1988). The involvement of serotonin in psychiatric disorders and behaviour. *British Journal of Psychiatry*, **153**, Suppl., 26–39.

López-Ibor Jr., J. J., Sáiz-Ruiz, J., and Moral-Iglesias, L. (1989). Neuroendocrine challenges in the diagnosis of depressive disorders. *British Journal of Psychiatry*, **154**, Suppl 4., 73–6.

López-Ibor Jr., J. J., Lana, F., and Sáiz-Ruiz, J. (1990). Serotonin, impulsivity and suicidal behaviour. In *Proceedings of the VIII World Congress of Psychiatry*. Athens, in press.

Meltzer, H. Y., Wiita, B., Tricou, B. J., *et al.* (1982). Effect of serotonin precursors and serotonin agonists on plasma hormone levels. In *Serotonin in biological psychiatry*, (ed. B. T. Ho, J. C. Schooler, and E. Usdin). Raven Press, New York.

Moreno, I., Sáíz, J., and López-Ibor Jr., J. J. (1990). Serotonin and gambling dependence. *Abstracts of the International Symposium on Serotonin and behavioural disturbances*, Lisbon.

Müller, E. E., Locatelli, V., Cella, S., Peñalva, A., Novelli, A., and Cocchi, D. (1983). Prolactin-lowering and -releasing drugs. Mechanisms of action and therapeutic applications. *Drugs*, **25**, 399–432.

Murphy, D. L., Mueller, E. A., Garrick, N. A., and Aulakh, C. S. (1986). Use of serotonergic agents in the clinical assessment of central serotonin function. *Journal of Clinical Psychiatry*, **47**, Suppl. 4, 9–15.

Parati, E. A., Zarnadi, P., Cocchi, D., Caraceni, T., and Muller, E. E. (1987). Neuroendocrine effects of Quipazine in man in healthy state or with neurological disorders. *Journal of Neurological Transmission*, **47**, 273–97.

Preziosi, P. (1983). Serotonin control of prolactin release: an intriguing puzzle. *Trends in Pharmacological Sciences*, **40**, 171–4.

Siever, L. J., Murphy, D. L., Slater, S., de la Vega. E., and Lipper, S. (1984). Plasma prolactin changes following fenfluramine in depressed patients compared to controls: an evaluation of central serotonergic responsivity in depression. *Life Sciences*, **34**, 1029–39.

Takahasi, S., Kondo, H., Yoshimura, H., Oshi, Y., and Yoshimi, U. (1973). Growth hormone response to administration of L-5-Hydroxytryptophan (5-HTp) in manic-depressive psychosis. *Folia Psychiatrica et Neurologica Japanica*, **27**, 197–206.

van Praag, H. M., Lemus, C., and Kahn, R. (1987). Hormonal probes of central serotonin activity: do they really exist? *Biological Psychiatry*, **22**, 86–98.

Discussion

GLOVER: Amongst psychiatrists there is an argument about whether endogenous, neurotic, or any of the other diagnostic subgroups of depression lie on a continuous spectrum or whether they are distinct diseases. Does your test give us a biochemical way of answering that question?

LÓPEZ-IBOR: The score on the Newcastle scale and the concentrations of prolactin correlate beautifully. It looks like a continuum, but the number of the subjects is too small to see if there is a bimodal or otherwise skewed distribution. Therefore, we cannot be sure.

MELTZER: It is crucial to do a placebo control for each of these neuroendocrine challenges because you can see surprising differences in placebo responses. The placebo response can cause plasma hormone levels to drop far below the baseline in certain groups of subjects. That makes an apparent blunted response quite normal in relationship to that group's baseline. Another general principle is that one must correct for blood levels. Dennis Murphy has shown that with *m*-chlorophenylpiperazine, and we have some similar data with 5-hydroxytryptophan (5-HTP) and fluoxetine; blood levels achieved in the different groups can change before and after treatment.

LINNOILA: I agree with that, but Bill Potter's observations, which were placebo controlled, certainly support Professor López-Ibor's results. Dr Potter used intravenous infusions of clomipramine (10 or 20 mg) and also showed blunted responses in melancholic patients.

MENDLEWICZ: Most patients we see are generally on medication such as benzodiaze-pines or tricyclic antidepressants. How long should the drug-free period be before one does such a challenge test?

LÓPEZ-IBOR: The wash-out period was two weeks, except for patients on neuroleptic medication when it was extended to four weeks.

MELTZER: Was that determined by careful withdrawal studies or decided arbitrarily?

LÓPEZ-IBOR: We decided arbitrarily, taking into account what is known about the pharmacokinetics of psychotropic drugs.

COWEN: Nobody knows how long this period should be. We try to work in primary care so that we can study patients who have not been treated with psychotropic drugs.

LINNOILA: There are changes in urinary catecholamine metabolites after up to four weeks of wash-out. Some healthy volunteers treated with monoamine oxidase inhibitors (MAOIs) showed changes in urinary catecholamine metabolite excretion up to three months after the treatment was stopped. Assuming that urinary catecholamines are related to what happens in the sympathetic nervous system and in noradrenergic transmission, this shows that we should wait for months, at least after MAOIs, before we can establish a baseline and interpret the results. With tricyclic antidepressants, three to four weeks is the minimum drug-free period.

MELTZER: We have been using 5-HTP and MK 212 as neuroendocrine challenges before and after fluoxetine in patients with obsessive-compulsive disorder and in depressed patients. With fluoxetine, but not with clomipramine or the other antidepressants, there is a tremendous enhancement of the cortisol response to 5-HTP and MK 212. This is not a blood level phenomenon, at least with 5-HTP; if anything, the 5-HTP levels have decreased significantly. We are seeing both pre- and post-synaptic enhancement of serotonergic function selectively with fluoxetine. I saw the same thing with sertraline in a small number of patients. Why are these drugs not better antidepressants than the tricyclics, if they are really producing more enhancement of the endocrine responses and if that is a relevant marker for post-synaptic serotonergic function?

COWEN: It is an enhanced response to a $5\text{-}HT_2$ receptor-mediated neuroendocrine challenge.

MELTZER: Or $5\text{-}HT_{1C}$—I cannot distinguish that yet.

COWEN: From Bill Deakin's theory about the relationship between $5\text{-}HT_1$ and $5\text{-}HT_2$ receptors in depression, increased $5\text{-}HT_2$ receptor function would not necessarily be advantageous.

DEAKIN: They are not very good antidepressants because they do not decrease function in the $5\text{-}HT_2$ receptor family.

LINNOILA: How does this theory fit with lithium enhancement of antidepressant efficacy?

COWEN: There is evidence for decreased $5\text{-}HT_2$ receptor function in humans after lithium treatment because slow-wave sleep is increased (Friston *et al.* 1989). And lithium enhances the L-tryptophan prolactin response, which is $5\text{-}HT_1$-mediated (Glue *et al.* 1986). So lithium seems to fit in the general pattern that antidepressants increase $5\text{-}HT_1$ receptor function but decrease responses mediated by $5\text{-}HT_2$ receptors.

MELTZER: I did not mean to imply that fluoxetine is not as good an antidepressant as typical tricyclic antidepressants; the evidence is strong that it is at least as good.

DEAKIN: I have to disagree. The evidence from the controlled trials comparing the selective 5-HT re-uptake blockers and the standard tricyclics is that the former take longer to work, and in some trials they did not work as well.

CARLSSON: It is dangerous to think along a monorail type of hypothesis, believing that if serotonin is involved in depression there are no other relevant factors, and therefore that a serotonergic agent should be better than anything else. Depression involves many neurotransmitters. Therefore, one can use many agents acting on different receptors. I am not surprised that serotonin does not do more than it does.

MELTZER: I certainly do not subscribe to a single monoamine hypothesis of affective disorders. In particular, I believe that dopamine, and perhaps noradrenaline, also play a critical role in depression. However, even if there are many factors contributing to depression, and unless serotonin is the rate-limiting factor, when you affect one component of a multifactorial system, you should see a more potent effect from an agent that is more potent for that particular component.

References

Friston, K. J., Sharpley, A. L., Solomon, R. A., and Cowen, P. J. (1989). Lithium increases slow wave sleep: possible mediation by brain 5-HT$_2$ receptors. *Psychopharmacology*, **98**, 139–40.

Glue, P.W., Cowen, P. J., Nutt, D. G., Kolakowska, T., and Grahame-Smith, D. G. (1986). The effect of lithium on 5-HT-mediated neuroendocrine responses and platelet 5-HT receptors. *Psychopharmacology*, **90**, 398–402.

15. Serotonin in anxiety: evidence from animal models

Mike Briley and Philippe Chopin

Benzodiazepines have been shown since the early 1970s to cause some reduction of 5-hydroxytryptamine (5-HT, serotonin) turnover (Chase *et al.* 1970), but in view of similar effects on other neurotransmitters these results did not generate any major interest in serotonin as a transmitter in anxiety. The probability of a close link between serotonin and anxiety was highlighted a few years ago by the demonstration of the anxiolytic properties of buspirone. Buspirone has a variety of pharmacological activities involving serotonin, noradrenaline, and dopamine, but its anticonflict properties are lost after serotonergic lesion, suggesting the importance of serotonin in anxiety (Eison *et al.* 1986). The anxiolytic activity in man of two close derivatives of buspirone, gepirone and ipsapirone, both of which lack the dopaminergic component of buspirone, further implicated serotonin in the control of anxiety (Csanalosi *et al.* 1987; Traber and Glaser 1987).

At the same time, advances in the classification of serotonin receptor subtypes have provided the tools for a better understanding of this involvement of serotonin. As is discussed elsewhere in this book, an ever increasing number of subtypes of serotonin receptors is being reported. Initially, radioligand binding studies revealed two serotonin recognition sites in the rat brain. These were designated 5-HT_1 and 5-HT_2 (Bradley *et al.* 1986), having high affinity for $^3\text{H-5-HT}$ and [^{3}H]spiperone respectively. The ability of spiperone to displace $^3\text{H-5-HT}$ in a biphasic manner subsequently led to the division of 5-HT_1 sites into 5-HT_{1A} and 5-HT_{1B} subtypes. A further subtype of 5-HT_1 receptor, designated 5-HT_{1C}, has been proposed, based on the high-affinity inhibition of $^3\text{H-5-HT}$ binding by mesulergine. Another $^3\text{H-5-HT}$-binding site has been named 5-HT_{1D} (Herrick-Davis and Titeler 1988). Finally (for the moment), a 5-HT_{1E} receptor has been discovered in human brain (Leonhardt *et al.* 1989). A third subtype of serotonin receptor, designated 5-HT_3, which is widely distributed throughout the peripheral nervous system, has also been found in brain (Kilpatrick *et al.* 1987; Peroutka and Hamik 1988).

5-HT_{1A} receptors appear to be located partly on cell bodies and dendrites of neurones in the raphe nuclei and partly post-synaptically. The serotonin autoreceptors on the nerve terminals have been shown, at least in rodents, to be of the 5-HT$_{1B}$ subtype (Hibert and Middlemiss 1986). Autoreceptors would appear, however, to represent only a very small proportion of the 5-HT$_{1B}$ receptors which are principally located post-synaptically (Offord *et al.* 1988; Brown *et al.* 1989). The 5-HT$_2$ receptors appear to be essentially post-synaptic (Dumbrille-Ross *et al.* 1982) and the synaptic localization of 5-HT$_3$ receptors has not yet been fully elucidated.

Thus a new architectural setting for serotonin neurotransmission is slowly appearing. In addition, many compounds have been described that modify serotonin neurotransmission in a variety of ways. Many of these have been used in different animal models of anxiety with apparently confusing results. In this review, we summarize these data and show that with some simplification and a few reasonable assumptions a coherent hypothesis for the involvement of serotonin in anxiety can be developed. For those unfamiliar with animal tests of anxiety, the principal tests are described in the Appendix.

Effect of compounds that reduce serotonin neurotransmission

Non-selective serotonin receptor antagonists, such as metergoline (Meert and Colpaert 1986*a*; Pellow *et al.* 1987), cinanserin (Becker 1986), bromolysergic acid (Graeff and Schoenfeld 1970), cyproheptadine (Meert and Colpaert 1986*a,b*; Becker 1986), and methysergide (Meert and Colpaert 1986*a,b*; Graeff and Schoenfeld 1970) (Table 15.1), and relatively selective 5-HT$_2$ receptor antagonists, such as pirenperone (Colpaert *et al.* 1985), R-56413 (3-[2-[4[bis(4-fluorophenyl)methylene]-1-piperidinyl]ethyl]-2-methyl-4H-pyrido[1,2-a]pyrimidine-4-one) (Meert and Colpaert 1986*a*; Colpaert *et al.* 1985; Critchley and Handley 1986), ritanserin, and ketanserin (Critchley and Handley 1986; Handley and Mithani 1984) (Table 15.2), all show anti-anxiety effects in rats in several tests, including various conflict procedures, the elevated plus-maze test and the two-compartment exploratory test. Unlike the effects of benzodiazepines, however, the anxiolytic activities of these compounds are weak and confined to a narrow dose range. Furthermore, as seen in Tables 15.1 and 15.2, anxiolytic activities have not been consistently observed by all authors (Deacon and Gardner 1986; File 1981; Becker 1986; Petersen and Lassen 1981; Critchley *et al.* 1987; Handley and Mithani 1984), although the narrow active dose range may be an explanation for this. Interestingly, none of the compounds tested was active in the social interaction test in the rat (Critchley *et al.* 1987; File 1981) nor the two-compartment test in the mouse (Costall *et al.* 1988*c*).

At present, information on the anxiolytic activity of drugs acting on central 5-HT$_3$ receptors is limited (Table 15.3). The 5-HT$_3$ antagonists, GR 38032F (1,2,3,9-tetrahydro-9-methyl-3-[2-methyl-1H-imidazol-1-yl)methyl]-4H-carbazol-4-one), BRL 43694 ((endo)-N-[9-methyl-9-azabicyclo(3,3,1)non-3-

TABLE 15.1. *Effects of non-selective 5-HT receptor antagonists in anxiety tests in rats*

Drugs	Tests	Anxiolytic responses
Metergoline	Conflict test	+/0
	Shock probe test	+
	Elevated plus-maze	+
	Social interaction	0
	Two-compartment test (mouse)	0
Cinanserin	Conflict test	+/0
Bromolysergic acid	Conflict test	+
Cyproheptadine	Conflict test	+/0
	Shock probe test	+
	Two-compartment test (mouse)	0
Methysergide	Conflict test	+/0
	Shock probe test	+
	Social interaction	0
	Two-compartment test (mouse)	0

+, anxiolytic effects; −, anxiogenic activity; 0, inactive.

yl]-1-methyl-indazole-3-carboxamide), ICS 205-930 ((3α-tropanyl)-1H-indole-3-carboxylic acid ester), and zacopride all exhibit anxiolytic activity in the social interaction test in rats (Jones *et al.* 1988; Piper *et al.* 1988; Costall *et al.* 1987*a*,*b*, 1988*b*) and the two-compartment test in mice (Costall *et al.* 1987*b*, 1988*a*,*b*) but not in the water-lick conflict test in rats (Jones *et al.* 1988). 5-HT$_3$ receptor antagonists, however, appear to be inactive in the elevated plus-maze test (File and Johnston 1989). In addition, File and Johnston (1989) reported a lack of anxiolytic effect of these compounds in the social interaction test, although another 5-HT$_3$ antagonist, MDL 72222 ((1αH,3α,5αH-tropan-3-yl)3,5-dichlorobenzoate) has shown anxiolytic activity in this test (Tyers *et al.* 1987). In the monkey and the marmoset, GR 38032F has been reported to reduce anxiety-related symptoms (Costall *et al.* 1987*a*).

p-Chlorophenylalanine (*p*-CPA), which reduces serotonin neurotransmission by inhibition of tryptophan hydroxylase, shows anxiolytic effects in the social interaction test (File and Hyde 1977) and conflict procedures (Engel 1986). This behaviour is closely correlated with the pharmacological time course of 5-HT depletion (Tye *et al.* 1977). In addition, lesions produced by intraventricular or local stereotaxic administration of the serotonergic neurotoxins, 5,6-dihydroxytryptamine (5,6-DHT) (Stein *et al.* 1975*a*) or

TABLE 15.2. *Effects of 5-HT$_2$ receptor antagonists in anxiety tests in rats*

Drugs	Tests	Anxiolytic responses
Pirenperone	Conflict test	+
	Elevated plus-maze	0
	Two-compartment test	+
R-56413	Conflict test	+
	Shock probe test	+
	Elevated plus-maze	+
	Two-compartment test	+
Ritanserin	Conflict test	+/0
	Shock probe test	+
	Elevated plus-maze	+/−
	Two-compartment test	+
	Two-compartment test (mouse)	0
	Social interaction	0
Ketanserin	Elevated plus-maze	+
	Social interaction	0

+, anxiolytic effects; −, anxiogenic activity; 0, inactive.

5,7-dihydroxytryptamine (5,7-DHT) (Tye *et al.* 1977) result in anxiolytic effects in conflict tests. 5,7-DHT lesions of the dorsal raphe nucleus also produce anxiolytic effects in the social interaction test (File *et al.* 1979), while intraventricular 5,7-DHT produced an anxiolytic effect in the elevated plus-maze test (M. Briley, P. Chopin, and C. Moret, unpublished results). However, the situation is complex because Critchley and Handley (1989) reported that 5,7-DHT lesions of the dorsal raphe which spared the median raphe did not alter elevated plus-maze activity whereas they did reverse the anxiogenic effects of 8-hydroxy-*N,N*-dipropyl-2-aminotetralin (8-OH-DPAT) and the anxiolytic effects of ipsapirone (see below).

Effects of 5-HT$_{1A}$ agonists, partial agonists, and antagonists

The results of studies of 5-HT$_{1A}$ receptor agonists and partial agonists and antagonists in tests of anxiety have not been particularly consistent (Table 15.4). For example, 8-OH-DPAT has shown anxiolytic, anxiogenic, and no activity, depending on the test and the authors (Engel 1986; Critchley and Handley 1987*b*; Meert and Colpaert 1986*b*; Pellow *et al.* 1987; Carli and Samanin 1988; Critchley and Handley 1989; P. Moser, unpublished paper, *Behavioural pharmacology of 5-HT*, Amsterdam, November 1987). The 5-HT$_{1A}$ full agonists, 5-methoxy-*N,N*-dimethyltryptamine (5-MeO-DMT), LY

TABLE 15.3. *Effects of 5-HT₃ receptor antagonists in anxiety tests in rats*

Drugs	Tests	Anxiolytic responses
GR 38032F	Conflict test	0
	Social interaction	+/0
	Two-compartment test (mouse)	+
	Elevated plus-maze	0
BRL 43694	Social interaction	+/0
	Two-compartment test (mouse)	+
	Elevated plus-maze	0
ICS 205-930	Social interaction	+
	Two-compartment test (mouse)	+
MDL 72222	Social interaction	+
Zacopride	Social interaction	+/0
	Two-compartment test (mouse)	+
	Elevated plus-maze	0

+, anxiolytic effects; −, anxiogenic activity; 0, inactive.

165163 ((1-(*m*-trifluoromethylphenyl)-4-*p*-aminophenylethyl)piperazine), and (−) and (+)-MDL 72832 (8-[4-(1,4-benzodioxan-2-yl-methylamino)butyl] 8 azaspiro [4,5]decane-7,9-dione), on the other hand, have been reported to be anxiogenic in various tests (Critchley and Handley 1986; Critchley *et al.* 1987; Stein *et al.* 1975*b*; P. Moser, unpublished paper, *Behavioural pharmacology of 5-HT*, Amsterdam, November 1987).

Buspirone, which amongst its other activities is a 5-HT$_{1A}$ partial agonist, has anxiolytic activity in man (Goldberg and Finnerty 1979). It reduces aggression and produces anticonflict activity in both rodents and primates (Merlo Pich and Samanin 1986; Geller and Hartmann 1982). The level of activity is, however, low and the active dose range very narrow. Similar results were obtained with rodents in the two-compartment test (Merlo Pich and Samanin 1986; Costall *et al.* 1988*c*). Other groups, however, have been unable to find anticonflict effects in various models (Meert and Colpaert 1986*a*; Budhram *et al.* 1986; Goldberg *et al.* 1983). Results in the social interaction and elevated plus-maze tests have also been inconsistent (Chopin and Briley 1987; File 1984; Gardner and Guy 1985; Pellow *et al.* 1987).

Interestingly, both buspirone and ipsapirone are strong inhibitors of foot-shock-induced aggression in mice (Goldberg and Finnerty 1979; Traber *et al.* 1984). It is not clear whether the effects on aggressive behaviour are related to anxiolytic activity, but it is generally thought that an enhancement of serotonin neurotransmission results in an inhibition of aggressive behaviour

TABLE 15.4. *Effects of 5-HT$_{1A}$ receptor agonists and partial agonists in anxiety tests in rats*

Drugs	Tests	Anxiolytic responses
8-OH-DPAT	Conflict test	+/0
	Shock probe test	+
	Elevated plus-maze	0/−
	Social interaction	+/−
	Two-compartment test	+
5-MeO-DMT	Elevated plus-maze	−
	Social interaction	−
	Conflict test	−
LY 165163	Elevated plus-maze	−
(+) or (−) MDL 72832	Elevated plus-maze	−
Buspirone	Conflict test	+/0
	Shock probe test	0
	Social interaction	+/0
	Elevated plus-maze	0/−
	Two-compartment test	+
Gepirone	Conflict test	+
Ipsapirone	Conflict test	+/0
	Shock probe test	0
	Elevated plus-maze test	+/0/−
	Inhibition of passive avoidance behaviour	+
	Social interaction	+
MDL 73005EF	Conflict test	+
	Elevated plus-maze	+

+, anxiolytic effects; −, anxiogenic activity; 0, inactive; 8-OH-DPAT, 8-hydroxy,-*N,N*-dipropyl-2-aminotetralin; 5-MeO-DMT, 5-methoxy-*N,N*-dimethyltryptamine.

(Broderick and Lynch 1982). Olivier *et al.* (1986) reported potent anti-aggressive activity with the 5-HT$_{1A}$ receptor agonists, 8-OH-DPAT and 5-MeO-DMT, the preferential 5-HT$_{1B}$ receptor agonists, RU 24969 and 1-(*m*-trifluoromethylphenyl)piperazine (TFMPP), and the 5-HT$_2$ receptor agonist, quipazine. One has to assume that these agonists are acting essentially post-synaptically if one is to maintain the hypothesis that low 5-HT stimulation leads to aggression.

TABLE 15.5. *Effects of 5-HT$_{1B}$ and 5-HT$_2$ receptor agonists in anxiety tests in rats*

Drugs	Tests	Anxiolytic responses
RU 24969	Conflict test	0/−
	Shock probe test	−
	Elevated plus-maze	−
	Social interaction	−
TFMPP	Shock probe test	−
Quipazine	Elevated plus-maze	−
α-Methyltryptamine	Conflict test	−

−, anxiogenic activity; 0, inactive; TFMPP, 1-[3-(trifluoromethyl)phenyl] piperazine.

Other 5-HT$_{1A}$ partial agonists, such as ipsapirone, gepirone, and MDL 73005EF (8-[2-[(2,3-dihydro-1,4-benzodioxin-2-yl)methylamino]ethyl]-8-azaspiro[4,5]decan-7,9-dionemethane sulphonate), have been found active in several models of anxiety, including conflict tests (Traber *et al.* 1984; Young *et al.* 1987; Moser *et al.* 1988), the social interaction test (Critchley *et al.* 1987; Higgins *et al.* 1987), and the elevated plus-maze test (Critchley and Handley 1987*a*, 1989), although other groups have failed to find any activity (Deacon and Gardner 1986; Chopin and Briley 1987; Meert and Colpaert 1986*b*).

(−)-Propranolol, which, amongst other activities, is an antagonist at the 5-HT$_{1A}$ receptor in the raphe nucleus (Middlemiss 1984) and would thus be expected to increase the firing of serotonergic neurones, has anxiogenic activity in the elevated plus-maze test (Pellow *et al.* 1987). In man propranolol has an anti-stress activity, but it is not considered to be anxiolytic (Hayes and Schulz 1987).

Effects of compounds that increase serotonin neurotransmission

RU 24969 and TFMPP, agonists that are selective for 5-HT$_{1B}$ receptors, show anxiogenic activity in the shock probe conflict procedure (Table 15.5) (Meert and Colpaert 1986*b*). RU 24969 is also anxiogenic in the elevated plus-maze (Pellow *et al.* 1987) and social interaction tests, although results in conflict tests (Deacon and Gardner 1986; Carli *et al.* 1988) are somewhat inconsistent. Although the 5-HT autoreceptor appears to be of the 5-HT$_{1B}$ type (Engel *et al.* 1986), the majority of 5-HT$_{1B}$ receptors are located post-synaptically (Brown *et al.* 1989).

TABLE 15.6. *Effects of inhibitors of 5-HT uptake and monoamine oxidase in anxiety tests in rats*

Drugs	Tests	Anxiolytic responses
5-Hydroxytryptophan	Conflict test	$+/-$
	Shock probe test	0
Fenfluramine	Elevated plus-maze	−
Fluoxetine	Conflict test	−
Paroxetine	Elevated plus-maze	−
Indalpine	Elevated plus-maze	−
Imipramine	Elevated plus-maze	0
Amitriptyline	Elevated plus-maze	0
Milnacipran	Elevated plus-maze	0
Clorgyline	Shock probe test	0
	Elevated plus-maze	0
Toloxatone	Elevated plus-maze	0
Pargyline	Shock probe test	0
	Elevated plus-maze	0
Selegiline	Shock probe test	0
(deprenyl)	Elevated plus-maze	0

The 5-HT$_2$ agonist, α-methyltryptamine, and the 5-HT$_2$/5-HT$_3$ agonist, quipazine, have been found to possess weak anxiogenic activity in the elevated plus-maze test (Handley and Mithani 1984; Chopin and Briley 1987; Pellow *et al.* 1987) and in a conflict test (Stein *et al.* 1975*b*). The serotonin precursor, 5-hydroxytryptophan (5-HTP), had varying effects in a conflict test depending on the doses used (Hjorth *et al.* 1987), whereas the serotonin releaser, fenfluramine, and the specific serotonin uptake inhibitors, paroxetine and indalpine, all increased anxiety in the elevated plus-maze test (Table 15.6) (Chopin and Briley 1987). Similar anxiogenic activity was found in a conflict test with fluoxetine (R. S. Feldman and L. F. Quenzer, unpublished results), another specific inhibitor of serotonin uptake. Interestingly, compounds that inhibit the uptake of both serotonin and noradrenaline, such as milnacipran (Moret *et al.* 1985) and the tricyclic antidepressants, imipramine and amitriptyline, have no specific effects on anxiety (Chopin and Briley 1987), suggesting that simultaneous stimulation of the noradrenergic system may attenuate the anxiogenic effect of serotonergic stimulation. Similarly, monoamine oxidase inhibitors, whether selective for the A or B form of the enzyme, appear to have no effect in animal models of anxiety (Meert and Colpaert 1986*a*; Chopin and Briley 1987).

Discussion

The data summarized here support a role for serotonin neurotransmission in the control of anxiety. In general, compounds that decrease serotonin neurotransmission produce anxiolytic effects whereas those that increase serotonin stimulation tend to increase anxiety. Unlike the actions of the benzodiazepines, however, these effects are relatively weak and often confined to a narrow dose range. The complicated situation found with compounds that act on 5-HT_{1A} receptors probably stems from the pre- and post-synaptic locations of these receptors which leads to opposing effects when the same compound is tested under different conditions.

Most of the animal tests of anxiety were developed, and thus optimized, for the benzodiazepines. What is considered to be an 'anxiolytic' activity may, in fact, be composed of any combination of anxiolytic, sedative, amnesic, anticonvulsant or myorelaxant elements. Any 'pure' anxiolytic compound may thus compare unfavourably with the benzodiazepines in these tests.

Despite an overall coherency, conflicting results have often been found. The narrow active dose range and the limited magnitude of the effect may explain some of the discrepancies between laboratories because small changes in experimental conditions may be enough to 'lose' an effect. Serotonin is known to play a major role in pain perception, aggression, and eating behaviour; these factors may contribute to the conflicting results obtained in tests that rely on the suppression of behaviour by conditioned fear of a specific painful punishment and disruptive factors such as electric shock, and food or water deprivation. The situation may also be complicated by the presence of functionally distinct serotonin pathways which may be involved in the control of anxiety. Furthermore, the general lack of selectivity of the currently available drugs inevitably complicates any mechanistic interpretation. This lack of selectivity may contribute to a weakening of the effect when a compound produces diametrically opposed effects (for example, at pre- or post-synaptic sites or as an agonist or antagonist). Thus the behavioural actions of drugs acting on the serotonin system may be very dependent on the experimental conditions (test, dose, time scale, species, etc.).

Finally, although the data show that drugs which act on the serotonin system can have significant effects in animal models of anxiety, the significance of this in predicting an effect on anxiety states in man remains, in most cases, to be demonstrated. Of the drugs discussed, only buspirone is marketed as an anxiolytic, its anxiolytic activity in man having been observed clinically before it was 'confirmed' by animal tests. Related compounds, such as ipsapirone and gepirone, have been shown in clinical trials to be potentially anxiolytic.

If the results of the animal tests presented here are predictive of an action in humans, one might expect anxiolytic or anxiogenic activities to be reported as side-effects for at least some of these drugs that are used clinically. However, an anxiolytic activity, especially if it is not accompanied by sedation, is not a side-effect of which patients would spontaneously complain. Most of the drugs for which one might predict an anxiogenic effect are prescribed as antidepressants (either experimentally or recently introduced) and are often co-administered with benzodiazepines. Nevertheless, anxiety and nervousness is one of the common side-effects of fluoxetine, a recently marketed antidepressant.

The involvement of serotonin in anxiety thus seems to be fairly certain. Furthermore, increased serotonergic neurotransmission appears to result in an increased level of anxiety. This obvious over-simplification presents a useful working hypothesis. Both clinical and fundamental research are providing new evidence that will enable us to define more accurately the nature of the involvement of serotonin in the control of anxiety.

Acknowledgement

The authors are grateful to Martine Dehaye for expert secretarial assistance.

References

Becker, H. C. (1986). Comparison of the effects of the benzodiazepine midazolam and three serotonin antagonists on a consummatory conflict paradigm. *Pharmacology Biochemistry and Behavior*, **24**, 1057–64.

Bradley, P. B., Engel, G., Feniuk, W., Fozard, J. R., Humphrey, P. A., Middlemiss, D. N., *et al.* (1986). Proposals for the classification and nomenclature of functional receptors for 5-hydroxytryptamine. *Neuropharmacology*, **25**, 563–76.

Broderick, P. and Lynch, V. (1982). Behavioral and biochemical changes induced by lithium and L-tryptophan in muricidal rats. *Neuropharmacology*, **21**, 671–80.

Brown, L. M., Smith, D. L., Williams, G. M., and Smith, D. J. (1989). Alterations in serotonin binding sites after 5,7-dihydroxytryptamine treatment in the rat spinal cord. *Neuroscience Letters*, **102**, 103–7.

Budhram, P., Deacon, R., and Garner, C. R. (1986). Some putative non-sedating anxiolytics in a conditioned licking conflict. *British Journal of Pharmacology*, **88**, 331P.

Carli, M. and Samanin, R. (1988). Potential anxiolytic properties of 8-hydroxy-2-(di-N-propylamino) tetralin, a selective serotonin$_{1A}$ receptor agonist. *Psychopharmacology*, **94**, 84–91.

Carli, M., Invernizzi, R., Cervo, L., and Samanin, R. (1988). Neurochemical and behavioural studies with RU-24969 in the rat. *Psychopharmacology*, **94**, 359–64.

Chase, T. N., Katz, R. I., and Kopin, I. J. (1970). Effect of diazepam on fate of intracisternally injected serotonin-C^{14}. *Neuropharmacology*, **9**, 103–8.

Chopin, P. and Briley, M. (1987). Animal models of anxiety: the effect of compounds that modify 5-HT neurotransmission. *Trends in Pharmacological Sciences*, **8**, 383–8.

Colpaert, F. C., Meert, T. F., Niemegeers, C. J. E., and Janssen, P. A. J. (1985). Behavioural and 5-HT antagonist effects of ritanserin: a pure and selective antagonist of LSD discrimination in rats. *Psychopharmacology*, **86**, 45–54.

Costall, B., Domeney, A. M., Kelly, M. E., Naylor, R. J., and Tyers, M. B. (1987*a*).

The behavioural consequences of treatment with selective 5-HT$_3$ receptor antagonists. *British Journal of Pharmacology*, **92**, 657P.

Costall, B., Domeney, A. M., Hendrie, C. A., Kelly, M. E., Naylor, R. J., and Tyers, M. B. (1987*b*). The anxiolytic activity of GR 38032F in the mouse and marmoset. *British Journal of Pharmacology*, **90**, 257.

Costall, B., Domeney, A. M., Kelly, M. E., Naylor, R. J., and Tyers, M. B. (1988*a*). Effects of the 5-HT$_3$ receptor antagonists GR 38023F, ICS 205–930 and BRL 43694 in tests for anxiolytic activity. *British Journal of Pharmacology*, **93**, 195P.

Costall, B., Domeney, A. M., Gerrard, P. A., Kelly, M. E., and Naylor, R. J. (1988*b*). Zacopride: an anxiolytic profile in rodent and primate models of anxiety. *Journal of Pharmacy and Pharmacology*, **40**, 302–5.

Costall, B., Kelly, M. E., Naylor, R. J., and Onaivi, E. S. (1988*c*). Actions of buspirone in a putative model of anxiety in the mouse. *Journal of Pharmacy and Pharmacology*, **40**, 494–500.

Critchley, M. A. E. and Handley, S. L. (1986). 5-HT$_2$ receptor antagonists show anxiolytic activity in the X-maze. *British Journal of Pharmacology*, **89**, 646P.

Critchley, M. A. E. and Handley, S. L. (1987*a*). 5-HT$_{1A}$ ligand effects in the X-maze anxiety test. *British Journal of Pharmacology*, **92**, 660P.

Critchley, M. A. E. and Handley, S. L. (1987*b*). Effects in the X-maze anxiety model of agents acting at 5-HT$_1$ and 5-HT$_2$ receptors. *Psychopharmacology*, **93**, 502–6.

Critchley, M. A. E. and Handley, S. L. (1989). Dorsal raphe lesions abolish effects of 8-OH-DPAT and ipsapirone in X-maze. *British Journal of Pharmacology*, **96**, 309P.

Critchley, M. A. E., Njung'e, K., and Handley, S. L. (1987). 5-HT ligand effects in the social interaction test of anxiety. *British Journal of Pharmacology*, **92**, 659P.

Csanalosi, I., Schweizer, E., Case, W. G., and Rickels, K. (1987). Gepirone in anxiety: a pilot study. *Journal of Clinical and Psychopharmacology*, **7**, 31–3.

Deacon, R. and Gardner, C. R. (1986). Benzodiazepine and 5-HT ligands in a rat conflict test. *British Journal of Pharmacology*, **88**, 330P.

Dumbrille-Ross, A., Tang, S. W., and Coscina, D. V. (1982). Lack of effect of raphe lesions on serotonin S$_2$ receptor changes induced by amitriptyline and desmethylimipramine. *Psychiatry Research*, **7**, 145–51.

Eison, A. S., Eison, M. S., Stanley, M., and Riblet, L. A. (1986). Serotonergic mechanisms in the behavioural effects of buspirone and gepirone. *Pharmacology Biochemistry and Behavior*, **24**, 701–7.

Engel, J. A. (1986). Anticonflict effect of the putative serotonin receptor agonist 8-OH-DPAT. *Psychopharmacology*, **89**, S13.

Engel, G., Göthert, M., Hoyer, D., Schlicker, E., and Hillenbrand, K. (1986). Identity of inhibitory presynaptic 5-hydroxytryptamine (5-HT) autoreceptors in the rat brain cortex with 5-HT$_{1B}$ binding sites. *Naunyn-Schmiedeberg's Archives of Pharmacology*, **332**, 1–7.

File, S. E. (1980). The use of social interactions as a method for detecting anxiolytic activity of chlordiazepoxide-like drugs. *Journal of Neuroscience Methods*, **2**, 219–38.

File, S. E. (1981). Behavioural effects of serotonin depletion. In *Metabolic disorders of the nervous system*, (ed. E. Clifford Rose), pp. 429–445, Pitman, London.

File, S. E. (1984). The neurochemistry of anxiety. In *Drugs in psychiatry*, (ed. G. D. Burrows, T. R. Norman, and B. Davies), pp. 13–32. Elsevier, Amsterdam.

File, S. E. and Johnston, A. L. (1989). Lack of effects of 5-HT$_3$ antagonists in social interaction and elevated plus-maze tests of anxiety. *Psychopharmacology*, **99**, 248–51.

File, S. E. and Hyde, J. R. G. (1977). The effects of p-chlorophenylalanine and ethanolamine-O-sulphate in an animal test of anxiety. *Journal of Pharmacy and Pharmacology*, **29**, 735–8.

File, S. E., Hyde, J. R., and Macleod, N. K. (1979). 5,7-Dihydroxytryptamine lesions of dorsal and median raphe nuclei and performance in the social interaction test of anxiety and in a home-cage aggression test. *Journal of Affective Disorders*, **1**, 115–22.

Gardner, C. R. and Guy, A. P. (1985). Pharmacological characterisation of a modified social interaction model of anxiety in the rat. *Neuropsychobiology*, **13**, 194–200.

Geller, I. and Seifter, J. (1960). The effects of meprobamate, barbiturates, d-amphetamine and promazine on experimentally induced conflict in the rat. *Psychopharmacologia*, **1**, 482–92.

Geller, I. and Hartmann, R. J. (1982). Effects of buspirone on operant behaviour of laboratory rats and cynomolgus monkeys. *Journal of Clinical Psychiatry*, **43**, 25–32.

Goldberg, H. L. and Finnerty, R. J. (1979). The comparative efficacy of buspirone and diazepam in the treatment of anxiety. *American Journal of Psychiatry*, **136**, 1184–7.

Goldberg, M. E., Salama, A. I., Patel, J. B., and Malick, J. B. (1983). Novel non-benzodiazepine anxiolytics. *Neuropharmacology*, **22**, 1499–504.

Graeff, F. G. and Schoenfeld, R.I. (1970). Tryptaminergic mechanisms in punished and nonpunished behavior. *Journal of Pharmacology and Experimental Therapeutics*, **173**, 277–83.

Handley, S. L. and Mithani, S. (1984). Effects of alpha-adrenoceptor agonists and antagonists in a maze-exploration model of 'fear'-motivated behaviour. *Naunyn-Schmiedeberg's Archives of Pharmacology*, **327**, 1–5.

Hayes, P. E. and Schulz, S. C. (1987). Beta-blockers in anxiety disorders. *Journal of Affective Disorders*, **13**, 119–30.

Herrick-Davis, K. and Titeler, M. (1988). Detection and characterization of the serotonin 5-HT$_{1D}$ receptor in rat and human brain. *Journal of Neurochemistry*, **50**, 1624–31.

Hibert, M. and Middlemiss, D. N. (1986). Stereoselective blockade at the 5-HT autoreceptor and inhibition of radioligand binding to central 5-HT recognition sites by the optical isomers of methiothepin. *Neuropharmacology*, **25**, 1–4.

Higgins, G. A., Jones, B. J., and Oakley, N. R. (1987). Compounds selective for the 5-HT$_{1A}$ receptors have anxiolytic effects when injected into the dorsal raphe nucleus of the rat. *British Journal of Pharmacology*, **92**, 658P.

Hjorth, S., Söderpalm, B., and Engel, J.A. (1987). Biphasic effect of L-5HTP in the Vogel conflict model. *Psychopharmacology*, **92**, 96–9.

Jones, B. J., Costall, B., Domeney, A. M., Kelly, M. E., Naylor, R. J., Oakley, N. R., and Tyers, M. B. (1988). The potential anxiolytic activity of GR 38032F, a 5-HT$_3$ receptor antagonist. *British Journal of Pharmacology*, **93**, 985–93.

Kilpatrick, G. J., Jones, B. J., and Tyers, M. B. (1987). Identification and distribution of 5-HT$_3$ receptors in rat brain using radioligand binding. *Nature*, **330**, 746–8.

Leonhardt, S., Herrick-Davis, K., and Titeler, M. (1989). Detection of a novel serotonin receptor subtype (5-HT$_{1E}$) in human brain. Interactions with a GTP-binding protein. *Journal of Neurochemistry*, **53**, 465–71.

Meert, T. F. and Colpaert, F. C. (1986*a*). The shock probe conflict procedure. A new assay responsive to benzodiazepines, barbiturates and related compounds. *Psychopharmacology*, **88**, 445–50.

Meert, T. F. and Colpaert, F. C. (1986*b*). A pharmacological evaluation of the selected emotional defecation and micturation test. *Psychopharmacology*, **89**, S23.

Merlo Pich, E. and Samanin, R. (1986). Disinhibitory effects of buspirone and low doses of sulpiride and haloperidol in two experimental anxiety models in rats: possible role of dopamine. *Psychopharmacology*, **89**, 125–30.

Middlemiss, D. N. (1984). Stereoselective blockade at [³H]-5-HT binding sites and at the 5-HT autoreceptors by propranolol. *European Journal of Pharmacology*, **101**, 289–93.

Moret, C., Charveron, M., Finberg, J. P. M., Couzinier, J. P., and Briley, M. (1985). Biochemical profile of midalcipran (F 2207), 1-phenyl-1-diethyl-aminocarbonyl-2-aminomethyl-cyclopropane (Z) hydrochloride, a potential fourth generation antidepressant drug. *Neuropharmacology*, **12**, 1211–19.

Moser, P., Hibert, M., Middlemiss, D. N., Mir, A. K., Tricklebank, M. D., and Fozard, J. R. (1988). Effects of MDL 73005EF in animal models predictive of anxiolytic activity. *British Journal of Pharmacology*, **93**, 3P.

Offord, S. J., Ordway, G. A., and Frazer, A. (1988). Application of ¹²⁵I iodocyano-pindolol to measure 5-hydroxytryptamine (1B) receptors in the brain of the rat. *Journal of Pharmacology and Experimental Therapeutics*, **244**, 144–53.

Olivier, B., Schipper, J., and Tulp, M. Th. M. (1986). 5-Hydroxytryptamine agonists: neurochemical profile and effects on agressive behaviour. *British Journal of Pharmacology*, **89**, 648P.

Pellow, S., Chopin, P., File, S. E., and Briley, M. (1985). Validation of open:closed arm entries in an elevated plus-maze as a measure of anxiety in the rat. *Journal of Neuroscience Methods*, **14**, 149–67.

Pellow, S., Johnston, A. L., and File, S. E. (1987). Selective agonists and antagonists for 5-hydroxytryptamine receptor subtypes and interactions with yohimbine and FG 7142 using the elevated plus-maze test in the rat. *Journal of Pharmacy and Pharmacology*, **39**, 917–28.

Peroutka, S. J. and Hamik, A. (1988). ³H-Quipazine labels 5-HT₃ recognition sites in rat cortical membranes. *European Journal of Pharmacology*, **148**, 297–9.

Petersen, E. N. and Lassen, J. B. (1981). A water lick conflict paradigm using drug experienced rats. *Psychopharmacology*, **75**, 236–9.

Piper, D., Upton, N., Thomas, D., and Nicholass, J. (1988). The effects of the 5-HT₃ receptor antagonists BRL 43694 and GR 38032F in animal behavioural models of anxiety. *British Journal of Pharmacology*, **94**, 314P.

Stein, L., Wise, C. D., and Belluzzi, J. D. (1975a). Effects of benzodiazepines on central serotonergic mechanisms. In *Mechanism of action of benzodiazepines* (ed. E. Costa and P. Greengard), pp. 29–44. Raven Press, New York.

Stein, L., Wise, C. D., and Belluzzi, J. D. (1975b). Effects of benzodiazepines on central serotonergic mechanisms. *Advances in Biochemistry and Psycopharmacology*, **14**, 29–44.

Traber, J. and Glaser, T. (1987). 5-HT₁ₐ receptor-related anxiolytics. *Trends in Pharmacological Sciences*, **8**, 432–7.

Traber, J., Davies, M. A., Dompert, W. U., Glaser, T., Schuurman, T., and Seidel, P. R. (1984). Brain serotonin receptors as a target for the putative anxiolytic TVXQ 7821. *Brain Research Bulletin*, **12**, 741–4.

Treit, D. (1985). Animal models for the study of anti-anxiety agents: a review. *Neuroscience Behavioral Reviews*, **9**, 203–22.

Tye, N. C., Everitt, B. J., and Iversen, S. D. (1977). 5-Hydroxytryptamine and punishment. *Nature*, **268**, 741–3.

Tyers, M. B., Costall, B., Domeney, A. M., Jones, B. J., Kelly, M. E., Naylor, R.

J., and Oakley, N. R. (1987). The anxiolytic acitivities of 5-HT$_3$ antagonists in laboratory animals. *Neuroscience Letters*, **29**, S68.

Vogel, J. R., Beer, D., and Clody, D. E. (1971). A simple and reliable conflict procedure for testing anti-anxiety agents. *Psychopharmacologia*, **21**, 1–7.

Young, R., Urbancic, A., Emrey, T. A., Hall, P. C., and Metcalf, G. (1987). Behavioural effects of several new anxiolytics and putative anxiolytics. *European Journal of Pharmacology*, **143**, 361–71.

Appendix: Animal models of anxiety

Conflict tests

In a typical conflict test (Geller and Seifter 1960), food-deprived animals are trained to press a bar to obtain food. Food is given during either a 'non-conflict period', where responses are rewarded with food, or a 'conflict period', which is signalled by a lamp and/or buzzer and where responses are both rewarded with food and punished with an electric shock in the foot. Typically there is a selective inhibition of behaviour and rats confine most of their responses to the non-conflict period. Other conflict paradigms involve inhibition of drinking by electric shock in water-deprived rats (Vogel *et al.* 1971). Benzodiazepines and related compounds attentuate the response inhibition. It has been reported that benzodiazepines have stimulatory effects on appetitive and ingestive behaviour. Thus, the 'anticonflict' effects of benzodiazepines can arise from a specific inhibition of fear motivation (electric shock), a specific facilitatory effect on food or water motivation, an effect on the sensitivity to pain, or from any combinations of these factors (Treit 1985).

Shock probe conflict test   Rats are placed in a novel environment which contains a probe (Meert and Colpaert 1986*a*). The exploration of the probe is reduced when the probe is electrified. Benzodiazepines block this inhibition. This procedure has the advantage that it requires no food or water deprivation and is thus insensitive to changes in appetite.

Social interaction test

Two male rats are placed in a neutral area and the time they spend in active social interaction (e.g., sniffing, following, grooming the partner) is scored. The inhibition of social interaction observed when the experimental area is unfamiliar or brightly lit is attenuated by anxiolytic drugs (File 1980), such as benzodiazepines. In this test, sedation interferes seriously with the measurement of anxiolytic activity.

Two-compartment exploration test

This test uses the aversion of mice and rats to large, brightly lit areas. A cage is separated into two compartments, one dark, the other brightly lit. Rodents show a clear preference for the dark area. Anxiolytic drugs increase the crossings between the two compartments.

Elevated plus-maze test

This test is based on the fact that exposure to an elevated and open maze arm leads to an approach-avoidance conflict that is considerably stronger than that evoked by exposure to an enclosed maze arm. The apparatus consists of a plus-maze elevated to a height of 50 cm with two open and two (opposite) closed arms. The number of entries into the open arms as a percentage of the total entries provides a measure of fear-induced inhibition of exploratory activity. This value is increased by anxiolytics and reduced by anxiogenic compounds (Pellow *et al.* 1985).

Most animal tests of anxiety have only been subjected to pharmacological validation. Their ability to predict a clinical effect has usually been limited to a single chemical class, the benzodiazepines. Thus, while certain tests may reliably detect compounds with benzodiazepine-like activity, they might not be useful for selecting anxiolytic compounds with other profiles. A test only validated with benzodiazepines may, in fact, reflect any one of the different behavioural effects of the benzodiazepines.

The social interaction test and the elevated plus-maze test possess several clear advantages over other paradigms. They are based on spontaneous behaviour and therefore do not require training or the use of noxious stimuli, such as electric shock, or manipulation of appetitive behaviours, such as food or water deprivation. Moreover, they have been the subject of pharmacological, behavioural, and physiological validation.

Discussion

SULSER: I understand that in animal tests increased serotonergic activity is anxiogenic and a decreased synaptic availability is usually anxiolytic. I was taught by Manfred Bleuler 30 years ago that anxiety is a core symptom of depression. If this is true, it is difficult to reconcile animal data with the available clinical data. For example, how can fluoxetine be a good antidepressant if from animal data it is thought to increase anxiety? According to animal studies, *para*-chlorophenylalanine (*p*-CPA) is quite anxiolytic. However, Shopsin *et al.* (1976) reported that in man *p*-CPA nullifies the therapeutic activity of tricyclic antidepressants and monoamine oxidase (MAO) inhibitors, with Hamilton scores showing an increase in anxiety. Obviously, it is difficult to extrapolate from the animal studies to man.

BRILEY: There may be different types of anxiety; generalized anxiety or anxiety alone may not be exactly analogous to anxiety in depression.

MURPHY: Anxiety and irritability are side-effects in about 20 per cent of patients treated with fluoxetine. However, anxiety as a component of the depressive syndrome responds as well to fluoxetine as it does to conventional tricyclic and other antidepressants.

CURZON: I have often wondered how it could be that drugs that are supposed to act on depression by releasing 5-hydroxytryptamine (5-HT, serotonin) or inhibiting

5-HT re-uptake are not also markedly anxiogenic if anxiety occurs when a post-synaptic 5-HT-dependent site is activated. Indeed, acute treatment with fenfluramine (Targum and Marshall 1989) or clomipramine (see discussion in Zohar *et al.* 1988) is reported to increase symptoms in patients with panic disorder and obsessive-compulsive disorder, respectively. One factor to be considered is that the 5-HT site at which activation is anxiogenic can be desensitized when 5-HT release is increased. Thus, chronic clomipramine treatment decreased the anxiogenic effect of *m*-chlorophenylpiperazine (*m*-CPP) (Zohar *et al.* 1988).

LINNOILA: When we try to relate these animal models to human conditions, the time course of treatment is important. In humans, 5-HT$_{1A}$ agonists do not work acutely. If the animal model mimics the human condition there should be a better response after chronic rather than acute use of the drug. It amazes me that decisions about whether these drugs are anxiolytic are based on single administration.

In his studies of the startle response in rats as a model of anxiety, Dr M. Davis can, with the same receptor-active drugs, potentiate or block the startle response, depending on whether he applies the drugs to spinal cord or in certain areas of the brain. Thus it might be better not to administer drugs systemically.

Patients with panic disorder tolerate fluoxetine, like the tricyclic antidepressants, very poorly. However, by using a sub-threshold dose (as low as 2.5 mg per day) which does not produce anxiety and increasing the dose gradually, as one would with tricyclic antidepressants, one can get genuine antipanic efficacy. Thus, down-regulation phenomena are probably involved in the anxiolytic effects, especially the antipanic effects, of these drugs.

A controlled double-blind study of specific 5-HT re-uptake inhibitors in generalized anxiety should be done in a similar way to the studies which showed that the long-term efficacy of imipramine and amitriptyline, even in generalized anxiety, is greater than that of the benzodiazepines.

COPPEN: I have been using tryptophan in the treatment of depression for about 30 years. Tryptophan significantly enhances the antidepressant effect of MAO inhibitors (Coppen *et al.* 1963). Many of us, certainly in the UK, have continued this strategy in patients over many years and we have rarely seen increased anxiety. In this treatment the CNS is flooded with 5-HT.

SULSER: Does lithium, which also enhances serotonergic activity and can enhance the therapeutic efficacy of tricyclic antidepressants, enhance anxiety?

COPPEN: No, lithium does not increase anxiety.

BRILEY: MAO inhibitors are neither anxiogenic nor anxiolytic. Professor Coppen, presumably you were using drugs that were not selective between 5-HT and noradrenaline?

COPPEN: Yes; we originally used tranylcypromine.

BRILEY: From the results with the uptake inhibitors it seems that a noradrenergic component in a drug cancels the anxiogenic effects of the 5-HT stimulation. I don't understand this, but an equilibrium between the two systems appears to attentuate any anxiogenic effect.

COPPEN: It would be interesting to look at one of the more specific MAO inhibitors with augmentation.

MENDLEWICZ: In a controlled study on the use of the MAO-B inhibitor, deprenyl, with 5-hydroxytryptophan, we showed antidepressant efficacy without anxiogenesis.

YOUDIM: But l-deprenyl increases human brain dopamine (Riederer and Youdim 1986). Perhaps there is a counterbalance because of effects on the dopamine system.

GUARDIOLA-LEMAITRE: Tianeptine enhances 5-HT uptake with an antidepressant activity but also has anxiolytic effects.

LÓPEZ-IBOR: We don't know how many different types of anxiety there are. Generalized anxiety, as currently defined, might be described as a waste basket of conditions. The mixed depression/anxiety syndrome is an even more difficult category. The action of drugs differs in these syndromes. MAO inhibitors may be anxiogenic in endogenous and severe major depressive patients, but they are effective anxiolytics in so-called atypical depression.

We have been training our students to diagnose the levels of anxiety and inhibition in depressed patients and to prescribe more sedative or less sedative antidepressants accordingly. But every study has shown that after two or three weeks of treatment the outcome is not related to how anxious the depression was or what kind of tricyclic antidepressants was prescribed (Beckman 1981). So the time course is important.

I agree with Dr Linnoila's comment about using small doses. My impression is that most selective 5-HT re-uptake blockers are too specific for current clinical practice. Therefore, if high doses are used, many problems may arise. This is similar to treatment of endocrinological disorders where titration of a hormone is a delicate matter. Whereas giving twice the dose of a tricyclic antidepressant is not critical, with some of the newer drugs, such as buspirone in patients with generalized anxiety, too high an initial dose will often lead to anxiety.

SULSER: Are you saying that the 'dirty' drugs are better?

LÓPEZ-IBOR: Yes and no. Yes, taking into account current clinical practice and the expectations of both clinicians and patients. No, because the practice will change as more is known about the physiopathology of the disorder. A patient might not respond to buspirone because he was previously on benzodiazepines. This is a difficult problem. The animal experiments are valid for acute effects, but we need to know what happens after two or three weeks or even months of treatment, and how that depends on the basic condition of the patient.

MURPHY: Not only with anxiety but also with readily measured physiological responses, one can sometimes see dose-dependent reversal of the response. For example, low doses of non-selective 5-HT agonists, such as 5-methoxy-N,N-dimethyltryptamine (5-MeO-DMT), elicit hyperthermia, whereas medium doses have no temperature effect, and high doses produce hypothermia. More selectivity is seen by comparing the temperature changes induced by 8-hydroxy-N, N-dipropyl-2-aminotetralin (8-OH-DPAT) and m-CPP in rodents. With m-CPP, one sees a dose-dependent increase in temperature, which we also found in humans. However, a dose-dependent hypothermia is seen in both rodents and humans with buspirone and other 5-HT$_{1A}$ agonists. By careful titration of doses of agents that are only relatively selective, it seems possible to obtain opposite physiological and perhaps psychological changes.

MAÎTRE: Is it possible to recognize a systematic biological pattern for substances that are active in punished behaviour test systems compared with substances that are active in tests using positive rewards?

BRILEY: There does not seem to be a generalized effect. In the past everybody talked about test selectively, but as more drugs are used on more systems the only test selectivity that seems to stand up is that the 5-HT$_3$ antagonists do not work on the elevated plus-maze, which is based on inherent behaviour rather than positive or negative reward.

LINNOILA: There are confounding factors in the punish and reward paradigms with these drugs, particularly the 5-HT$_{1A}$ agonists. The analgesic activity will confound the electric shock, and even very small intracerebroventricular doses of 8-OH-DPAT produce hyperglycaemia in the rat, which makes the animal less likely to seek sucrose. If one ignores these factors one gets misleading results.

EVENDEN: These drugs have effects in almost any test that is used. It is not true to say that the effects on anxiety are selective. There are conflicting results in all sorts of tests. For example, Dr Linnoila has just suggested that rats should be less interested in food when treated with 8-OH-DPAT, but both Professor Curzon's group (Dourish *et al.* 1985) and I (unpublished data) have found that 8-OH-DPAT increases feeding. So there is a difference between the effect of the drug suggested by a biochemical aspect of its action and the results of other behavioural tests. We should study the interactions between various tests, and the many different effects of the drugs across these tests.

DEAKIN: It has been suggested that excessive 5-HT neurotransmission is associated with anxiety and that deficient 5-HT neurotransmission is associated with depression. In fact, the symptoms of anxiety and depression go together; symptoms of anxiety point to a high probability of symptoms of depression, and vice versa. In community surveys of minor affective morbidity, anxiety and depression cannot be separated. It is a real paradox. The best treatment for both conditions is a tricyclic antidepressant. Benzodiazepines have short-term effects. How does that fit with your concept of 5-HT in anxiety, Dr Briley? How does a tricyclic antidepressant dampen the 5-HT system? My answer is that we have to look at the different 5-HT subsystems. We must consider the dorsal raphe nucleus 5-HT$_2$ system as distinct from the median raphe nucleus 5-HT$_1$ system. Everything that you discuss can be explained by anxiogenesis arising from excessive stimulation of the 5-HT$_2$ family of receptors and anxiolysis arising from damping down the 5-HT$_2$ family in the dorsal raphe nucleus system.

BRILEY: I am not sure that 5-HT deficiency causes depression. We are confusing acute and chronic effects. We tend to say that antidepressants are 5-HT stimulants, in the general sense of the term, and that therefore depression must involve a lack of 5-HT. But these drugs work after chronic administration; we are getting down-regulation. So perhaps we can say that depression is an excess of 5-HT, in which case the paradox disappears.

DEAKIN: But Claude de Montigny's work showed that all antidepressants given long-term enhance rather than down-regulate function in the 5-HT$_1$ receptor family (de Montigny and Aghajanian 1978).

MELTZER: We shall jeopardize the credibility of psychopharmacology if we do not try to reconcile some of the inconsistencies and paradoxes in our theories of antidepressant drug action! Claude de Montigny has tried to explain the actions of all antidepressants by a serotonergic model. He suggests that buspirone and gepirone shut down the raphe acutely, and that chronic treatment produces desensitization of this effect, leading to enhanced serotonergic activity from post-synaptic receptor stimulation. That is inconsistent with the role of 5-HT in anxiety where more 5-HT should worsen anxiety. We cannot have it both ways. Dr Linnoila made the point that if we increase the dose of fluoxetine slowly we get down-regulation and less serotonergic activity. But it seems from the antidepressant effect and the neuroendocrine data that there is tremendous potentiation, at least in some systems, from fluoxetine. So either we are going to say that the drugs are doing diametrically opposite things in the same person at different times in different regions, which may be the case, or we have to reject one or more of these conclusions about antidepressant action.

LINNOILA: Nobody expected panic disorder patients to experience increased anxiety after low doses of 5-HT re-uptake inhibitors; the hypotheses were heavily weighted towards the noradrenaline system, and it was thought that panic patients were particularly supersensitive to desipramine or imipramine. Something must be subsensitive over time; some adaptation takes place. Panic disorder is the purest form of anxiety disorder. Most patients with panic disorder show suppression in dexamethasone suppression tests and do not have altered monoamine functions. Biochemical abnormalities in these systems are known biological correlates of certain kinds of depression which often respond to treatment with specific 5-HT re-uptake inhibitors and specific noradrenaline re-uptake inhibitors. This is particularly true for endogenous depression or major unipolar depression with melancholia. Thus, we cannot get away from the fact that the drugs that affect relatively specifically either the serotonin system or the noradrenaline system seem to have efficacy in both anxiety and depression, even when the disorders exist in their purest forms.

ROBINSON: I wonder whether this paradox might be explained by a concentration or dose phenomenon. Some partial agonists are on a spectrum between agonism and antagonism. It is conceivable that de Montigny's results, for example, reflect the fact that he studied a limited range of doses in the animal models. If the pathophysiology of anxiety disorders is some kind of a serotonin excess, it is conceivable that at the right dose the partial agonist would start to produce anxiolytic activity. The reverse could be true, for example, in depressive disorders, where there may be a relative functional deficiency.

Perhaps the anxiety symptoms of depressive disorders ought to be differentiated pathophysiologically, if it were possible, from anxiety symptoms of anxiety disorders. These seemingly paradoxical effects might depend on the underlying pathophysiology.

DEAKIN: There is evidence that panic disorder is different from other forms of anxiety, although it does seem to emerge in the course of depressive illness. I don't think that other symptoms of anxiety are distinct from depressive symptoms. They are all symptoms of minor affective disturbance. Very few people have generalized anxiety without symptoms of depression, either at the same time or emerging during the course of their lifetime disturbance.

MENDLEWICZ: The tricyclic antidepressants are efficient in treating these anxiety disorders in the long term. But one of the acute, rapid effects of these drugs is improvement in sleep, even before there is an improvement in the depression. But one would not say that the tricyclics should be used as hypnotics. By the same reasoning, lithium, which is one of the most efficient mood-stabilizing drugs, would be efficient in generalized anxiety disorders. But lithium has not been shown to be efficient against anxiety.

DEAKIN: I am not sure what lithium does to 5-HT$_1$ and 5-HT$_2$ neurotransmission.

MENDLEWICZ: But, as Arvid Carlsson has said, we cannot discuss anxiety simply in terms of serotonin.

DEAKIN: I agree; we have to bring in other neurotransmitters or look at the receptor subtypes.

CARLSSON: One cause of our confusion is that we are discussing certain drugs as if they are tools. We do not know for sure how the tricyclic antidepressants work, although there are some likely hypotheses, such as uptake inhibition. They are excellent drugs but they cannot be used to identify mechanisms. This is true for many other drugs; even buspirone is a 'dirty' drug. However, buspirone and the related drugs are the only ones that we can use in man at present. We are waiting for more specific 5-HT$_{1A}$ agonists.

GLOVER: The evidence, as I see it, is that in anxiety there is over-activity of a serotonergic system in the hippocampus; in depression, from the challenge tests, there is under-activity of a serotonergic system in the hypothalamus. Could there be two different serotonergic pathways, with over-activity in one causing feedback inhibition in the other? This model could explain the paradox of the coexistence of anxiety and depression, the former associated with excessive 5-HT neurotransmission, the latter with under-activity. It could also explain how one drug could help both types of symptom.

MURPHY: There certainly is evidence (Murphy, this volume) for at least two serotonin subsystems, but how they interact is not clear.

FRAZER: The site-specific injection approach in both behavioural and neurochemical experiments might be important in clarifying some of the disparate results. The plasma levels of these drugs achieved in animals tend to be much higher than those usually achieved clinically; some systems might be affected in preclinical experiments and yet hardly be altered clinically. Also, drugs given systemically reach many sites and the effect measured is likely to be a composite of all the actions. Site-specific injection could give us a more precise picture of the effects mediated by particular areas of the brain.

We also need more information from clinicians as to specific effects of drugs on psychiatric syndromes. Behaviourally, for example, how do antidepressants improve depression? On which components of this syndrome must antidepressants work to cause an overall improvement in depression? Do these various components improve simultaneously, or are there some which improve early and are necessary to initiate total improvement? We could then consider whether there are important target symptoms for drug action. In the NIMH-sponsored collaborative study of the psychobiology of depression, Dr M. Katz found that it was the early improvement in anxiety and hostility that differentiated those patients who ultimately had a good response to amitriptyline from those who did not. In contrast, sleep improved regardless of the ultimate response. A consistent body of such data would be helpful for studying the underlying mechanism of action of antidepressants.

DOOGAN: We have not properly addressed in animal experimentation the complex interaction between dose and time. The result is a series of observations which lead to partial truth and perhaps partial progress. When a compound is presented to me for development I don't know whether to study it in anxiety, depression, or panic disorder. In clinical studies I find that the predictions from animal experiments do not hold true. When we investigate whether a drug is a sedative antidepressant or a sedative anxiolytic, we find that after four weeks of therapy with some of these drugs the sedative action is tolerated. Fluvoxamine and fluoxetine cause anxiety after acute administration but the effect becomes tolerated. The tricyclic antidepressants are sedative initially. I think that is why the insomnia is resolved rapidly, which explains why the onset of action of these antidepressants is quicker than for specific non-sedative drugs. A new compound must be tried clinically under all these conditions before we can say that the human results have confirmed the animal experiments.

LINNOILA: Protriptyline and desipramine are both non-sedative tricyclics that work on depression and panic disorder.

References

Beckman, H. (1981). Die medicamentose Therapie der Depressionen. *Der Nerven-artz*, **2**, 135–46.

Coppen, A., Shaw, D., and Farrell, J. P. (1963). The potentiation of the antidepressant effect of monoamine oxidase inhibitors by tryptophan. *Lancet*, **i**, 79–81.

Dourish, C. T., Hutson, P. H., and Curzon, G. (1985). Low doses of the putative serotonin agonist 8-hydroxy-2-(di-*N*-propylamino)tetralin (8-OH-DPAT) elicit feeding in the rat. *Psychopharmacology*, **86**, 197.

de Montigny, C. and Aghajanian, G. K. (1978). Tricyclic antidepressants: long term treatment increases responsivity of rat forebrain neurons to serotonin. *Science*, **202**, 1203–6.

Murphy, D. L. (1991). An overview of serotonin neurochemistry and neuroanatomy. In *5-Hydroxytryptamine in psychiatry: a spectrum of ideas*, (ed. M. Sandler, A. Coppen and S. Harnett), pp. 23–36. Oxford University Press.

Riederer, P. and Youdim, M. B. H. (1986). Monoamine oxidase activity and monoamine metabolism in brains of Parkinson patients treated with l-deprenyl. *Journal of Neurochemistry*, **46**, 1359–65.

Shopsin, B., Friedman, E., and Gershon, S. (1976). *Para*-chlorophenylalanine reversal of tranylcypromine effects in depressed patients. *Archives of General Psychiatry*, **33**, 811–19.

Targum, S. D. and Marshall, L. E. (1989). Fenfluramine provocation of anxiety in patients with panic disorder. *Psychiatry Research*, **28**, 295–306.

Zohar, J., Insel, T. R., Zohar-Kadouch, R. C., Hill, J. L., and Murphy, D. L. (1988). Serotonergic responsivity in obsessive-compulsive disorders. Effects of chronic clomipramine treatment. *Archives of General Psychiatry*, **45**, 167–72.

16. Anxiogenic effect of the 5-HT$_{1C}$ agonist m-chlorophenylpiperazine

G. Curzon, G. A. Kennett, and P. Whitton

Introduction

The earlier literature on 1-(3-chlorophenyl)piperazine (m-CPP) and 1-[3-(trifluoromethyl)phenyl]piperazine (TFMPP) describes these compounds mainly as agonists at the 1B subtype of 5-hydroxytryptamine (5-HT, serotonin) receptors (e.g. Sills *et al*. 1984; McKenny and Glennon 1986). However, many findings suggest that their hypolocomotor (Kennett and Curzon 1988*a*) and hypophagic (Kennett and Curzon 1988*b*; Curzon, this volume) effects are mediated by stimulation of 5-HT$_{1C}$ receptors.

As m-CPP causes anxiety in humans (Mueller *et al*. 1985; Charney *et al*. 1987) we investigated whether m-CPP and TFMPP had anxiogenic-like effects in rats. The results indicate that this occurs and is mediated by hippocampal 5-HT$_{1C}$ receptors.

Materials and methods

Male Sprague-Dawley rats (200–250 g, Charles River, UK) were individually housed under a 12 h light/dark cycle (lights on at 06.00) at 20 ± 2 °C, with free access to food and water for at least five days before the drugs were given. The rats were injected in their holding rooms and tested in a separate, quiet room as follows.

Social interaction was scored under red light in a box with opaque walls on three sides and a glass front and top (height 30 cm; depth 27 cm; length 60 cm; base divided into six rectangles, 13.5 cm × 20 cm). On each of the two days immediately before experimentation, the rats were individually habituated to the box for ten minutes. On the third day they were injected subcutaneously in weight-matched pairs (difference < 10 g) between 10.00 and 13.30 with a 5-HT receptor antagonist or vehicle and returned to their home cages. Twenty minutes later they were injected intraperitoneally (i.p.) with m-CPP or 0.9 per cent NaCl, and again returned to their home cage. After a further 20 min, they were placed with their pair-mate in the social interaction box, and their behaviour over the next 15 min was recorded (camera and video-recorder). The total interaction times were measured using stopwatches and hand-held counters. Their locomotion (numbers of rectangles crossed) was also measured.

When *m*-CPP was given centrally, the procedure was as above except that the rats were anaesthetized (pentobarbitone, Sagatal, May and Baker, 60 mg kg^{-1} i.p.) and a guide cannula was implanted 1 mm above one of the following sites of infusion (coordinates from Paxinos and Watson 1982): third ventricle, -1.3 mm (bregma), L 0.0 mm, H 3.8 mm below dura; hippocampus, -4.0 mm (bregma), L 2.9 mm, H 3.0 mm below dura; amygdala (central nucleus), -1.8 mm, (bregma), L 3.8 mm, H 7.0 mm below dura. The guides were fitted with dummy cannulae and the rats were placed in perspex individual cages (26 cm cube) and allowed five days to recover before further experimentation. On the experimental day the dummy cannulae were removed and infusion cannulae were inserted so that they projected 1 mm past the tip of the guide cannula.

Pairs of rats were infused at 1 μl min^{-1} for 1 min with 0.9 per cent NaCl or *m*-CPP dissolved in 0.9 per cent NaCl at the amounts indicated in Tables 16.1 and 16.2. The needles were left in place for a further minute to allow the infusate to diffuse away. The two rats were immediately transferred to the box and their behaviour was recorded as above. The rats were then killed by an overdose of pentobarbitone and 1 μl indian ink was infused at the injection site. The brains were removed, fixed in formal-saline, and sectioned on a microtome. A few rats had injection sites further than 0.3 mm from the intended site, and the results on the pairs containing these rats were rejected.

Drugs—1-(3-chlorophenyl)piperazine dihydrochloride (*m*-CPP), 1-naphthylpiperazine (both Research Biochemicals Inc., Wayland, MA, USA), ICS 205-930 (Sandoz Ltd., Basel), and chlordiazepoxide hydrochloride (Roche Products Ltd., England)—were dissolved in 0.9 per cent saline and injected intraperitoneally (*m*-CPP and chlordiazepoxide) or subcutaneously (ICS 205-930) at the nape of the neck. ($-$)-Propranolol hydrochloride (ICI, Macclesfield, UK) was also dissolved in 0.9 per cent saline and injected subcutaneously after being brought to pH 6.5. Metergoline (Farmitalia), ($+$)-cyanopindolol (Sandoz Ltd, Basel), ketanserin tartrate and ritanserin (Janssen, Beerse, Belgium), mianserin hydrochloride (Organon Laboratories Ltd., Newhouse, England), and cyproheptadine (Merck, Sharp, and Dohme, Harlow, UK) were dissolved in 100–200 μl of 10 per cent acetic acid made up to almost the required volume with 0.9 per cent saline and brought to pH 6.5 before subcutaneous injection. All drugs were administered in volumes of 1 ml kg^{-1}.

Results and discussion

The effects of *m*-CPP given intraperitoneally on social interaction are shown in Table 16.1. Social interaction was substantially decreased at a dose that

TABLE 16.1. *Effects of* m-*CPP on social interaction and locomotion*

m-CPP (μg kg^{-1})	Social interaction time (s per 15 min)	Locomotion (crossings/15 min)
Intraperitoneal injection		
0	542 ± 40	204 ± 10
200	352 ± 44	190 ± 10
500	232 ± 38*	210 ± 24
Intracerebroventricular injection		
0	461 ± 27	186 ± 16
2.0	309 ± 18***	205 ± 23
4.0	215 ± 14**	154 ± 7
Hippocampal injection		
0	429 ± 64	180 ± 22
0.25	271 ± 32	161 ± 32
1.0	164 ± 15**	143 ± 30
Amygdala injection		
0	456 ± 54	204 ± 36
1.0	494 ± 114	160 ± 34

Means ± S.E.M., n = 3–9 pairs.
Significant differences from 0.9% NaCl controls: *, $p < 0.05$; **, $p < 0.02$; ***, $p < 0.01$ (Mann-Whitney U test following significant Kruskal-Wallis analysis of variance).
Results from Kennett *et al.* (1989), Whitton and Curzon (1990).

TABLE 16.2. *Effect of 5-HT antagonists on inhibition of social interaction by* m-*CPP (0.5 mg kg^{-1} i.p.)*

Treatment	Dose	Blockade	Interpretation
Metergoline	2.5 mg kg^{-1} s.c.	Yes	5-HT receptor
Ketanserin	0.2 mg kg^{-1} s.c.	No	Not 5-HT$_2$
Ritanserin	0.6 mg kg^{-1} s.c.	No	Not 5-HT$_2$
Mianserin	2 mg kg^{-1} s.c.	Yes	5-HT$_{1C}$, 5-HT$_2$
Cyproheptadine	2 mg kg^{-1} s.c.	Yes	5-HT$_{1C}$, 5-HT$_2$
Cyanopindolol	6 mg kg^{-1} s.c.	No	Not 5-HT$_{1A}$ or 5-HT$_{1B}$
(−)-Propranolol	16 mg kg^{-1} s.c.	No	Not 5-HT$_{1A}$ or 5-HT$_{1B}$
ICS 205-930	0.05 mg kg^{-1} i.p.	Yes	
Chlordiazepoxide	5 mg kg^{-1} per day i.p. × 5	Yes	

Results from Kennett *et al.* (1989).

did not affect locomotion. TFMPP gave similar results. *m*-CPP was also potent in another anxiety model, the light/dark box test (Kennett *et al.* 1989). Data on punished responding in the pigeon also suggest that *m*-CPP has anxiogenic properties (Gleeson *et al.* 1989).

The social interaction time was significantly decreased when *m*-CPP was infused into the third ventricle; by 33 per cent with 2 μg and 53 per cent with 4 μg. The drug was more potent on hippocampal infusion; the interaction decreased by 37 per cent with 0.25 μg and 62 per cent with 1.0 μg, although only the larger dose had a statistically significant effect ($p < 0.02$). This dose did not decrease the interaction when infused into the amygdala. None of the central treatments significantly affected locomotion.

An approximate ED_{50} of 400 μg kg^{-1} *m*-CPP for the decrease of social interaction after intraperitoneal injection can be calculated from Table 16.1, although more recent work in our laboratory gives values of about 1 mg kg^{-1}. The corresponding approximate ED_{50} values of 4 and 0.5 μg for ventricular and hippocampal infusion respectively point to a central site of action with a major role for the hippocampus.

The results in Table 16.2 strongly suggest that the a xiogenic effect of *m*-CPP is mediated by 5-HT$_{1C}$ receptors and inhibited by the anxiolytic benzodiazepine drug chlordiazepoxide and the putatively anxiolytic 5-HT$_3$ antagonist ICS 205-930. The evidence in general points to hippocampal 5-HT$_{1C}$ receptors as biological substrates of anxiety. Although 5-HT$_{1C}$ receptors are most dense in the choroid plexus, they also occur in numerous regions of the rat (Pazos and Palacios 1985) and human (Pazos *et al.* 1987) brain, including the hippocampus. Our present results suggest that highly selective 5-HT$_{1C}$ antagonists might be effective anxiolytics. While such drugs are not yet available, less selective antagonists with high affinity for 5-HT$_{1C}$ and 5-HT$_2$ sites (Hoyer 1988) have anxiolytic properties. Such compounds include metergoline, cyproheptadine, methysergide, and cinanserin, although these anxiolytic effects are not manifest using a social interaction test (Chopin and Briley 1987; Briley and Chopin, this volume).

In view of the above findings, it is of interest that the anxiolytic benzodiazepine drug diazepam reduced 5-HT synthesis specifically in the hippocampus when injected systemically and also reduced it on hippocampal injection at coordinates similar to those used in this study (Nishikawa and Scatton 1986). Similarly, benzodiazepines decreased hippocampal 5-HT release on both local and systemic injection (Pei *et al.* 1989).

These findings provide a possible link with the anxiolytic properties of 5-HT$_{1A}$ agonists which may arise from activation of autoreceptors on the raphe nuclei so that 5-HT release at terminals is reduced (Dourish *et al.* 1986). As *in vivo* release of rat hippocampal 5-HT decreased when the 5-HT$_{1A}$ agonist 8-hydroxy-*N*,*N*,-dipropyl-2-aminotetralin was infused into the dorsal raphe (Hutson *et al.* 1989; Sharp *et al.* 1989), 5-HT$_{1A}$ agonists may cause anxiolysis by decreasing 5-HT availability to hippocampal 5-HT$_{1C}$ sites.

Conversely, abnormaility of these or other 5-HT$_{1C}$ sites or increased release of 5-HT to them could have a causal role in pathological anxiety and other possibly related disorders such as panic (Kahn *et al.* 1988), obsessive-compulsive disorder (Insel, this volume) and migraine (Brewerton *et al.* 1988, Curzon *et al.* 1990).

Acknowledgement

This work was supported by the Medical Research Council.

References

Brewerton, T. D., Murphy, D. L., Mueller, E. A., and Jimerson, D. C. (1988). Induction of migrainelike headaches by the serotonin agonist m-chlorophenylpiperazine. *Clinical Pharmacology and Therapeutics*, **43**, 605–9.

Briley, M. and Chopin, P. (1991). Serotonin in anxiety: evidence from animal models. In *5-hydroxytryptamine in psychiatry: a spectrum of ideas*, (ed. M. Sandler, A. Coppen, and S. Harnett), pp. 177–197. Oxford University Press.

Charney, D. S., Woods, S. W., Goodman, W. K., and Heninger, G. R. (1987). Serotonin function in anxiety. II. Effects of the serotonin agonist mCPP in panic disorder patients and healthy subjects. *Psychopharmacology*, **92**, 14–24.

Chopin, P. and Briley, M. (1987). Animal models of anxiety: the effect of components that modify 5-HT neurotransmission. *Trends in Pharmacological Sciences*, **8**, 383–8.

Curzon, G. (1991). 5-Hydroxytryptamine in the control of feeding and its possible implications for appetite disturbance. In *5-Hydroxytryptamine in psychiatry: a spectrum of ideas*, (ed. M. Sandler, A. Coppen, and S. Harnett), pp. 279–302. Oxford University Press.

Curzon, G., Kennett, G. A., Shah, K., and Whitton, P. (1990). Behavioural effects of *m*-chlorophenylpiperazine (*m*-CPP), a reported migraine precipitant. In *Migraine: a spectrum of ideas*, (ed. M. Sandler and G. Collins), pp. 173–81. Oxford University Press.

Dourish, C. T., Hutson, P. H., and Curzon, G. (1986). Putative anxiolytics, 8-OH-DPAT, buspirone and TVXQ 7821 are agonists at 5-HT$_{1A}$ autoreceptors in the raphe nuclei. *Trends in Pharmacological Sciences*, **7**, 212–14.

Gleeson, S., Ahlers, S. T., Mansbach, R. S., Foust, J. M., and Barrett, J. E. (1989). Behavioural studies with anxiolytic drugs. VI. Effects on punished responding of drugs interacting with serotonin receptor subtypes. *Journal of Pharmacology and Experimental Therapeutics*, **250**, 809–17.

Hoyer, D. (1988). Functional correlates of serotonin 5-HT$_1$ recognition sites. *Journal of Receptor Research*, **8**, 59–81.

Hutson, P. H., Sarna, G. S., O'Connell, M. T., and Curzon, G. (1989). Hippocampal 5-HT synthesis and release in vivo is decreased by infusion of 8-OH-DPAT into the nucleus raphe dorsalis. *Neuroscience Letters*, **100**, 276–80.

Insel, T. R. (1991). Serotonin in obsessive-compulsive disorder: a causal connection or more monomania about a major monoamine? In *5-hydroxytryptamine in psychiatry: a spectrum of ideas*, (ed. M. Sandler, A. Coppen, and S. Harnett), pp. 228–257. Oxford University Press.

Kennett, G. A. and Curzon, G. (1988*a*). Evidence that mCPP may have behavioural effects mediated by 5-HT$_{1C}$ receptors. *British Journal of Pharmacology*, **94**, 137–47.

Kennett, G. A. and Curzon, G. (1988*b*). Evidence that hypophagia induced by mCPP and TFMPP requires 5-HT$_{1C}$ and 5-HT$_{1B}$ receptors: hypophagia induced by RU 24969 only requires 5-HT$_{1B}$ receptors. *Psychopharmacology*, **96**, 93–100.

Kennett, G. A., Whitton, P., Shah, K., and Curzon, G. (1989). Anxiogenic-like effects of mCPP and TFMPP in animal models are opposed by 5-HT$_{1C}$ receptor antagonists. *European Journal of Pharmacology*, **164**, 445–54.

Kahn, R. S., Asnis, G. M., Wetzler, S., and van Praag, H. M. (1988). Neuroendocrine evidence for serotonin receptor hypersensitivity in panic disorder. *Psychopharmacology*, **96**, 360–4.

McKenny, J. D. and Glennon. R. A. (1986). TFMPP may produce its stimulus effect via a 5-HT$_{1B}$ mechanism. *Pharmacology Biochemistry and Behaviour*, **24**, 43–7.

Mueller, E. A., Murphy, D. L., and Sunderland, T. (1985). Neuroendocrine effects of m-chlorophenylpiperazine, a serotonin agonist in humans. *Journal of Clinical Endocrinology and Metabolism*, **61**, 1179–84.

Nishikawa, T. and Scatton, B. (1986). Neuroanatomical site of the inhibitory influence of anxiolytic drugs on central serotonergic transmission. *Brain Research*, **371**, 123–132.

Paxinos, G. and Watson, C. (1982). *The rat brain in stereotaxic coordinates*. Academic Press, New York.

Pazos, A. and Palacios, J. M. (1985). Quantitative autoradiographic mapping of serotonin receptors in the rat brain. I. Serotonin-1 receptors. *Brain Research*, **346**, 205–30.

Pazos, A., Probst, A., and Palacios, J. M. (1987). Serotonin receptors in the human brain. III. Autoradiographic mapping of serotonin-1 receptors. *Neuroscience*, **21**, 97–122.

Pei, Q., Zetterstrom, T., and Fillenz, M. (1989). Both systemic and local administration of benzodiazepine agonists inhibit the *in vivo* release of 5-HT from ventral hippocampus. *Neuropharmacology*, **28**, 1061–6.

Sharp, T. Bramwell, S. R., Clark, D., and Grahame-Smith, D. G. (1989). In vivo measurement of extracellular 5-hydroxytryptamine in hippocampus of the anaesthetized rat using microdialysis: changes in relation to 5-hydroxytryptaminergic neuronal activity. *Journal of Neurochemistry*, **53**, 234–40.

Sills, M. A., Wolfe, B. B., and Frazer, A. (1984). Determination of selective and non-selective compounds for the 5-HT$_{1A}$ and 5-HT$_{1B}$ receptor subtypes in rat frontal cortex. *Journal of Pharmacology and Experimental Therapeutics*, **231**, 480–7.

Whitton, P. and Curzon, G. (1990). Anxiogenic-like effect of infusing 1-(3-chlorophenyl) piperazine (mCPP) into the hippocampus. *Psychopharmacology*, **100**, 138–40.

Discussion

SANDLER: Dr Peroutka, do you accept the the anxiogenic effect of *m*-CPP observed by Professor Curzon is mediated by 5-HT$_{1C}$ receptors?

PEROUTKA: Ritanserin is an equally potent antagonist at 5-HT$_{1C}$ and 5-HT$_2$ sites. Ketanserin is about 40 to 50-fold more potent at 5-HT$_2$ sites than at 5-HT$_{1C}$ sites. The most potent site of action of *m*-CPP in the human brain is the 5-HT$_3$ receptor (about 15 nM). It is slightly less potent at 5-HT$_{1C}$ sites, and even less potent at 5-HT$_2$ sites. Mianserin is also moderately potent (15–30 nM) at 5-HT$_3$ sites. Thus, because ritanserin and ketanserin do not block the action of *m*-CPP, whereas mianserin does, I would say that the evidence suggests a major 5-HT_3 component to the action of *m*-CPP. The effect of metergoline, however, does not agree with this conclusion.

CURZON: How does the potency of mianserin at 5-HT_{1C} sites compare with that at 5-HT_3 sites?

PEROUTKA: Mianserin is more potent by an order of magnitude at 5-HT_{1C} sites than at 5-HT_3 sites.

CURZON: Is *m*-CPP an agonist or an antagonist at 5-HT_3 sites?

MURPHY: In the rat vagus, *m*-CPP is a 5-HT_3 antagonist (Ireland and Tyers 1987).

PEROUTKA: The fact that ICS 205-930 blocks the effect of *m*-CPP suggests that 5-HT_3 receptors are involved in the behavioural effect of *m*-CPP.

CURZON: ICS 205-930 (like benzodiazepines) is anxiolytic and certainly blocks *m*-CPP action at some stage of the anxiolytic process. But the balance of evidence from effects of antagonists and from our limited knowledge of interactions between 5-HT_3 sites and *m*-CPP favours the mediation of its anxiogenic properties by 5-HT_{1C} sites. The metergoline data are particularly suggestive. However, evidence on the whole is not as solid as that on the involvement of 5-HT_{1C} sites in the hypophagic effect of *m*-CPP (Curzon, this volume).

SULSER: Dr Peroutka, are there regional differences in the potency of a drug such as ritanserin, which is a potent 5-HT_{1C} antagonist in the choroid plexus?

PEROUTKA: Nobody has studied regional differences. Ritanserin and cinanserin blocked 5-HT_2 receptor-mediated neuronal excitation (Davies *et al.* 1987). In retrospect, perhaps we were looking at a 5-HT_{1C} receptor-mediated physiological effect. There may be excitatory putative 5-HT_2-mediated effects which ritanserin blocks and spiperone does not. We should re-evaluate all the 5-HT_2 models to determine the role of 5-HT_{1C} receptors.

SULSER: Are these data on potency based on radioligand displacement or on blockade of phosphoinositide (PI) hydrolysis?

PEROUTKA: Both. PI turnover effects correlate significantly with the binding data. The binding is very predictive of the functional affinity of the drugs.

MURPHY: *m*-CPP has anxiogenic effects in humans which seem to be differentiated by dose. Our first studies with 0.5 mg kg^{-1} orally produced modest anxiogenesis, but smaller doses (0.1 mg kg^{-1}) given intravenously had more marked anxiogenic effects (Murphy *et al.* 1989). A dose (0.25 mg kg^{-1}) that did not produce anxiety in healthy controls induced panic episodes in panic disorder patients (Kahn *et al.* 1988). Obsessive-compulsive disorder (OCD) patients are more sensitive to the anxiogenic effects and also show increases in OCD symptomatology when they receive *m*-CPP orally rather then intravenously.

In a comparison of oral and intravenous (i.v.) administration of *m*-CPP the concentrations in the blood reached similar plateau levels after the rapid infusion phase. A small increase in anxiety ratings was seen with oral *m*-CPP (0.5 mg kg^{-1}). After i.v. *m*-CPP the anxiety peaked at 30 min and disappeared after 60 min. Anxiety was measured using our NIMH anxiety self-rating scale which picks up both physical symptoms and subjective elements, such as tension and nervousnesss. We found essentially equivalent peak increases in plasma cortisol after intravenous and oral *m*-CPP, although the time courses were different. Similar results were obtained for plasma prolactin responses and for temperature changes.

Thus, it is the anxiogenic response that differs between oral and i.v. administration. Professor Curzon raised the possibility that *m*-CPP was different in terms of its behavioural reactivity, rather than in some other systems. In our hypotheses about clinical disorders and their treatment, we should explore the consequences of the idea that there are different 5-HT subsystems using different 5-HT receptors. Not all systems may respond equally. This may also apply to antagonist effects.

From the subcomponents of our NIMH self-rating scale we can see that *m*-CPP has other behavioural effects that are more marked after intravenous rather than oral administration. For example, functional deficit, a composite subscale including difficulty in concentrating and performing routine tasks, and feeling slowed down, is greatly affected by *m*-CPP.

CARLSSON: How does *m*-CPP act at 5-HT receptors?

PEROUTKA: This drug is a 5-HT_{1C} agonist, a 5-HT_2 antagonist, and a 5-HT_3 antagonist.

MELTZER: Clineschmidt (1979), who developed this series of drugs, showed that there are large discrepancies between affinities and intrinsic activity: *m*-CPP had more affinity than MK 212 for 5-HT_2 receptors but MK 212 was more active.

CURZON: We know from human data that *m*-CPP is anxiogenic. We know from rat data that its anxiogenic-like properties are not easily explicable by 5-HT_{1A}, 5-HT_{1B}, 5-HT_2 or 5-HT_3 effects and that available evidence is strongly in favour of 5-HT_{1C} sites. That does not mean that *m*-CPP does not also act at other sites.

PEROUTKA: In molecular modelling studies it is seen that *m*-CPP is very small and theoretically will fit into the 'docking site' of almost any biogenic amine receptor.

MURPHY: However, despite *m*-CPP's promiscuous affinity for multiple 5-HT sites, drug discrimination studies clearly show that *m*-CPP's interoceptive cue is different from that of agents acting at 5-HT_{1A} sites (Cunningham and Appel 1986; McKenny and Glennon 1986). Other pharmacological studies, including antagonist studies, suggest that *m*-CPP is not acting for the most part at 5-HT_{1A} sites, although its *in vitro* affinity for 5-HT_{1A} sites is nearly as high as its affinity for 5-HT_{1C} and 5-HT_{1B} sites.

FRAZER: Potency and intrinsic activity are two very separate characteristics of a drug. We have found, using inhibition of cyclase in the hippocampus, which is a 5-HT_{1A}-mediated effect, that *m*-CPP is much weaker in terms of its ability to produce this effect (EC_{50} = 9000 mM) than its affinity obtained in binding assays using ^{3}H-DPAT (K_i = 100 mM). This underscores the importance of using functional measures, and not just binding data, as measures of selectivity.

LINNOILA: We cannot use drug discrimination paradigms to say that *m*-CPP does not have activity at the 5-HT_{1A} site. The drug discrimination paradigm tells us that when we teach an animal to discriminate to 5-HT_{1A} drugs and then give it a non-specific drug which affects multiple receptor sites the animal finds it different. That does not mean that the drug would not have the 5-HT_{1A} affinity.

Substitution of benzodiazepine treatment by partial 5-HT_{1A} agonists is not efficient against anxiety. This is not surprising. Particularly with patients with somatic anxiety, we are probably dealing with people who are extremely sensitive to interoceptive cues. We are changing to a drug which gives totally different cues. This becomes a type of human drug discrimination. Clinically, many patients are reassured by the slight 'rush' that they get from diazepam, which gets to their brain very quickly and calms then down. Harban Lal has shown slight generalization from 5-HT_{1A} drugs to the pentylenetetrasol cue which generalizes to alcohol and benzodiazepine withdrawals. If you immediately substitute a benzodiazepine with a 5-HT_{1A} partial agonist, given that the available drugs are fairly non-specific, and if it is a drug which an animal equates with the benzodiazepine withdrawal cue, then you could be making the situation worse.

MELTZER: Before we become too focused on *m*-CPP in anxiety it is important to remember that it was first reported to make obsessives more obsessive and panic patients more panicked. Dennis Charney's group found that all eight schizophrenic patients studied had an increase in positive symptoms of psychosis when given *m*-CPP. Markku Linnoila has some similar data for alcoholics. One could say that *m*-CPP makes you more of whatever you are! This speaks to Markku Linnoila's point about interoceptive cues.

MK 212, which has a somewhat parallel profile to *m*-CPP, although weaker in most regards, and is clearly blocked by ritanserin in all the animal experiments, has very small anxiogenic effects.

References

Clineschmidt, B. V. (1979). MK-212: a serotonin-like agonist in the CNS. *General Pharmacology*, **10**, 287–90.

Cunningham, K. A. and Appel, J. R. (1986). Possible 5-hydroxytryptamine$_1$ (5-HT$_1$) receptor involvement in the stimulus properties of 1-(*m*-trifluoromethyl-phenyl)piperazine (TFMPP). *Journal of Pharmacology and Experimental Therapeutics*, **237**, 369–77.

Curzon, G. (1991). 5-Hydroxytryptamine in the control of feeding and its possible implications for appetite disturbance. In *5-Hydroxytryptamine in psychiatry: a spectrum of ideas*, (ed. M. Sandler, A. Coppen, and S. Harnett), pp. 279–302 Oxford University Press.

Davies, M. F., Diez, R. A., Prince, D., and Peroutka, S. J. (1987). Two distinct effects of 5-hydroxytryptamine on single cortical neurons. *Brain Research*, **423**, 347–52.

Ireland, S. J. and Tyers, M. B. (1987). Pharmacological characterization of 5-hydroxytryptamine-induced depolarization of the rat isolated vagus nerve. *British Journal of Pharmacology*, **90**, 229–38.

Kahn, R. S., Wetzler, S., van Praag, H. M. *et al.* (1988). Behavioural indications for serotonin hypersensitivity in panic disorder. *Psychiatry Research*, **25**, 101–4.

McKenny, J. D. and Glennon, R. A. (1986). TFMPP may produce its stimulus effects via a 5-HT$_{1B}$ mechanism. *Pharmacology, Biochemistry and Behaviour*, **24**, 1152–9.

Murphy, D. L., Mueller, E. A., Hill, J. L., Tolliver, T. J., and Jacobsen, F. M. (1989). Comparative anxiogenic, neuroendocrine and other physiologic effects of *m*-chlorophenylpiperazine given intravenously or orally to healthy volunteers. *Psychopharmacology*, **98**, 275–82.

17. Does 5-HT have a role in anxiety and the action of anxiolytics?

Michael G. Palfreyman and John H. Kehne

Introduction

In our quest for better treatments for anxiety it is essential first to ask, what is the anxiety syndrome we are trying to treat? Anxiety is a perfectly normal response to a stressful situation, such as speaking in public. The somatic manifestations of this 'situational' anxiety are well controlled with β-adrenoceptor blockers, such as propranolol. However, this form of anxiety is rarely incapacitating and obviously is self limiting. It is also a moot point that it needs 'treating'. On the other hand, it has been estimated that 2–4 per cent of the population suffers from anxiety disorders which are so severe and prolonged that they can become incapacitating (Schweitzer and Adams 1979).

Anxiety disorders

Anxiety, as the symptom, appears associated with a number of different affective disorders, and each syndrome may respond to different pharmacological treatments (Table 17.1).

Anxiety associated with generalized anxiety disorder responds well to benzodiazepines whereas anxiety associated with depression responds poorly. It is also probable that a significant proportion of generalized anxiety disorder is treated by self-medication with ethanol. Patients withdrawing from benzodiazepines and alcohol often experience anxiety reactions and these do not respond to treatment with buspirone. Panic disorders, phobias, and post-traumatic stress disorders, with their components of anxiety, respond best to monoamine oxidase (MAO) inhibitors and tricyclic antidepressants and only poorly to benzodiazepines. Additionally, the anxiety associated with obsessive-compulsive disorders decreases when the compulsive behaviour is controlled with 5-hydroxytryptamine (5-HT, serotonin) uptake inhibitors. These varied treatments imply, but do not prove, that anxiety is a symptom with many causes and that no single treatment is likely to be a panacea.

Onset of action of anxiolytics

A second important issue is the timing of the onset of anxiolytic activity. The anti-anxiety effects of buspirone have consistently not been apparent until

TABLE 17.1.   *Types of anxiety and their treatment*

Anxiety associated with	Possible treatments
Generalized anxiety disorder	Benzodiazepines, buspirone
Benzodiazepine withdrawal	Benzodiazepine with long half-life
Panic disorders	Tricyclic antidepressants, MAO inhibitors
Phobias	Tricyclic antidepressants, MAO inhibitors
Obsessive-compulsive disorder	5-HT uptake inhibitors
Mixed anxiety/depression syndrome	Tricyclic antidepressants, 5-HT uptake inhibitors, MAO inhibitors, buspirone?
'Atypical' depression	MAO inhibitors
Post-traumatic stress disorder	Tricyclic antidepressants, MAO inhibitors

MAO, monoamine oxidase

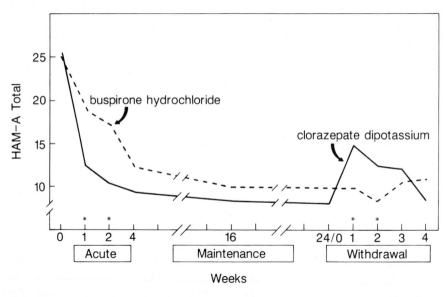

FIG. 17.1.   Comparison of the anxiolytic effects of buspirone and the benzodiaze-pine, clorazepate on generalized anxiety disorder. Mean response of 61 patients (buspirone, *n* = 21; clorazepate, *n* = 40) on the Hamilton Anxiety scale (HAM-A). *, significant difference between groups. Redrawn with permission from Fig. 1, Rickels *et al.* 1988 (Copyright, American Medical Association).

after two to three weeks of treatment (Fig. 17.1). Although many patients report that benzodiazepines rapidly relieve the symptoms of anxiety, much of this response may be due to the muscle relaxant/sedative actions of this class of drugs. When the underlying 'feelings' of anxiety, rather than the somatic symptoms, are studied, it appears that benzodiazepines do have a delayed onset of therapeutic effect. This contrasts with the rapid development of symptoms of anxiety after withdrawal from benzodiazepines (see Fig. 17.1).

Animal models

Also important in the development of new therapies are the animal models used to predict anxiolytic activity of a new agent (Table 17.2). Nearly all the most frequently used models have been developed and validated with benzodiazepines, such as diazepam, as the reference drugs. Many of the tests are relatively insensitive to buspirone and related compounds (even after chronic administration), and the responses seen with 5-HT$_2$ and 5-HT$_3$ antagonists are at best very slight when compared to the robust responses seen with benzodiazepines. A critical question is whether a given model is selectively detecting anxiolytic activity of a compound, or are the sedative/muscle relaxant properties more salient cues? Muscle relaxation may contribute to the overall *Gestalt* of anxiolysis in humans, but if we hope to develop new, more selective therapeutic approaches to treating anxiety, we need to identify appropriate models.

Given that animal models are at best only approximations to human conditions, we nevertheless believe that models for anxiety disorders should fulfil several criteria. First, the end-point should be sensitive to known benzodiazepine and buspirone-like anxiolytics. Second, the end-point should be robust, making it possible within a reasonable time scale to carry out sophisticated pharmacological studies. Third, the end-point should have ethological significance or at least be reliably elicited by 'natural' anxiety-provoking stimuli. Fourth, the end-point should be sensitive to anxiogenic as well as anxiolytic agents.

We are using and developing several models of anxiety that satisfy these criteria, although each model has its particular strengths and weaknesses. When a pre-weaning rat pup is separated from its litter, it emits a series of ultrasonic vocalizations. These 'separation-induced vocalizations' (SIV), also referred to as 'isolation calls' or 'distress cries', have adaptive value in that they signal to the mother that the pup has strayed from the litter and elicit from her a stereotypic retrieval response. We can measure and quantify these vocalizations with an ultrasonic detector (QMC Bat Detector) tuned to the appropriate frequency range (approximately 32–52 kHz). Pretreatment with diazepam or with the 5-HT$_{1A}$ partial agonists, buspirone or MDL 73005EF, produced a dose-related suppression of these responses (Fig. 17.2). These drugs are approximately equipotent in suppressing SIV, which parallels their reported clinical efficacies. We also tested the *N*-methyl-D-aspartate (NMDA) receptor antagonist, AP5 (Meldrum 1985) and the strychnine-insensitive glycine antagonist, 5,7-dichlorokynurenic acid (Baron *et al.* 1990). Both these compounds, which work at the glutamate receptor-operated ion channel, were effective at blocking the separation-induced vocalization,

TABLE 17.2.   *Anxiety models and their responses to anxiolytics*

Model	Drug response	References
Geller/Seifter	Benzodiazepines, barbiturates, p-CPA, 5, 7-DHT lesions, cyproheptadine, cinanserin	Geller and Seifter (1960), Dalterio *et al.* (1988), Kettelaars and Bruinvels (1989), Geller *et al.* (1974)
Vogel drinking test	Benzodiazepines, buspirone?, MDL 73005EF	Vogel *et al.* (1971), Higgins *et al.* (1988), Hibert *et al.* (1988), Moser *et al.* (1990)
Elevated plus-maze	Benzodiazepines, buspirone, MDL 73005EF, 5-HT$_3$ antagonists	File and Johnston (1989), Stephens *et al.* (1986), Moser *et al.* (1990)
Social interaction studies	Benzodiazepines, 5-HT$_3$ antagonists, 5-HT$_{1A}$ partial agonists	File and Johnston (1989), File *et al.* (1979), Jones *et al.* (1988), Johnston and File (1988), File and Hyde (1978), Collins (1979)
Rat pup ultrasonic vocalization	Benzodiazepines, 5-HT$_{1A}$ partial agonists, 5-HT uptake inhibitors, MDMA, glutamate antagonists, strychnine-insensitive glycine antagonists	Gardner (1985, 1988), Insel *et al.* (1986), Kehne *et al.* (unpublished), Mos *et al.* (1988)
Potentiated startle paradigm	Benzodiazepines, 8-OH-DPAT?, buspirone, gepirone, ipsapirone	Davis (1979, 1986), Kehne *et al.* (1988), Mansbach and Geyer (1988)
Conflict testing (pigeons)	Benzodiazepines, buspirone, 8-OH-DPAT	Barrett *et al.* (1986), Barrett *et al.* (1988), Witkin *et al.* (1987), Gleeson *et al.* (1989)
Conditioned suppression of drinking	Benzodiazepines, chronic buspirone	Kilts *et al.* (1981), Cowen *et al.* (1987), McCloskey *et al.* (1987), Schefke *et al.* (1989)

p-CPA, p-chlorophenylalanine; 5,7-DHT, 5,7-dihydroxytryptamine; MDMA, 3,4-methylene dioxymethamphetamine; 8-OH-DPAT, 8-hydroxy-N,N-dipropyl-2-aminotetralin.

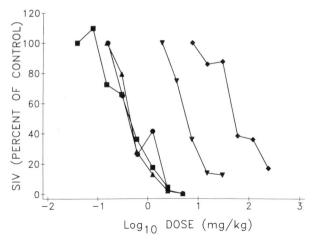

FIG. 17.2. Suppressant effects of intraperitoneal administration of: ■, diazepam (0.078–2.5 mg kg⁻¹; $n = 8$ per dose); ●, buspirone (0.313–5.0 mg kg⁻¹; $n = 5$ per dose); ▲, MDL 73005EF (0.313–5.0 mg kg⁻¹; $n = 5$ per dose); ▼, AP5 (3.75–30 mg kg⁻¹; $n = 4$ per group); ♦, 5,7-dichlorokynurenic acid (15–240 mg kg⁻¹; $n = 10$ per dose) on separation-induced ultrasonic vocalizations (SIV) in 8–10 day-old rat pups. After injection, pups were returned to the home cage and 30 min later were placed into isolated sound-attenuated chambers and tested for 10 min. Each point represents mean number of total vocalizations emitted during the first 3 min of testing, expressed as percentage of vehicle-injected control mean. All drugs produced suppresant effects on SIV that were linearly related to the doses used ($p < 0.00005$).

albeit at fairly high doses (Fig. 17.2). In a parallel test run on the same rat pups, buspirone, MDL 73005EF, and 5,7-dichlorokynurenic acid were devoid of muscle relaxant/sedative effects, whereas diazepam and the competitive glutamate antagonist AP5 produced clear sedative effects. MDL 11939, a potent and highly selective 5-HT₂ antagonist with hundredfold or greater selectivity for the 5-HT₂ receptor relative to effects on the 5-HT₁C receptor, the α_1, α_2, and β-adrenergic receptors, and the dopamine DA₂, histamine H₁, and muscarinic receptors (Dudley *et al.* 1988), was devoid of activity against the vocalization, as was the very selective 5-HT₃ antagonist, MDL 73147EF (Gittos and Fatmi 1989; Sorensen *et al.* 1989).

The clear-cut dose-response curves for anxiolytics in this model suggest that it will be amenable to pharmacological evaluation. For example, we could study whether propranolol or pindolol is able to antagonize the anxiolytic effects of the 5-HT₁A partial agonists, buspirone and MDL 73005EF.

A major consideration in interpreting data gathered with this model is that drug effects in the infant may be very different from those in the adult. In one respect we are attempting to capitalize on this immaturity by viewing the rat pup nervous system as a simplified version of a more complex adult CNS, which is analogous to a decerebrate preparation being considered a 'reduced' preparation. The striking degree to which the pup ultrasonic vocalization response can be turned off by 5-HT_{1A} anxiolytics suggests a pivotal role for serotonergic neurones. Electrophysiological studies using iontophoretic application on to 5-HT cell bodies of the dorsal raphe indicate that excitatory α_1-adrenergic modulation and inhibitory 5-HT modulation are fully functional soon after the birth (Smith and Gallager 1989). Thus, the rat pup vocalization response may be a behavioural manifestation of a phylogenetically primitive anxiety system that is 'uncomplicated' by the more complex modulatory circuits in the mature adult. The discrepancy between clinical reports of the delayed onset of buspirone anxiolysis and the exquisite sensitivity of vocalizations to acute 5-HT_{1A} agonist administration may be a consequence of using the pup rather than the adult. Interestingly, noradrenergic regulation of behaviour is not fully developed in the pup, as seen by a profound developmental shift in the pharmacological effect of clonidine from an α_1 to an α_2 agonist (Reinstein and Isaacson 1977; Kehoe and Harris 1989; Nomura *et al.* 1980). Given the α_1-adrenergic excitatory modulation of the dorsal raphe (Smith and Gallager 1989), we are addressing the possibility of a noradrenergic/serotonergic interaction in the regulation of vocalizations, and how this relationship might differ between the infant and the adult.

Another important consideration is the level of maturity of the blood–brain barrier. Drugs that fail to cross the blood–brain barrier in adults might readily achieve central access in the neonate. A unique characteristic of the separation vocalization response is that it is present from postnatal Day 1 to approximately Day 15 (Insel *et al.* 1988). Thus, testing at an early age (e.g., Day 3) could detect potential anxiolytic activity of compounds that do not readily cross the blood–brain barrier in adults, and testing at a later age (e.g., Day 10), when the barrier is mature, would allow a simple determination of central bioavailability. It should be acknowledged that developmental differences in drug metabolism could complicate the interpretation.

Finally, the limited ontogenetic appearance of the separation vocalization response (two weeks) limits the use of chronic drug designs. This limitation might be overcome by dosing the mother with drugs that cross the placenta, thus allowing long-term exposure of the offspring. In addition, conditioned and unconditioned ultrasonic vocalization responses to certain stressors are seen in adult animals, and these responses may be useful end-points for assessment of psychotherapeutic agents (see, for example, Tonoue *et al.* 1986). Further experiments to validate the ultrasonic model are under way.

A second model of anxiety that we are developing uses a simple reflex behaviour—a startle response elicited by a loud noise or an airpuff—as the behavioural end-point. Although the startle response is a primitive reflex involving a relatively simple neural pathway from the brainstem to the spinal cord (Davis *et al.* 1982), the reflex can be markedly enhanced by fear-induced activation of limbic system pathways (Davis 1986; Hitchcock and Davis 1986). Personal experience reminds us that we startle more easily when we are in frightening situations, for example walking down a dark alley. In fact, exagerrated startle responses are listed (American Psychiatric Association 1980) as one of the diagnostic criteria for generalized anxiety disorder. Some of the most consistent findings in people with 'post-traumatic stress disorder' are the heightened startle responses (American Psychiatric Association 1980; Kinzie *et al.* 1984; Ross *et al.* 1989; Creamer 1989).

Using an automated system for quantifying acoustic and tactile startle reflexes in rodents, we are refining various models for discovering novel anxiolytic agents. In one model, rodents are exposed to a classical conditioning procedure in which a light conditioned stimulus is paired with a shock unconditioned stimulus. In a subsequent test session the animal exhibits heightened startle responses in the presence (but not in the absence) of the conditioned stimulus, presumably because the animal is in a heightened fear state. Consistent with this interpretation, a corticotropin-releasing factor (CRF) antagonist, α-CRF, blocks potentiated startle (Swerdlow *et al.* 1989). Furthermore, administration of an anxiogenic β-carboline enhances potentiated startle (Hijzen and Slangen 1989), an important attribute for a valid animal model of anxiety. The potentiated startle response can be blocked by acute administration of benzodiazepines (Davis 1979, 1986) and buspirone and related compounds (Kehne *et al.* 1988; Davis *et al.* 1988; Mansbach and Geyer 1988). However, the role of 5-HT in the response to buspirone is unclear in that 5-HT antagonists or combined lesions of the dorsal and median raphe nuclei failed to block potentiated startle *per se*, and failed to attenuate buspirone's anxiolytic effect in this model (Davis *et al.* 1988). Further work is needed to clarify the neurotransmitter substrates underlying the blockade of potentiated startle by buspirone and related compounds.

As with other models that employ classically conditioned fear procedures, potentiated startle is tightly linked to the presentation of the conditioned stimulus, that is, the anxiety is transitory and unsustained. Thus, the anxiety could be considered more situation-specific than generalized. Perhaps more suitable models for chronic anxiety states would involve prior exposure to chronic stressors (see Ottenweller *et al.* 1989) which might induce more general chronic neurochemical and behavioural changes.

The coexistence of anxiety as a key symptom in affective disorders is harder to model in animal studies (Table 17.1). None of the existing models (including potentiated startle; see Cassella and Davis 1985) used to study anxiety responds consistently to MAO inhibitors or tricyclic antidepressants, and yet these classes of drugs are very effective at reducing anxiety when it coexists with depression. Again, the use of chronic stressors might allow a closer approximation of these disorders, in this case possibly by incorporating the element of 'uncontrollability' (see, for example, Weiss and Simson 1986).

Another approach to models for chronic anxiety would be to use animals that have been bred specifically for high levels of anxiety, for example the Maudsley Reactive strains of rat (see Broadhurst 1975 for review). The study of these strains might provide new insights and new directions for the development of anti-anxiety treatments and, in addition, might allow a better understanding of the 'adaptive' responses that occur after repeated administration of anxiolytic drugs such as buspirone. The two behavioural end-points described (separation vocalizations and startle reflexes) have been studied to a limited extent in Maudsley Reactive strains. Relative to the 'non-reactive' controls, Maudsley Reactive adult rats exhibit heightened unconditioned startle responses (Commissaris *et al.* 1988) and Maudsley Reactive neonates exhibit enhanced rates of separation vocalizations (Insel and Hill 1987), suggesting that these models can serve as sensitive indicants of chronic anxiety. Potentiated startle has not yet been assessed in Maudsley Reactive adults. Such conditioning might produce a profound anxiety response in an animal that is genetically predisposed to exhibit high emotional reactivity.

Mode of action of anxiolytic drugs

A major issue in the development of improved treatments for anxiety is a better understanding of how the effective drug treatments actually work. Briley and Chopin (this volume) have discussed the evidence for a possible interaction of benzodiazepines with the serotonergic system. Buspirone, a $5\text{-}HT_{1A}$ partial agonist, obviously has a serotonergic component in its action, but what is the exact mechanism by which buspirone produces its anxiolytic effect in man? Buspirone and other $5\text{-}HT_{1A}$ partial agonists depress the serotonergic system by inhibiting the firing of dorsal raphe neurones via the somatodendritic autoreceptor (Sprouse and Aghajanian 1987). Such an inhibition of neuronal activity reduces the output of serotonin (Sharp *et al.* 1989). However, this acute response to the drug may not be related to its delayed clinical effects. An additional factor to consider is, as always, the dose. The median raphe is not as sensitive to inhibition as the dorsal raphe, although buspirone acts as a full agonist in both (Sinton and Fallon 1988). Thus, different serotonin systems with different projection areas may be selectively affected by buspirone, depending on the dose used.

In the terminal field, buspirone and MDL 73005EF act as partial agonists. For example, forskolin-stimulated adenylate cyclase in the rat hippocampus is inhibited by 5-HT, 8-hydroxy-*N,N*-dipropyl-2-aminotetralin (8-OH-DPAT), buspirone, and MDL 73005EF (Cornfield *et al.* 1989). However, MDL 73005EF and, to a lesser extent, buspirone antagonize the effects of 8-OH-DPAT and 5-HT. This is a post-synaptic response and it is not clear if a partial agonist would increase or decrease transmission of the serotonergic message. Because a partial agonist acts as an antagonist when the serotonergic tone is high and as an agonist when the tone is low, the baseline activity of the serotonergic system ultimately affects the pharmacology of the drug under study. When a patient is anxious is the serotonergic drive increased or decreased from normal levels and, therefore, do we need to develop better agonists or better antagonists? Of equal importance is the question of whether the somatodendritic and/or post-synaptic 5-HT_{1A} receptors adapt to the continued presence of the agonist/antagonist. A better understanding of adaptive responses will clarify the main question—do we need to increase or decrease serotonergic activity to produce an anxiolytic affect?

We must also consider what other neurotransmitter systems or other types of serotonergic receptors are modified after repeated administration of 5-HT_{1A} partial agonists. For example, do 5-HT_2 or 5-HT_3 receptors change in responsiveness after repeated administration of buspirone? Are there adaptive changes in noradrenergic or dopaminergic systems? Dudley and Baron (Abstract 12, *Proceedings of the XXII Winter Conference on Brain Research*, Snowbird, Utah, 1989) and Fandeleur and Jones (1989) have shown that four-day administration of 8-OH-DPAT or buspirone in combination with desipramine will down-regulate β-adrenoceptors and isoproterenol-stimulated adenylate cyclase. The down-regulation does not occur in this short time with either drug given alone. It will also be important to study the adaptive responses to repeated benzodiazepine treatment. Studies conducted during benzodiazepine withdrawal may give insight into the anxiety that this state engenders.

Evaluation of the role of 5-HT in anxiety

What evidence is there that a derangement of 5-HT is of aetiological significance in anxiety states? The fact that certain drugs that affect serotonergic systems are able to alleviate some of the symptoms of anxiety does not imply that derangements of the serotonergic system cause anxiety; the data supporting such a causal relationship are essentially non-existent. How might such data be accumulated? In which patients should such studies be conducted (see above) and can we define patients in terms of a state of, or a trait for, anxiety? We shall make several suggestions for experiments we consider worthy of discussion but, of course, leave it to our clinical colleagues to advise us on the feasibility of such approaches.

Many agents provoke anxiety and/or panic responses in man: infusion or ingestion of lactate, caffeine, inverse benzodiazepine agonists, yohimbine, and *m*-CPP. Only for the last compound is a serotonergic component evident. Do the other anxiogenic agents modulate serotonergic systems in man, and how does *m*-CPP work in man? Several modes of action for *m*-CPP have been discussed elsewhere in this volume. We also have to deal with the confounding variable that it is anxiogenic after intravenous but not oral administration. Answers to these questions may give insights into state anxiety. Analysis of the role of serotonin in the anxious trait may be amenable to investigation with the new and more selective serotonergic receptor agonists and antagonists. 5-HT_{1A} partial agonists, such as buspirone, produce a number of endocrine responses that have been discussed in detail in other chapters of this book. 5-HT_2 agonists also produce responses that in some instances are similar. Are endocrine responses to 5-HT agonists a valid way of investigating anxiety? A largely neglected, and easily quantified, response is the change in body temperature produced by serotonergic agonists. In animals, 5-HT_{1A} agonists decrease, whereas 5-HT_2 agonists increase, body temperature (Gudelsky *et al.* 1986). Do anxious patients respond differently to the thermoregulatory effect of serotonergic agents, such as MDL 73005EF or *m*-CPP? 5-HT potentiates the aggregatory response of platelets by activating the 5-HT_2 receptor (Dudley *et al.* 1988). Receptor binding using ^{125}I-labelled lysergic acid diethylamide ($[^{125}$I]LSD) has been performed (Cowen *et al.* 1987). Do 5-HT_2 receptors on platelets from anxious patients differ from those from normals?

Millson *et al.* (1988) demonstrated that the 5-HT_2 receptor antagonist, ICI 160,369, caused a decrease in mean pupil diameter in healthy volunteers. 5-HT precursors and 5-HT-releasing agents such as fenfluramine also produce changes in pupil diameter (Kramer *et al.* 1973). Based on these observations, Paul Schechter, at our institute, has devised a non-invasive way to assess the effects of selective 5-HT_2 antagonists. This method uses variable light intensity and photography of pupil diameter to quantify the response to 5-HT_2 receptor blockade. Pilot studies on MDL 11939 are under way. In future could these be used to compare pupillary response in normal and anxious patients?

5-HT_2 antagonists have consistently been shown to prolong slow-wave sleep in animals and man (Adam and Oswald 1989). Could these studies also be conducted in anxious patients to assess the sensitivity of the 5-HT_2 system? Deakin *et al.* (this volume) described preliminary studies on ritanserin which suggest that 5-HT_2 antagonists might have anxiolytic effects. However, ritanserin also potently antagonizes 5-HT_{1C} receptors, so the question of the importance of 5-HT_2 antagonism in anxiety remains open.

The 5-HT_3 system is more difficult to study in anxiety. Briley and Chopin (this volume) presented data suggesting that 5-HT_3 antagonists display anxiolytic-like activity in certain animal models. Direct assessment of central 5-HT_3 function is not available in man but peripheral indices might be obtained by studying the skin flare response to intradermal injections of 5-HT (Orwin and Fozard 1986) or the pain response to application of 5-HT to a blister base (Richardson *et al.* 1985). Both responses appear to be mediated by activation of 5-HT_3 receptors. Do anxious patients display different sensitivity to 5-HT_3 activation?

We do not yet have tests to probe the function in man of the recently described 5-HT_{1D} receptor at which sumatriptan is a potent agonist (Peroutka and Schmidt, this volume) and the 5-HT_3 receptor at which various benzamides, including zacopride, are partial agonists (Clarke *et al.* 1989). Might the action of these drugs be exploited to probe the serotonin system in man?

Another strategy for probing the role of 5-HT in anxiety and anti-anxiety agents would be to re-evaluate the consequences of inhibition of serotonin synthesis. Pioneering studies by Shopsin *et al.* (1975, 1976) demonstrated that the tryptophan hydroxylase inhibitor, *p*-chlorophenylalanine (*p*-CPA) reversed the antidepressant effect of imipramine and tranylcypromine. If it were possible to repeat these types of experiments, which is unlikely now, an important question would be whether the anxiolytic effect also disappears. It would certainly be worthwhile studying whether pindolol or propranolol could block the anxiolytic effect of buspirone or other anxiolytic drugs. Dennis Charney's group has developed an interesting strategy to produce an acute tryptophan depletion; they administer a cocktail of amino acids at high concentrations without tryptophan. The amino acids compete for the uptake of endogenous tryptophan and, in theory, produce a brief depletion of brain serotonin. Some of their preliminary data suggest that such a cocktail reverses the antidepressant effect of several compounds (Delgado *et al.* 1989).

Could we extend this approach, looking at the effect of this cocktail with anxiolytic drugs, and ask similar questions? As selective antagonists of different 5-HT receptor subtypes are developed, specific questions of the involvement of 5-HT in the mode of action of anxiolytics and the role of 5-HT in the aetiology of anxiety can be answered. Selective 'tools', such as MDL 11939, MDL 73005EF, and MDL 73147EF, may also be useful in such investigations.

Final comments

A constantly recurring theme in anxiety is its relationship to depression. How are these two phenomena linked? Anxiety and depression frequently coexist; drugs used to treat depression are effective anxiolytics and the converse is probably true for buspirone. We do not know if the mechanism of the anxiolytic and antidepressant actions of these compounds are the same, but the interrelationship begs the question, are anxiety and depression part of a spectrum of pathological responses that form part of a continuum of responses to stress? Or are there anxiety disorders which are distinct and separate from depression? We suspect that we shall be able to delineate distinct syndromes. Some will be of the 'spectrum-related' type; others will be anxiety which stands alone from other behavioural phenomena. As patients withdraw from benzodiazepines, now a frequent occurrence, shall we have the opportunity to evaluate a role for 5-HT in the emergent anxiety symptoms? How will this syndrome differ from idiopathic anxiety states? And, most crucially, can we develop therapeutic modalities that are directed towards the disease rather than the symptoms?

Acknowledgements

The authors thank Tim McCloskey for his major contribution to development of the separation-induced vocalization model, Jeffrey Sprouse for his valuable suggestions and discussion, and Mary Dooley for her skill and patience in preparing this manuscript.

References

Adam, K. and Oswald, I. (1989). Effects of repeated ritanserin on middle-aged poor sleepers. *Psychopharmacology*. **99**, 219–21.

American Psychiatric Association. (1980). *Diagnostic and statistical manual of mental disorders*, (3rd edn). American Psychiatric Association, Washington DC.

Baron, B. M., Harrison, B. L., Miller, F. P., McDonald, I. A., Salituro, F. G., Schmidt, C. J., *et al.* (1990). Activity of 5,7-dichlorokynurenic acid, a potent antagonist at the N-methyl-D-aspartate receptor-associated glycine binding site. *Molecular Pharmacology*, **38**, 454–61.

Barrett, J. E., Witkin, J. M., Mansbach, R. S., Skolnick, P., and Weissman, B. A. (1986). Behavioural studies with anxiolytic drugs, III. Antipunishment actions of buspirone in the pigeon do not involve benzodiazepine receptor mechanisms. *Journal of Pharmacology and Experimental Therapeutics*, **238**, 1009–13.

Barrett, J. E., Fleck-Kandath, C., and Mansbach, R. S. (1988). Effects of buspirone differ from those of gepirone and 8-hydroxy-2-(di-n-propylamino)tetralin (8-OH-DPAT) on unpunished responding of pigeons. *Pharmacology Biochemistry and Behaviour*, **30**, 723–7.

Briley, M. and Chopin, P. (1991). Serotonin in anxiety: evidence from animal models. In *5-Hydroxytrptamine in psychiatry: a spectrum of ideas*, (ed. M. Sandler, A. Coppen, and S. Harnett), pp. 177–197. Oxford University Press.

Broadhurst, P. L. (1975). The Maudsley reactive and nonreactive strains of rats: a survey. *Behaviour Genetics*, **5**, 299–319.

Cassella, J. V. and Davis, M. (1985). Fear-enhanced acoustic startle is not attenuated by acute or chronic imipramine treatment in rats. *Psychopharmacology*, **87**, 278–82.

Clarke, D. E., Craig, D. A. and Fozard, J. R. (1989). The 5-HT$_4$ receptor: naughty, but nice. *Trends in Pharmacological Sciences*, **10**, 385–6.

Collins, G. G. (1979). The effects of 5,7-dihydroxytryptamine lesions of the median and of the dorsal raphe nuclei on social interaction in the rat. *British Journal of Pharmacology*, **66**, 114–15.

Commissaris, R. L., Harrington, G. M., Baginski, T. J., and Altman, H. J. (1988). MR/Har and MNRA/Har Maudsley rats strains: differences in accoustic startle habituation. *Behaviour Genetics*, **18**, 663–9.

Cornfield, L. J. Nelson, D. L., Taylor, E. W., and Martin, A. R. (1989). MDL 73005EF: partial agonist at the 5-HT$_{1A}$ receptor negatively linked to adenylate cyclase. *European Journal of Pharmacology*, **173**, 189–92.

Cowen, P. J., Charig, E. M., Fraser, S., and Elliott, J. M. (1987). Platelet 5-HT receptor binding during depressive illness and tricyclic antidepressant treatment. *Journal of Affective Disorders*, **13**, 45–50.

Creamer, M. (1989). Post-traumatic stress disorder: some diagnostic and clinical issues. *Australian and New Zealand Journal of Psychiatry*, **4**, 517–22.

Dalterio, S. L., Wagner, M. J., Geller, I., and Hartmann, R. J. (1980). Ethanol and diazepam interactions on conflict behaviour in rats. *Alcohol*, **5**, 471–6.

Davis, M. (1979). Diazepam and flurazepam: effects on conditioned fear as measured with the potentiated startle paradigm. *Psychopharmacology*, **62**, 1–7.

Davis, M. (1986). Pharmacological and anatomical analysis of fear conditioning using the fear-potentiated startle paradigm. *Behavioural Neuroscience*, **100**, 814–24.

Davis, M., Gendelman, D. S., Tischler, M. D., and Gendelman, P. M. (1982). A primary acoustic startle circuit; lesion and stimulation studies. *Journal of Neuroscience*, **6**, 791–805.

Davis, M., Cassella, J. V., and Kehne, J. H. (1988). Serotonin does not mediate anxiolytic effects of buspirone in the fear-potentiated startle paradigm: comparison with 8-OH-DPAT and ipsapirone. *Psychopharmacology*, **94**, 14–20.

Deakin, J. F. W., Guimaraes, F. S., Wang, M., and Hensmen, R. (1991). Experimental tests of the 5-HT receptor imbalance theory of affective disturbance. In *5-Hydroxytryptamine in psychiatry: a spectrum of ideas*, (ed. M. Sandler, A. Coppen, and S. Harnett), pp. 143–156. Oxford University Press.

Delgado, P. L., Charney, D. S., Price, L. H., Goodman, W. K., Aghajanian, G. K., and Heninger, G. F. (1989). Behavioral effects of acute tryptophan depletion in psychiatric patients and healthy subjects. *Society for Neuroscience Abstracts*, **15**, 166.13.

Dudley, M. W., Wiech, N. L., Miller, F. P., Carr, A. A., Cheng, H. S., Roebel, L. E., *et al.* (1988). Pharmacological effects of MDL 11939: a selective, centrally acting antagonist of 5-HT$_2$ receptors. *Drug Development Research*, **13**, 29–43.

Fandeleur, P. C. and Jones, C. R. (1989). Additive effects of desipramine and 8-OHDPAT on β-adrenoceptor down-regulation. *British Journal of Pharmacology*, **98**, 918P.

File, S. E. and Hyde, J. R. (1978). Can social interaction be used to measure anxiety? *British Journal of Pharmacology*, **62**, 19–24.

File, S. E. and Johnston, A. L. (1989). Lack of effects of 5-HT$_3$ receptor antagonists in the social interaction and elevated plus-maze tests of anxiety in the rat. *Psychopharmacology*, **99**, 248–51.

File, S. E., Hyde, J. R., and MacLeod, N. K. (1979). 5,7-dihydroxytryptamine lesions of dorsal and median raphe nuclei and performance in the social interaction test of anxiety and in a home-cage aggression test. *Journal of Affective Disorders*, **1**, 115–22.

Gardner, C. R. (1985). Distress vocalization in rat pups. A simple screening method for anxiolytic drugs. *Journal of Pharmacological Methods*, **14**, 181–7.

Gardner, C. R. (1988). Potential use of drugs modulating 5-HT activity in the treatment of anxiety. *General Pharmacology*, **19**, 347–56.

Geller, I. and Seifter, J. (1960). The effects of meprobamate, barbiturates, d-amphetamine and promazine on experimentally induced conflict in the rat. *Psychopharmacology*, **1**, 482–92.

Geller, I., Hartmenn, R. J., and Croy, D. J. (1974). Attenuation of conflict behavior with cinanserin, a serotonin antagonist: reversal of the effect with 5-hydroxytryptophan and α-methyltryptamine. *Research Communications in Chemical Pathology and Pharmacology*, **7**, 165–74.

Gittos, M. W. and Fatmi, M. (1989). Potent 5-HT$_3$ receptor antagonists incorporating a novel bridged pseudopelletierine ring system. *Actualité de Chimie Therapeutique*, **16**, 187–98.

Gleeson, S., Ahlers, S. T., Mansbach, R. S., Foust, J. M., and Barrett, J. E. (1989). Behavioral studies with anxiolytic drugs. VI. Effects on punished responding of drugs interacting with serotonin receptor subtypes. *Journal of Pharmacology and Experimental Therapeutics*, **250**, 809–17.

Goa, K. L. and Ward, A. (1986). Buspirone, a preliminary review of its pharmacological properties and therapeutic efficacy as an anxiolytic. *Drugs*, **32**, 114–29.

Gudelsky, G. A., Koenig, J. I., and Meltzer, H. Y. (1986). Thermoregulatory responses to serotonin (5-HT) receptor stimulation in the rat. *Neuropharmacology*, **25**, 1307–13.

Hibert, M., Mir, A., Maghiros, G., Moser, P., Middlemiss, M., Tricklebank, M., and Fozard, J. (1988). The pharmacological properties of MDL 73,005EF: a potent and selective ligand at 5-HT_{1A} receptors. *British Journal of Pharmacology*, **93**, 2.

Higgins, G. A., Bradbury, A. J., Jones, B. J., and Oakley, N. R. (1988). Behavioural and biochemical consequences following activation of 5-HT_1-like and GABA receptors in the dorsal raphe nucleus of the rat. *Neuropharmacology*, **27**, 993–1001.

Hijzen, T. H. and Slangen, J. L. (1989). Effects of midazolam, DMCM and lindane on potentiated startle in the rat. *Psychopharmacology*, **99**, 362–5.

Hitchcock, J. and Davis, M. (1986). Lesions of the amygdala, but not of the cerebellum or red nucleus, block conditioned fear as measured with the potentiated startle paradigm. *Behavioral Neuroscience*, **100**, 11–22.

Insel, T. R. and Hill, J. L. (1987). Infant separation distress in genetically fearful rats. *Biological Psychiatry*, **22**, 786–9.

Insel, T. R., Hill, J. L., and Mayor, R. B. (1986). Rat pup ultrasonic isolation calls: possible mediation by the benzodiazepine receptor complex. *Pharmacology Biochemistry and Behavior*, **24**, 1263–7.

Insel, T. R., Miller, L., Gelhard, R., Hill, J. (1988). Rat pup ultrasonic isolation calls and the benzodiazepine receptor. In *The physiological control of mammalian vocalization*, (ed. J. D. Newman), pp. 331–42. Plenum Press, New York.

Johnston, A. L. and File, S. E. (1988). Profiles of the antipanic compounds, triazolobenzodiazepines and phenelzine, in two animal tests of anxiety. *Psychiatry Research*, **25**, 81–90.

Jones, B. J., Costall, B., Domeney, A. M., Naylor, R. J., Oakley, N. R., and Tyers, M. B. (1988). The potential anxiolytic activity of GR38032F, a 5-HT_3-receptor antagonist. *British Journal of Pharmacology*, **93**, 985–93.

Kehne, J. H., Cassella, J. V., and Davis, M. (1988). Anxiolytic effects of buspirone and gepirone in the fear-potentiated startle paradigm. *Psychopharmacology*, **94**, 8–13.

Kehoe, P. and Harris, J. C. (1989). Ontogeny of noradrenergic effects on ultrasonic vocalizations in rat pups. *Behavioral Neuroscience*, **103**, 1099–107.

Kettelaars, C. E. and Bruinvels, J. (1989). The anti-conflict effect of cyproheptadine is not mediated by its 5-hydroxytryptamine antagonistic property. *Life Sciences*, **44**, 1743–9.

Kilts, C. D., Commissaris, R. L., and Rech, R. H. (1981). Comparison of anti-conflict drug effects in three experimental animal models of anxiety. *Psychopharmacology*, **74**, 290–6.

Kinzie, J. D., Fredrickson, R. H., Ben, R., Fleck, J., and Karls, W. (1984). Posttraumatic stress disorder among survivors of Cambodian concentration camps. *American Journal of Psychiatry*, **141**, 645–50.

Kramer, R., Rubieck, M., and Turner, P. (1973). The role of norfenfluramine in fenfluramine-induced mydriasis. *Journal of Pharmacy and Pharmacology*, **25**, 575–6.

Mansbach, R. S. and Geyer, M. A. (1988). Blockade of potentiated startle responding in rats by $5\text{-hydroxytryptamine}_{1A}$ receptor ligands. *European Journal of Pharmacology*, **156**, 375–83.

McCloskey, T. C., Paul, B. K., and Commissaris, R. L. (1987). Buspirone effects in an animal conflict procedure: comparison with Diazepam and Phenobarbital. *Pharmacology Biochemistry and Behavior*, **27**, 171–5.

Meldrum, B. (1985). Possible therapeutic applications of antagonists of excitatory amino acid neurotransmitters. *Clinical Science*, **68**, 113–22.

Millson, D. S., Harry, J. D., Haworth, S. J., and Wilkerson, D. (1988). Effects of a 5-HT$_2$ antagonist (ICI 169,369) on human pupillary responses. *British Journal of Clinical Pharmacology*, **26**, 625P.

Moser, P. C., Tricklebank, M. D., Middlemiss, D. N., Mir, A. K., Hibert, M. F., and Fozard, J. R. (1990). Characterization of MDL 73005EF as a 5-HT$_{1A}$ selective ligand and its effects in animal models of anxiety: comparison with buspirone, 8-OH-DPAT and diazepam. *British Journal of Pharmacology*, **99**, 343–9.

Mos, J., Bevan, P., and Olivier, B. (1988). Ultrasonic vocalizations by rat pups as an animal model for anxiolytic activity. *Society for Neuroscience Abstracts*, **14**, 404.8.

Nomura, Y., Oki, K., and Segawa, T. (1980). Pharmacological characterization of central α-adrenoceptors which mediate clonidine-induced locomotor hypoactivity in the developing rat. *Naunyn-Schmiedeberg's Archives of Pharmacology*, **311**, 41–4.

Orwin, J. M. and Fozard, J. R. (1986). Blockade of the flare response to intradermal 5-hydroxytryptamine in man by MDL 72,222, a selective antagonist at neuronal 5-hydroxytryptamine receptors. *European Journal of Clinical Pharmacology*, **30**, 209–12.

Ottenweller, J. E., Natelson, B. H., Pitman, D. L., and Drastal, S. D. (1989). Adrenocortical and behavioral responses to repeated stressors: toward an animal model of chronic stress-related mental illness. *Biological Psychiatry*, **26**, 829–41.

Peroutka, S. J. and Schmidt, A. W. (1991). An overview of 5-hydroxytryptamine receptor families. In *5-Hydroxytryptamine in psychiatry: a spectrum of ideas*, (ed. M. Sandler, A. Coppen, and S. Harnett), pp. 2–22. Oxford University Press.

Reinstein, D. K. and Isaacson, R. L. (1977). Clonidine sensitivity in the developing rat. *Brain Research*, **135**, 378–82.

Richardson, B. P., Engel, G., Donatsch, P., and Stadler, P. A. (1985). Identification of serotonin receptor subtypes and their specific blockade by a new class of drugs. *Nature*, **316**, 126–31.

Rickels, K., Schweizer, E., Csanalosi, I., Case, W. G., and Chung, H. (1988). Long-term treatment of anxiety and risk of withdrawal. *Archives of General Psychiatry*, **45**, 444–50.

Ross, R. J., Ball, W. A., Sullivan, K. A., and Caroff, S. N. (1989). Sleep disturbance as the hallmark of posttraumatic stress disorder. *American Journal of Psychiatry*, **146**, 697–707.

Schefke, D. M., Fontana, D. J., and Commissaris, R. L. (1989). Anti-conflict efficacy of buspirone following acute versus chronic treatment. *Psychopharmacology*, **99**, 427–9.

Schweitzer, L. and Adams, G. (1979). The diagnosis and management of anxiety for primary care physicians. In *Phenomenology and treatment of anxiety*, (ed. W. E. Fann, I. Karacan, A. D. Parkorny, and R. L. Williams), pp. 19–42. Spectrum, New York.

Sharp, T., Bramwell, S. R., Hjorth, S., and Grahame-Smith, D. G. (1989). Pharmacological characterization of 8-OH-DPAT-induced inhibition of rat hippocampal 5-HT release *in vivo* as measured by microdialysis. *British Journal of Pharmacology*, **98**, 989–97.

Shopsin, B., Friedman, E., and Gershon, S. (1976). Parachlorophenylalanine reversal of tranylcypromine effects in depressed patients. *Archives of General Psychiatry*, **33**, 811–19.

Shopsin, B., Gershon, S., Goldstein, M., Friedman, E., and Wilk, S. (1975). Use of synthesis inhibitors in defining a role for biogenic amines during imipramine treatment in depressed patients. *Psychopharmacology Communications*, **1**, 239–49.

Sinton, C. M. and Fallon, S. L. (1988). Electrophysiological evidence for a functional differentiation between subtypes of the 5-HT$_1$ receptor. *European Journal of Pharmacology*, **157**, 173–81.

Smith, D. A. and Gallager, D. W. (1989). Electrophysiological and biochemical characterization of the development of α_1 adrenergic and 5-HT$_1$ receptors associated with dorsal raphe neurons. *Developmental Brain Research*, **46**, 173–86.

Sorensen, S. M., Humphrey, T. M., and Palfreyman, M. G. (1989). Effect of acute and chronic MDL 73147EF, a 5-HT$_3$ receptor antagonist, on A9 and A10 dopamine neurons. *European Journal of Pharmacology*, **163**, 115–18.

Sprouse, J. S. and Aghajanian, G. K. (1987). Electrophysiological responses of serotoninergic dorsal raphe neurons to 5-HT$_{1A}$ and 5-HT$_{1B}$ agonists. *Synapse*, **1**, 3–9.

Swerdlow, N. R., Britton, K. T., and Koob, G. F. (1989). Potentiation of acoustic startle by corticotropin-releasing factor (CRF) and by fear are both reversed by α-helical CRF (9–41). *Neuropsychopharmacology*, **2**, 285–92.

Tonoue, T., Ashida, Y., Makino, H., and Hata, H. (1986). Inhibition of shock-elicited ultrasonic vocalization by opioid peptides in the rat: a psychotropic effect. *Psychoneuroendocrinology*, **11**, 177–84.

Vogel, J. R., Beer, B., and Clody, D. E. (1971). A simple and reliable conflict procedure for testing anti-anxiety agents. *Psychopharmacology*, **21**, 1–7.

Weiss, J. M. and Simpson, P. G. (1986). Depression in an animal model: focus on the locus ceruleus. In *Antidepressants and receptor function*, Ciba Foundation Symposium 123, pp. 191–215. Wiley, Chichester.

Witkin, J. M. Mansbach, R. S., Barrett, J. E., Bolger, G. T., Skolnick, P., and Weissman, B. (1987). Behavioral studies with anxiolytic drugs, IV. Serotonergic involvement in the effects of buspirone on punished behavior of pigeons. *Journal of Pharmacology and Experimental Therapeutics*, **243**, 970–7.

Discussion

ROBINSON: We have some information on the interaction between 5-HT$_{1A}$ agonists and benzodiazepines from a study of 750 patients in placebo-controlled three-arm trials of buspirone in generalized anxiety disorder. One third of the patients had taken benzodiazepines recently, one third had done so in the remote past, and one third had never received a benzodiazepine. Those discontinuing treatment one to four weeks before the trial showed marked improvement in the first week of the trial when benzodiazepine was re-instituted. Improvement involved a symptom cluster thought to be the typical withdrawal symptoms of sedative hypnotic (benzodiazepine) drugs. The first week improvement pattern differed from this in the other two treatment groups. Patients who had taken benzodiazepines remotely or never also did not show this first response pattern. However, by the end of the trial the treatment response was similar for all groups. Thus, as Rickels *et al.* (1983,

1988) have shown, patients who discontinue benzodiazepines may have manifestations of drug withdrawal for four weeks or longer.

The question whether this interaction could be serotonergically mediated is interesting. Those patients recently discontinuing a benzodiazepine who are assigned to buspirone and drop out in the first four weeks suffer significantly more light-headedness, which is a specific serotonergic side-effect of these drugs. They also have a higher incidence of insomnia, a typical benzodiazepine withdrawal symptom that may be mediated by other neurotransmitters.

INSEL: Professor Curzon suggested that benzodiazepines may in some way regulate the release of 5-hydroxytryptamine (5-HT, serotonin) in the hippocampus. We thought we could study one mechanism for that directly in the primate brain with lesions of the serotonin terminals. We reasoned that if benzodiazepine receptors were pre-synaptic at serotonin terminals, destruction of the terminals with repeated 3,4-methylene dioxymethamphetamine (MDMA) administration should be associated with a loss of benzodiazepine sites. We also investigated [³H]glutamate binding in the same regions. Much to our surprise, after extensive lesions of the 5-HT terminals there was absolutely no change in benzodiazepine or N-methyl-D-aspartate receptors. Using *in vitro* receptor autoradiography in adjacent sections, we know that in areas where there is about a 50 per cent loss of terminals (assessed with [³H]paroxetine binding) benzodiazepine sites (assessed with [³H]flunitrazepam binding) are conserved. Thus, benzodiazepines may regulate the release of serotonin, but not directly at the pre-synaptic terminal. There must be some interneurone involved in the regulation of 5-HT release.

COWEN: Green *et al.* (1985) treated rats with benzodiazepines for two or three weeks and found an increase in brain 5-HT₂ receptor density together with evidence of an increase in their functional responsiveness. If the same thing occurs with 5-HT₁ receptors located post-synaptically that might explain some of the effects of buspirone in patients who have recently withdrawn from benzodiazepines.

YOUDIM: I like the suggestion that we should consider manipulation of 5-HT release. Thalidomide was an important hypnotic but the mechanism of its action was unknown. Unlike thalidomide, the sister drug, supidimide, was not teratogenic. We examined the action of thalidomide and supidimide in various biogenic amine metabolic and behavioural systems in the rat. Both drugs inhibited the 5-HT behavioural syndrome in rats induced pre-synaptically with a monoamine oxidase inhibitor plus tryptophan, but not the behaviour induced post-synaptically with the 5-HT agonist, 5-methoxy-N,N-dimethyltryptamine. We attributed these effects to decreased 5-HT release, as evidenced by increased brain 5-HT without an altered 5-HT metabolism. Thalidomide and supidimide may be important new tools for studying the inhibition of 5-HT release. They are devoid of 5-HT₁ₐ agonistic property. Early studies indicated anxiolytic properties for these agents (Youdim and Ashkenazi 1985; Youdim *et al.* 1990).

Many years ago both Gerald Curzon and our group showed that yohimbine affects 5-HT-synthesis in the brain: it inhibits liver tryptophan pyrrolase, thus shunting tryptophan into the brain. That may explain why it is anxiogenic (Papeschi *et al.* 1971).

PALFREYMAN: Yohimbine may act on the serotonin heteroreceptor, the α_2 receptor that is on serotonergic terminals, which controls release (Feuerstein *et al.* 1985).

INSEL: The ultrasonic vocalization test measures a behaviour that is exquisitely sensitive to temperature changes. Could these apparent 5-HT drug effects be secondary to thermoregulatory changes?

PALFREYMAN: That is an important issue that we have not yet addressed. The pups will not vocalize if they are kept warm; it is definitely a temperature-sensitive response.

LÓPEZ-IBOR: I like the rat pup separation model because patients with panic disorders often have had a separation anxiety in the past (López-Ibor 1989). Current diagnostic criteria tend to neglect the natural history of the disorders. Besides, we should remember that anxiety and depression are both feelings and disorders. As feelings both are related to events, being the experience of the threat of an event (anxiety) or of the loss induced by it (depression). Both emotions are essential for the survival of the individual—depression to cope with a loss (Sartre 1939), anxiety to cope with a threat. Anxiety is an unspecific reaction that prepares the individual to face a yet unidentified threat. It is the psychological experience of what we call stress at the biological level. The individual is able to activate more specific mechanisms once the threat has been identified. But sometimes these coping mechanisms become self-destructive (Bakan 1968), as when they arise after minimal stimuli or spontaneously or when they persist longer than needed. From this point of view, anxiety and depressive disorders are forms of the adaptation disorders (Selye 1956).

MURPHY: Dr Palfreyman raised the question of the time delay in therapeutic responses to anxiolytic drugs. The results of Curzon *et al.* (this volume) suggest that one should study 5-HT_{1C} antagonists in anxiety. We have begun to address both issues. Chronic administration of *m*-chlorophenylpiperazine (*m*-CPP) to six depressed patients for two weeks led to decreased anxiety and depression in several of the patients with mixed anxiety/depression. We are now doing longer term studies. One way to get a 5-HT_{1C} antagonist, or at least an 'anti-*m*-CPP' effect, is to administer that very compound in gradually increasing doses over time. This illustrates some of the complexities associated with comparison of acute and chronic studies.

BELMAKER: The largest group of people exposed to *m*-CPP are the tens, if not hundreds, of thousands of depressed patients who have been treated with trazodone. Although fluoxetine is anxiogenic, trazodone is not; it is a highly sedative antidepressant. These patients have significant blood levels of *m*-CPP, which is a metabolite of trazodone. Why isn't *m*-CPP anxiogenic here?

   Another finding that may be related to a subtle timing effect is the lithium enhancement of serotonin release induced by tricyclic antidepressants. This only occurs if the tricyclic antidepressant is given to patients for three weeks before the lithium is given. If imipramine is given simultaneously with lithium for three weeks, there is no greater improvement than with imipramine alone (Lingjaerde *et al.* 1974).

COWEN: The parent compound, trazodone, blocks 5-HT_2 receptors and might also block 5-HT_{1C} receptors, thus attenuating the action of *m*-CPP *in vivo*.

MURPHY: This difference cannot be explained by differences in plasma levels. When *m*-CPP is given orally at doses of 0.5 mg kg^{-1}, the plasma levels are about 38 ng ml^{-1}. When single doses of trazodone are given, the *m*-CPP levels are around 22 or 18 ng ml^{-1}. Intravenous administration of *m*-CPP gives higher peak levels, but after oral doses, including those used in panic disorder patients (0.25 mg kg^{-1}; Kahn *et al.* 1988), the plasma levels would be similar to those seen during trazodone administration. Even patients receiving trazodone clinically, who may be given up to 600 mg per day, are more likely to be sedated than anxious. Thus, Dr Cowen's explanation that the parent drug is an antagonist is more likely to be correct. We think that with chronic administration, after the first dose, which may be covered by the antagonist effect, there may be some down-regulation with positive effects instead of an anxiogenic effect.

SULSER: How robust is the evidence that tricyclic antidepressants and monoamine oxidase (MAO) inhibitors are anti-anxiety agents?

MELTZER: The evidence that the tricyclics are anti-anxiety drugs is fairly strong.

LINNOILA: Phenelzine is more effective than imipramine in panic disorder. This may relate to the relative lack of anticholinergic effects of phenelzine. It has been claimed that for patients with classical atypical depression a history of even one panic attack is predictive of a superior response to an MAO inhibitor compared to the tricyclic antidepressants. I think that can be contested.

ROBINSON: In the 1970s at Vermont, we studied about 170 patients who were randomly assigned to a fixed dose of either a tricyclic antidepressant, amitriptyline, or the MAO inhibitor, phenelzine. The entry criterion was that the patients must be diagnosed as suffering from primary depression; it covered a fairly broad spectrum of depressive disorders. The depressive symptoms improved almost equally, but there was a statistically significantly greater improvement with the MAO inhibitor in all the anxiety (psychic and somatic) measures, both self-rated and observer-rated. I would argue that there are some specific anxiolytic properties of MAO inhibitors. In panic disorder there is a trend in the same direction.

COPPEN: I am fairly convinced that depressive disorder is a pathological disorder. We know quite a lot about its natural history: it is a chronic relapsing condition in about 60 per cent of cases; it has a high ongoing morbidity and increased mortality through suicide. I am less convinced about anxiety.

Professor López-Ibor made the point that anxiety and depression are appropriate normal responses to life events. Phobic anxiety and panic attacks are inappropriate and severe responses to life events. What happens to these people as they get older? For how long do we need to treat them? We have some answers to these questions in depression. We all suffer to a certain degree from anxiety, but some people who experience acute anxiety ask their doctors for help. I am unhappy about the concept of a general anxiety illness. Many actors say that if they do not feel anxiety they will not give a good performance. Whom should we be treating?

LINNOILA: Panic disorder has a devastating course with a high risk of suicide and great social disability if the disorder is not treated. As you say, many competent performers feel that anxiety is necessary. At the same time, it seems that the performance of marksmen can be improved by low doses of β-blockers which block the cardiovascular responses to anxiety. Thus, this issue has not been resolved.

LÓPEZ-IBOR: We have done follow-up studies of patients who were seen during the 1950s for anxiety disorders (López-Ibor 1989). According to current criteria, two thirds were panic disorder patients and one third had generalized anxiety. Patients with panic disorder tend to have mild depression, sometimes with melancholia, and they often become alcoholics. This does not happen so often with generalized anxiety patients, but later on in life they all become chronic somatizers. They go frequently to their doctors complaining of different somatic symptoms—pains, aches, etc. They are severely affected by their disorder, leading very uninteresting lives; for many the only contact with the outside world is when they visit their physician.

COPPEN: What is the sex distribution among these people? Depression is predominantly suffered by females. Biopolar illness has an almost equal sex distribution.

LÓPEZ-IBOR: There are more females than males in our sample.

MENDLEWICZ: The categorization of anxiety disorders is rather recent, and most of these patients are already on various drugs, such as benzodiazepines, hypnotics, and antidepressants. We know little about the natural course of these syndromes. In affective disorder we benefited from long-term prophylactic studies, such as the lithium studies, which provided information on the course of the illness. In anxiety we lack important information.

COPPEN: Does chronic anxiety lead to alcohol abuse?

MENDLEWICZ: Yes.

DOOGAN: There is evidence that the 5-HT uptake inhibitors are effective in panic disorder. Westenberg and den Boer (1988) reported that the 5-HT$_2$ antagonist, ritanserin, which has some anxiolytic effects, has no effect in panic disorder. Has that finding been replicated?

DEAKIN: I don't think so, but I thought it was a decisive trial because they showed in the same study that fluvoxamine was effective on panic. This suggests that 5-HT$_2$ receptors may not be involved in panic, whereas we have evidence for anxiolytic effects of ritanserin in our trial (Deakin *et al.*, this volume).

LINNOILA: Ritanserin has been reported to make panic disorder worse in some patients, which may support that idea.

Co-morbidity with panic disorder is extremely common in middle-class individuals, at least in Washington DC, who seek treatment for alcoholism. Often they had been given low-dose benzodiazepines and then discovered that alcohol was helpful. That worsens the situation; each alcohol withdrawal produces panic-like symptoms.

SULSER: Can we come to a consensus on the clinical efficacy of the various drugs that are used in anxiety? How do benzodiazepines, 5-HT$_{1A}$ partial agonists, MAO inhibitors, tricyclic antidepressants, and even alcohol compare?

COWEN: The MAO inhibitors may have the broadest spectrum of action in many kinds of anxiety. Then there are more selective agents that work in fewer conditions, such as ritanserin, which does not work in panic disorder. The newer drugs may help us to understand the specific neuropharmacological changes that underlie therapeutic effects in distinct disorders.

LINNOILA: I disagree about the MAO inhibitors: there has not been a controlled trial in generalized anxiety disorders. Dr Robinson's study is excellent, but is on depressed patients and mixed anxiety/depression.

Alcohol has acute, effective anxiolytic action. But studies of its chronic use in humans show that alcohol significantly increases anxiety through the withdrawal effect.

MELTZER: In schizophrenics the short-acting benzodiazepines are effective anxiolytics. In our hands, the 5-HT$_{1A}$ partial agonists have been ineffective. In many parts of the world low-dose neuroleptics are the most widely used anxiolytic drugs. They are effective but produce tardive dyskinesia.

MENDLEWICZ: I agree that we have good data on the acute anxiolytic effects of benzodiazepines and the newer serotonergic drugs. However, if we agree that anxiety may be a chronic problem and cannot be limited to an acute reaction, we must acknowledge our need for information about the natural course of anxiety disorders. My feeling is that we have no proven efficient treatment of chronic anxiety.

References

Bakan, D. (1968). *Disease, pain and sacrifice. Towards a psychology of suffering.* University of Chicago Press.

Curzon, G., Kennett, G. A., and Whitton, P. (1991). Anxiogenic effect of the 5-HT$_{1C}$ agonist *m*-chlorophenylpiperazine, In *5-Hydroxytryptamine in psychiatry: a spectrum of ideas*, (ed. M. Sandler, A. Coppen, and S. Harnett), pp. 198–206. Oxford University Press.

Deakin, J. F. W., Guimaraes, F. S., Wang, M., and Hensman, R. (1991). Experimental tests of the 5-HT receptor imbalance theory of affective disturbance. In *5-Hydroxytryptamine in psychiatry: a spectrum of ideas*, (ed. M. Sandler, A. Coppen, and S. Harnett), pp. 143–156. Oxford University Press.

Green, A. R., Johnson, P., Mountford, J. A., and Nimgaonkar, V. L. (1985). Some anticonvulsant drugs alter monoamine mediated behaviour in mice in ways similar to electroconvulsive shock: implications for antidepressant therapy. *British Journal of Pharmacology*, **84**, 337–46.

Feuerstein, T. J., Hertting, G., and Jackisch, R. (1985). Endogenous noradrenaline as modulator of hippocampal serotonin (5-HT)-release. *Naunyn-Schmiedebergs's Archives of Pharmacology*, **329**, 216–21.

Kahn, R. S., Asnis, G. M., Wetzer, S., *et al.* (1988). Neuroendocrine evidence for serotonin receptor hypersensitivity in panic disorder. *Psychopharmacology*, **96**, 360–4.

Lingjaerde, O., Edlvna, A. H., Gorsen, C. A., Gottfries, C. G., Haugstad, A., Herman, I.L., *et al.* (1974). The effect of lithium carbonate in combination with tricyclic antidepressants in endogenous depression. *Acta Psychiatrica Scandinavica*, **50**, 233.

López-Ibor Jr., J. J. (1989). The classification of neurotic, anxiety and related disorders in light of ICD-10. In *Contemporary themes in psychiatry*, (ed. K. Davison and A. Kerr), pp. 156–66. Gaskell and the Royal College of Psychiatrists, London.

Papeschi, R., Sourkes, T. L., and Youdim, M. B. H. (1971). The effect of yohimbine on brain serotonin metabolism, motor behaviour and body temperature. *European Journal of Pharmacology*, **15**, 318–36.

Rickels, K., Case, W. G., Downing R. W., and Winokus, A. (1983). Long-term diazepam therapy and clinical outcome. *Journal of the American Medical Association*, **250**, 767–71.

Rickels, K., Schweizer, E., Csanalosi, I., Case, W. G., and Chung, H. (1988). Long-term treatment of anxiety and risk of withdrawal. *Archives of General Psychiatry*, **45**, 444–50.

Sartre, J. P. (1939). *Equisse d'une thérie des émotions.* Herman, Paris.

Selye, H. (1956). *The stress of life.* McGraw Hill, New York.

Westenberg, H. G. M. and den Boer, J. A. (1988). Serotonin uptake inhibitors and agonists in the treatment of panic disorders. *Psychopharmacology*, **96**, Suppl., 56.

Youdim, M. B. H. and Ashkenazi, R. (1985). Serotonergic involvement in pharmacological actions of anxiolytic sedatives thalidomide and supidimide. *European Journal of Pharmacology*, **119**, 39–47.

Youdim, M. B. H., Marmors, S., Aviram, M., and Gavish, M. (1990). The inhibition of platelet 5-HT release by 5-HT$_{1A}$ agonists and the binding of [^{3}H]8-OH-DPAT to platelet membranes. *Biogenic Amines*, **7**, 11–19.

18. Serotonin in obsessive-compulsive disorder: a causal connection or more monomania about a major monoamine?

Thomas R. Insel

Serotonin (5-hydroxytryptamine, 5-HT) has been implicated in a number of psychiatric syndromes, but it is obsessive-compulsive disorder (OCD) that currently provides the most compelling evidence of a connection between serotonin and psychopathology. The precise nature of this connection remains unclear—in spite of strong evidence implicating serotonin in the treatment of OCD, we still lack a clear model of serotonergic dysfunction to explain the pathophysiology of this syndrome. This paper reviews the current literature about serotonin and OCD to examine two questions: do OCD patients have an abnormality in serotonergic neurotransmission and, if so, what is the nature of this abnormality?

Obsessive-compulsive disorder

Obsessive-compulsive disorder is a chronic, disabling syndrome characterized by obsessions (intrusive ideas, images, or impulses which are reprehensible) and/or compulsions (repetitive behaviours often connected with an obsession). A typical obsession would be the relentless thought that one's hands are contaminated with 'germs', radioactivity, faeces, or some undefinable toxin. The related compulsion would be repetitive washing, often for hours at a time. Other patients may feel that they have injured someone and will compulsively check to reassure themselves that no damage has actually been done. Generally, patients recognize the senselessness of these intrusive ideas; it is the intrusive irrationality of these symptoms which may be most bothersome. Similarly, the compulsive behaviours have a stereotyped, ritualistic quality which in some cases includes both an intentional and an involuntary component.

Although this disorder is classified with other anxiety disorders, OCD has many features that are distinct from the phobias, panic disorder, and generalized anxiety. OCD patients are likely to present with as much dysphoria as anxiety; often with major complaints involving guilt, doubt, or despair. It should be noted that OCD patients share many of the physiological abnormalities associated with major depressive disorder, including changes in neuroendocrine, sleep electroencephalogram, and platelet measures (Insel *et al.* 1984). This relationship may be partly explained by the very high prevalence of depression in OCD; as many as 70 per cent of patients with OCD describe a history of a major depressive episode. In addition, the quality of the intrusive thoughts is often tic-like, raising the question of a relationship between OCD and Tourette's syndrome. The emerging literature on the co-morbidity and the familial patterns of these two syndromes suggests a considerable overlap in their genetics (Pauls *et al.* 1986).

The relationship to Tourette's syndrome, the presence of stereotypic behaviours, and the perseverative aspects of this disorder may suggest an abnormality in dopaminergic pathways. In fact, an OCD-like syndrome, known as klazomania, was described in association with post-encephalitic Parkinsonism earlier in this century. Nevertheless, dopamine receptor antagonists, such as the neuroleptics, have not been shown to reduce the symptoms of OCD, except in some cases of combined OCD and Tourette's syndrome (McDougle *et al.* 1989). Large, single doses of d-amphetamine acutely decrease OCD symptoms, but this effect may not be related to dopamine agonist effects (Insel *et al.* 1985). Chronic administration of d-amphetamine is associated with increased dopaminergic neurotransmission and does not appear to be a useful treatment for OCD (Insel *et al.* 1985).

The selectivity of anti-obsessional agents

From a neuropharmacological perspective, the most remarkable aspect of OCD is its high selectivity for drug response (Table 18.1) (Insel and Zohar 1987). Most drugs that reduce anxiety, depression, or psychosis are not effective against obsessions. While individual OCD patients may respond to antidepressants such as the tricyclic imipramine or the monoamine oxidase inhibitor tranylcypromine, thus far the only medications that appear consistently effective in studies of OCD are clomipramine (CMI) (Thoren *et al.* 1980*a*; Insel *et al.* 1983; Flament *et al.* 1985), fluvoxamine (Perse *et al.* 1987; Goodman *et al.* 1989), and fluoxetine (Fontaine and Chouinard 1985; Turner *et al.* 1985). These three compounds are all antidepressants, and yet they reduce obsessional symptoms in non-depressed OCD patients. For this reason, they have been described as anti-obsessional drugs, in addition to being antidepressants. Just as in the treatment of depression, therapeutic effects only emerge after chronic (> 5 weeks) administration of these drugs. What is surprising is that so many other excellent antidepressants, even those which are structurally related to these anti-obsessional drugs, appear ineffective for the symptoms of OCD. The salient difference may be that each·of the anti-obsessional drugs is a potent inhibitor of serotonin re-uptake.

T. R. Insel

TABLE 18.1. *Double-blind drug treatment studies in OCD patients*

Study	Treatment	Design, *n*	Result
Drugs vs placebo (P)			
Thoren *et al.* 1980*a*	CMI (150 mg) vs NOR (150 mg) vs P	Parallel, 35	CMI > P (5 wk), NOR not > P
Marks *et al.* 1980	CMI (183 mg) vs P	Parallel, 40	CMI > P (4 wk self-rating only)
Montgomery 1980	CMI (75 mg) vs P	Cross-over, 14	CMI > P (4 wk)
Mavissakalian *et al.* 1985	CMI (228 mg) vs P	Parallel, 15	CMI > P (6 wk)
Flament *et al.* 1985	CMI (141 mg) vs P	Cross-over, 19	CMI > P (5 wk) (Childhood OCD)
Perse *et al.* 1987	FLUV (300 mg) vs P	Cross-over, 16	FLUV > P (8wk)
Foa *et al.* 1987	IMI (233 mg) vs P	Parallel, 37	IMI = P (6 wk)
Goodman *et al.* 1989	FLUV (255 mg) vs P	Parallel, 42	FLUV > P (6–8 wk)
de Veaugh Geiss *et al.* 1989	CMI (100–250 mg) vs P	Parallel, 260	CMI > P (10 wk)
Drug vs drug			
Ananth *et al.* 1981	CMI (133 mg) vs AMI (197 mg)	Parallel, 20	CMI > baseline, AMI = baseline
Insel *et al.* 1983	CMI (236 mg) vs CLG (28 mg)	Cross-over, 13	CMI > CLG (4 + 6 wk)
Volavka *et al.* 1985	CMI (275 mg) vs IMI (265 mg)	Parallel, 16	CMI > IMI (6 wk)
Zohar and Insel 1987	CMI (235 mg) vs DMI (290 mg)	Cross-over, 10	CMI > DMI (6 wk)
Leonard *et al.* 1988	CMI vs DMI (3 mg kg^{-1} as tolerated)	Cross-over, 21	CMI > DMI (6 wk)
Pato *et al.* 1989	CMI (150–300 mg) vs BUSP (30–60 mg)	Parallel, 20	CMI = BUSP
Goodman *et al.* 1989	FLUV vs DMI	Parallel, 35	FLUV > DMI

CMI, clomipramine; NOR, nortriptyline; FLUV, fluvoxamine; AMI, amitriptyline; CLG, clorgyline; IMI, imipramine; DMI, desipramine; BUSP, buspirone; wk, weeks.

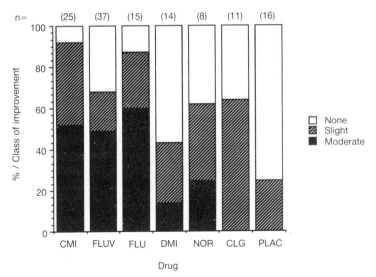

FIG. 18.1. Summary of various treatment studies in OCD patients shows percentage with moderate (> 40 per cent), slight (5–40 per cent), or no improvement at end-points compared to baseline. After chronic treatment with potent serotonin re-uptake blockers, about 50 per cent of patients are in the moderate improvement category: clomipramine (CMI) data from Insel and Zohar (1987); fluvoxamine (FLUV) data from Perse *et al.* (1987) and Goodman *et al.* (1989); fluoxetine (FLU) data from open studies by Fontaine and Chouinard (1985) and Turner *et al.* (1985). Clinical response to antidepressants without potent serotonin uptake blockade effects appears consider-ably less: desipramine (DMI) and clorgyline (CLG) data from Insel and Zohar (1987) and Insel *et al.* (1983); nortriptyline (NOR) data from Thoren *et al.* (1980*b*). Placebo (PLAC) is consistently ineffective for reducing OCD symptoms (Insel and Zohar 1987). Data from controlled trials with imipramine (Volavka *et al.* 1985; Foa *et al.* 1987) and amitriptyline (Ananth *et al.* 1981) are not included in this figure, but appear consistent with the observation that only potent serotonin re-uptake blockers are anti-obsessional as these drugs are less effective than clomipramine (Volavka *et al.* 1985; Ananth *et al.* 1981) or not more effective than placebo (Foa *et al.* 1987) for the relief of OCD symptoms.

Antidepressant drugs without effects on serotonin re-uptake, such as nortrip-tyline (Thoren *et al.* 1980*a*) and desipramine (Zohar and Insel 1987), and drugs with weaker effects on serotonin re-uptake, such as imipramine (Volavka *et al.* 1985; Foa *et al.* 1987), and amitriptyline (Ananth *et al.* 1981), have all been demonstrated to be either less effective than clomipramine or essentially ineffective in the treatment of OCD (Table 18.1, Fig. 18.1).

Clomipramine is not a particularly selective serotonin re-uptake inhibitor (Table 18.2). Its major metabolite, desmethylclomipramine, is extremely potent for blocking noradrenaline re-uptake while conserving much of the parent compound's effects on serotonin. As a result, clomipramine and

TABLE 18.2. *Comparison of clomipramine and imipramine*

	In vitro IC_{50} (nM)			In vivo
	Synaptosome uptake*		Platelet[†] ^{3}H-IMI binding	Serotonin syndrome[‡] Total intensity
	5-HT	NA		
Clomipramine	18	60	7	37
Desmethylclomipramine	120	2	10	
Imipramine	140	28	10	17
Desipramine	1100	3	120	2

* Ross and Renyi 1977.
[†] Paul *et al.* 1981.
[‡] Wozniak 1984.
5-HT, 5-hydroxytryptamine; NA, noradrenaline.

desmethylclomipramine combine to block serotonin re-uptake with greater potency than other tricyclic antidepressants in current use. In some studies (Insel *et al.* 1983; Stern *et al.* 1980), but not others (Thoren *et al.* 1980*a*; Flament *et al.* 1985), the improvement in obsessional symptoms correlates with the plasma level of clomipramine and not that of its less selective metabolite desmethylclomipramine.

Further evidence for a serotonergic mechanism mediating anti-obsessional effects comes from reports that L-tryptophan and lithium can augment the clomipramine response (Rasmussen 1984; Golden *et al.* 1988). Electrophysiological studies in rat hippocampus have demonstrated that lithium increases serotonergic responsiveness during long-term administration of tricyclic antidepressants (Blier and de Montigny 1985). Neither L-tryptophan or lithium have been shown to be effective anti-obsessional agents when administered alone.

Changes in serotonergic function have also been associated with clinical improvement during treatment with anti-obsessional drugs. With clomipramine treatment, the decrease in obsessional symptoms correlates ($r = 0.76$) with the decrease in the concentration of the serotonin metabolite 5-hydroxyindoleacetic acid (5-HIAA) in cerebrospinal fluid (CSF)—implicating the inhibition of uptake in the anti-obsessional effect (Thoren *et al.* 1980*b*). A similar result obtains with serotonin content in blood platelets. During clomipramine treatment, the decrease in platelet serotonin content correlates highly ($r = 0.87$) with the decrease in obsessional symptoms (Flament *et al.* 1987). It should be noted, however, that these measures—decreases in metabolite concentration and decreases in platelet content—reflect acute drug effects which might be expected to emerge early, weeks before the decrease in obsessional symptoms. In addition, decreases in platelet serotonin are generally so complete that the magnitude of the decrease is largely determined by individual differences in serotonin content before treatment. Thus, the reported correlation may actually reflect a relationship between baseline platelet serotonin content and improvement on drug.

In addition to this correlational evidence for a serotonergic mechanism underlying the anti-obsessional response, a recent study with metergoline, a 5-HT receptor antagonist (Benkelfat *et al.* 1989), has examined the effects of altering serotonin neurotransmission in OCD patients during long-term treatment. Metergoline (4 mg) was administered orally to OCD patients who had received clomipramine for four months and manifested on average a 40 per cent reduction in OC symptoms. The study was designed as a placebo-controlled cross-over with four days of placebo and four days of metergoline treatment in addition to the daily dose of clomipramine. Compared with the four-day placebo period, OCD patients became progressively more anxious and obsessional during the metergoline phase (Fig. 18.2). In a subsequent study with a different cohort of clomipramine-treated patients, a single 12 mg dose of metergoline was associated with a similar worsening of OC symptoms (Fig. 18.2). Although an identical treatment regimen has yet to be investigated in untreated OCD patients, a single dose of 4 mg of metergoline does not appear to increase OC symptoms in untreated patients (Zohar *et al.* 1987). Thus, the effects during clomipramine administration may reflect a reversal of serotonergic changes associated with treatment and not an intrinsic 'pro-obsessional' effect of metergoline. It seems likely that metergoline did, in fact, result in physiological serotonin antagonism in this study, because the drug lowered plasma prolactin concentration in clomipramine-treated patients.

In summary, the link between serotonin and anti-obsessional effects has been suggested by the selectivity of the serotonin re-uptake inhibitors, the correlations between clinical response and changes in serotonergic markers, and the recent evidence of a partial relapse of symptoms following metergoline administration in OCD patients who had improved with clomipramine treatment. Several aspects of this emerging story still need to be addressed. Inhibition of serotonin re-uptake occurs within minutes of the first dose of drug and yet anti-obsessional effects emerge only after several weeks of treatment. The clinical response may be related to some late, compensatory response to re-uptake inhibition. Recent evidence has suggested that some serotonin uptake inhibitors may not be anti-obsessional—a mixed set of results has been noted with zimelidine (Prasad 1985; Kahn *et al.* 1984; Insel *et al.* 1985; Fontaine *et al.* 1985). In one study (Insel *et al.* 1985), patients receiving zimelidine had a decrease in CSF 5-HIAA and yet failed to improve clinically. Clearly drugs differ in their regional selectivity; they may also have some interfering non-serotonergic effects or may lack effects on some essential serotonergic target. Perhaps blockade of serotonin re-uptake is necessary but not sufficient for anti-obsessional efficacy. Finally, anti-obsessional effects

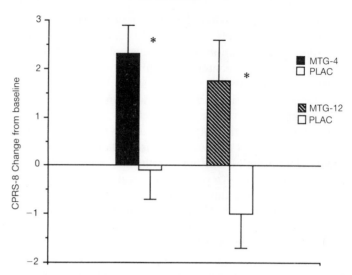

FIG. 18.2. Response to the serotonin receptor antagonist metergoline in OCD patients receiving chronic clomipramine treatment. In the first study, ten patients who were on average 40 per cent improved on clomipramine (CMI) received either placebo or metergoline (MTG, 4 mg) orally for four days in a double-blind, cross-over design. On the fourth day, changes in the OCD subscale of the Comprehensive Psychiatric Rating Scale (CPRS-8) indicated an increase in symptoms during metergoline compared to placebo treatment (* = $p < 0.05$). These data are modified from Benkelfat *et al.* (1989). In a subsequent study, five OCD patients showing similar improvement on CMI received a higher oral dose of metergoline (12 mg) or placebo using the same experimental design with only a single day of treatment. Results again demonstrate a significant increase in CPRS-8-rated symptoms after metergoline compared with placebo treatment (* = $p < 0.05$). Both studies indicate that serotonin receptor blockade may partially reverse the clinical response to clomipramine in OCD patients (data kindly provided by C. Benkelfat).

have been reported for the 5-HT$_{1A}$ partial agonist buspirone (Pato *et al.* 1989; although also see Jenike and Baer 1988). Undoubtedly, it is not re-uptake blockade *per se*, but indirect effects of re-uptake blockade on serotonergic function that are key to anti-obsessional drug action. We still do not know the nature of these indirect effects.

Evidence for serotonin involvement in the pathophysiology of OCD

The evidence from treatment studies of OCD has naturally led to a search for some abnormality in serotonin functioning in untreated OCD patients. This search has followed three paths: studies of serotonin function in blood elements; measurement of CSF concentrations of the serotonin metabolite

5-HIAA; and challenge of untreated OCD patients with serotonergic agents. Although the data are inconsistent, several observations are worth noting.

Peripheral studies

One early investigation (Yaryura-Tobias and Bhagavan 1977) reported a decrease in serotonin concentration in whole blood from OCD patients, but this has not been replicated by a careful study of platelet serotonin content in children with OCD (Flament *et al.* 1987). Platelets, which are the major reservoir of serotonin in blood, show normal uptake of serotonin in OCD patients (Insel *et al.* 1985; Weizman *et al.* 1986). Serotonin uptake sites on platelets, labelled with [^{3}H]imipramine, appear reduced by nearly 50 per cent in one study of 18 OCD adults and children (Weizman *et al.* 1986), but not in another study of 12 untreated OCD adults (Insel *et al.* 1985). As platelet [^{3}H]-imipramine binding may be reduced for several weeks following treatment with CMI, an extensive drug-free period is necessary before obtaining a baseline measurement. No studies of serotonin receptors in peripheral tissues (such as the 5-HT$_2$ receptor on platelets) in OCD patients have been published thus far.

Studies of cerebrospinal fluid

The serotonin metabolite in CSF, 5-HIAA, may serve as an indicator of central serotonin turnover. CSF 5-HIAA was 30 per cent higher in one small cohort ($n = 8$) of OCD patients compared to 23 controls (Insel *et al.* 1985). In a larger study, Thoren and co-workers (1980*b*) did not find a significant difference, although CSF 5-HIAA concentrations were 20 per cent higher in OCD patients than in healthy controls (Thoren *et al.* 1980*b*). No differences in other CSF monoamine metabolites have been noted in OCD patients (Insel *et al.* 1985), and the apparent 5-HIAA concentration differences cannot be explained by group differences in height, weight, diet, activity level, or season of sampling (Insel *et al.* 1985). Clearly, it is too early to conclude that OCD patients have increased central turnover of serotonin. There is, however, a curious contrast here with impulsive or aggressive sociopaths who tend to show low CSF 5-HIAA (Brown *et al.* 1982; Linnoila *et al.* 1983; Lidberg *et al.* 1985; Virkkunen *et al.* 1987). The contrast is of particular interest because, from a certain phenomenological perspective, OCD is the opposite of sociopathy. Patients with OCD are tormented by guilt for crimes they have never committed, whereas sociopaths, by definition, experience little if any guilt after criminal behaviour.

Challenge studies

To investigate further the possible role of 5-HT in the mediation of obsessional symptoms, several studies have examined either the behavioural or physiological responses to activation of the serotonergic system (Table 18.3).

Only one study, thus far, has used a precursor loading strategy in OCD patients. Charney *et al.* (1988) administered 7 g of L-tryptophan intravenously over 20 minutes to 21 OCD patients and 21 age-matched healthy controls. No differences were evident in the behavioural or neuroendocrine (cortisol, prolactin, growth hormone) responses comparing the two groups, although plasma prolactin concentrations at baseline were lower in female patients than in female controls. As a result, increases in prolactin following L-tryptophan were slightly higher in patients than in controls. These same investigators have used the inverse strategy, dietary tryptophan depletion, as a challenge test in OCD and depressed patients. Acute tryptophan depletion (lowering serum tryptophan by 90 per cent) does not appear to alter the symptoms of untreated OCD patients, although this same treatment is associated with relapse in depressed patients on chronic antidepressant treatment (Delgado *et al.* 1989).

The serotonin-releasing agent fenfluramine has also been given as a provocative test in OCD patients. In one study, fenfluramine (60 mg orally) appeared nearly identical to placebo in terms of behavioural responses (Hollander *et al.* 1988). In a larger study the same group (Hollander *et al.* 1989), as well as an independent group (Hewlett *et al.* 1989), reported a blunted prolactin response to fenfluramine in either female or both male and female OCD patients relative to controls. Preliminary results suggest that treatment with fluoxetine normalizes the endocrine response to fenfluramine (Hollander *et al.* 1989).

Several studies have used the substituted piperazine, *m*-chlorophenylpiperazine (*m*-CPP), a metabolite of the antidepressant trazodone. In animals, administration of *m*-CPP is associated with decreased food consumption (Samanin *et al.* 1979; Mennini *et al.* 1980); decreased locomotion (Vetulani *et al.* 1982); neuroendocrine responses such as increased prolactin, cortisol, and corticotropin levels (Maj and Lewandowska 1980); and physiological reactions such as hyperthermia (Aloi *et al.* 1984), all of which might be expected of a post-synaptic 5-HT receptor agonist. These changes are reversed by administration of the 5-HT receptor antagonist, metergoline, and are responsive to presumed alterations in 5-HT receptor sensitivity produced by lesions and drugs (Samanin *et al.* 1979; Maj and Lewandowska 1980; Aloi *et al.* 1984).

In the first study to investigate whether patients with OCD differ from healthy controls in their behavioural responses to *m*-CPP, responses to single oral doses (0.5 mg kg^{-1}) of *m*-CPP were compared with responses to placebo under double-blind, random assignment conditions on separate days (Zohar *et al.* 1987). Relative to healthy controls, the untreated patients with OCD became markedly more anxious and obsessional (Fig. 18.3A). The peak behavioural response was generally observed within three hours of *m*-CPP

TABLE 18.3. *Challenge studies in OCD patients*

Drug	Dose, route	Behavioural response	Physiological response	Reference
L-Tryptophan	7.0 g, i.v.	OCD=CON	OCD=CON for GH, PRL, CORT	Charney *et al.* 1988
L-Tryptophan depletion	Oral amino acid load	No effect	90% depletion of tryptophan	Delgado *et al.* 1989
Fenfluramine	60 mg, p.o. 60 mg, p.o.	FEN=PLAC	OCD < CON for CORT, PRL OCD < CON for PRL (females)	Hollander *et al.* 1988, 1989 Hewlett *et al.* 1989
m-CPP	0.5 mg kg⁻¹, p.o.	OCD>CON	OCD=CON for PRL, OCD<CON for CORT	Zohar *et al.* 1987
	0.5 mg kg⁻¹, p.o.	OC symptoms increased 123%		Hollander *et al.* 1988
	0.1 mg kg⁻¹, i.v. 0.1 mg kg⁻¹, i.v.	OCD=CON OCD=CON	OCD female < CON female for PRL	Charney *et al.* 1988 Pigott *et al.* 1989
Metergoline	4 mg, p.o.	MTG=PLAC		Zohar *et al.* 1987

CON, control; GH, growth hormone; PRL, prolactin; CORT, cortisol; FEN, fenfluramine; PLAC, placebo; *m*-CPP, *m*-chlorophenylpiperazine; MTG, metergoline; i.v., intravenously; p.o., orally.

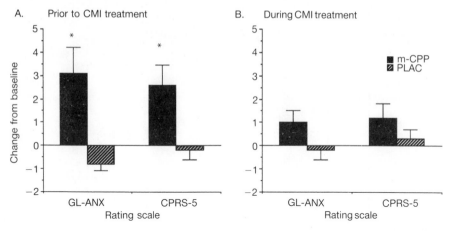

FIG. 18.3. Response to the serotonin agonist *m*-chlorophenylpiperazine (*m*-CPP) and placebo administered as a single oral dose under double-blind conditions. A. Untreated OCD patients ($n=12$) manifest a significant increase in anxiety (Global-anxiety scale, GL-ANX) and OC symptoms (Comprehensive Psychiatric Rating Scale, CPRS-5) after 0.5 mg kg^{-1} of *m*-CPP relative to placebo (*, $p < 0.05$). B. A subgroup of these same patients ($n = 9$) receiving chronic clomipramine treatment were re-challenged with *m*-CPP and placebo with only slight, non-significant increases in the same measures. These results suggest that clomipramine treatment confers a subsensitivity in the serotonin receptor mediating *m*-CPP's effects.

administration and the duration of the worsening ranged from several to 48 hours. Moreover, after *m*-CPP, but not placebo, approximately 50 per cent of the patients spontaneously described emergence of new obsessions or re-occurrence of obsessions that had not been present for several months. They also described themselves as being more depressed and dysphoric. The response to placebo as well as the side-effects in both groups were mild and did not differ significantly between the patients and the controls (Zohar and Insel 1987; Zohar *et al.* 1987). A second study by Hollander and colleagues (1988) using a similar paradigm described an exacerbation of OC symptoms in five of eight OCD patients receiving oral *m*-CPP. Patients in this study had a 123 per cent increase in symptoms after *m*-CPP as opposed to a 35 per cent reduction following placebo.

As oral administration of *m*-CPP has also been associated with anxiogenic effects in patients with panic disorders (Kahn *et al.* 1988), it seems possible that *m*-CPP is not increasing OC symptoms selectively; rather, it may cause a non-specific exacerbation of diverse psychopathological responses. Certainly, *m*-CPP affects several symptoms other than obsessions in the patients with OCD; thus, the drug might primarily increase anxiety or dysphoria, with OC symptoms increasing only as a secondary phenomenon. This possibility would be supported if patients with OCD were hypersensitive to other anxiogenic compounds. However, anxiogenic agents such as lactate (Gorman *et al.* 1985), yohimbine (Rasmussen *et al.* 1987), and caffeine (J. Zohar *et al.*, unpublished data) failed to increase either anxiety or OC symptoms in patients with OCD. It seems, therefore, that patients with OCD are not especially prone to respond to provocative agents that exacerbate symptoms in patients with non-OCD anxiety disorders.

It may seem paradoxical that OCD patients exhibit increased OC symptoms and anxiety in response to *m*-CPP and yet appear unresponsive to serotonin precursors such as L-tryptophan (Charney *et al.* 1988) or to serotonin-releasing agents such as fenfluramine (Insel *et al.* 1984; Hollander *et al.* 1988). These agents, while sharing some neuroendocrine and other physiological effects with *m*-CPP, also act at many other serotonin terminal fields and receptors that have been identified in preclinical studies. Some of these receptors (e.g., the 5-HT$_{1A}$ receptor) mediate a number of responses in animals that are opposite to those elicited by *m*-CPP. For example, agents acting at 5-HT$_{1A}$ receptors in rodent brain elicit hypothermia, hypotension, increased food intake, and 'anxiolytic' responses in some animal models of anxiety; in contrast, *m*-CPP has hyperthermic, hypertensive, anorectic, and 'anxiogenic' actions in rodents (reviewed in Murphy *et al.* 1989). Although *m*-CPP is, so far, the only agent that has been associated with exacerbation of OC symptoms in a placebo-controlled study (Zohar *et al.* 1987), the regional and pharmacological specificities of *m*-CPP in human brain need to be elucidated before we can formulate a mechanism for its apparent 'pro-obsessional' effects.

Aside from the questions of *m*-CPP's specificity, there has been a conflict in the literature regarding the drug's behavioural effects. Charney *et al.* (1988) reported that *m*-CPP given intravenously elicits equivalent responses in OCD patients and controls. Both OCD patients and controls developed marked anxiety and many other psychological and somatic symptoms, results similar to observations by Murphy *et al.* (1989) when comparing i.v. and oral administration of *m*-CPP in healthy volunteers. Pigott *et al.* (1989) also found that *m*-CPP given intravenously to OCD patients and controls failed to elicit OC symptoms in the patients. Observations of the patients and their own reports indicated that the abrupt, severe provocation of anxiety and many somatic symptoms of short duration were such an overwhelming experience that most patients were distracted from any obsessional thoughts or compulsive rituals they had experienced before i.v. *m*-CPP administration or during placebo administration. A probable interpretation of this is that intravenously administered *m*-CPP provides a considerably different experience from that following orally administered *m*-CPP. After oral *m*-CPP OC symptoms developed progressively over several hours, in a manner that corresponded quite closely to the duration of the neuroendocrine and temperature responses and also to the time course of the plasma concentrations of *m*-CPP (Mueller *et al.* 1985; Zohar and Insel 1987; Murphy *et al.*

1989). Perhaps most importantly, metergoline pre-treatment blocked the neuroendocrine responses to intravenous *m*-CPP, but did not significantly attenuate the behavioural response. Thus it appears that when given intravenously rather than orally *m*-CPP has qualitatively different behavioural effects that may not mediated by a serotonergic receptor.

Changes in serotonin sensitivity with treatment

As noted earlier, there is considerable evidence that the effects of anti-obsessional drugs may be mediated via serotonergic mechanisms. The apparent hypersensitivity to oral *m*-CPP in OCD patients has provided a novel approach for assessing changes in the responsiveness of serotonin receptors during treatment with serotonin uptake inhibitors. In one such study, *m*-CPP and placebo were given under double-blind conditions to nine patients with OCD before and after treatment with clomipramine (Zohar *et al.* 1988). Although there was a marked transient increase in obsessional symptoms and anxiety after *m*-CPP administration in patients before treatment, readministration of *m*-CPP after four months of treatment with clomipramine did not significantly increase obsessional symptoms and anxiety (Fig. 18.3B). Preliminary evidence has been reported for a similar 'normalization' of both the behavioural and neuroendocrine responses to *m*-CPP following fluoxetine treatment (Hollander *et al.* 1989). It must be noted that challenges before and after treatment are examining responses from different baselines. While these differences in responsiveness may look like receptor down-regulation, the behavioural pharmacology literature is replete with responses that are rate-dependent without underlying changes in receptors. Nevertheless, it will be of interest to determine whether similar decreases in serotonergic receptor responsiveness occur during the treatment of OCD patients with other serotonin-selective uptake inhibitors, such as fluvoxamine, sertraline, and paroxetine, and also during treatment with some structurally different serotonergic agents, such as buspirone and gepirone which act at 5-HT_{1A} sites.

Where is the lesion?

Although the studies are few and the sample sizes are small, it is never too early to speculate on a neurochemical lesion in OCD. The major findings thus far are the efficacy of the serotonin uptake inhibitors and the provocative effects of oral *m*-CPP. Whatever serotonin uptake inhibitors do, their therapeutic effects emerge over many weeks. There is no single, satisfying answer to the effect of these drugs on serotonin neurotransmission. Peroutka and Snyder (1980) were the first to report a decrease in cortical binding of [^{3}H]spiperone after chronic treatment with imipramine. More recent studies in rat brain have reported either a decrease (Stolz *et al.* 1983) or no change

(Hyttel *et al.* 1984) in 5-HT$_2$ receptors after chronic administration of potent serotonin uptake blockers as well as several other antidepressants. No consistent change in 5-HT$_1$ receptors, assayed by ^{3}H-5-HT binding, has been reported following chronic antidepressant treatment (reviewed by Willner 1985). From a functional perspective, de Montigny and his colleagues (1978, 1984) have described an increase in sensitivity to iontophoretically applied 5-HT in hippocampus following long-term administration of various antidepressants, including serotonin uptake inhibitors, to rats. However, Olpe (1981) noted no change in sensitivity to serotonin in cingulate and rostral cortical neurones following chronic clomipramine treatment. Results from behavioural studies have also been mixed, with serotonin uptake inhibitors sometimes yielding decreased responsiveness to the post-synaptic serotonin agonist 5-methoxy-*N*,*N*,-dimethyltryptamine whereas other antidepressants more consistently result in an increase in responsiveness (reviewed by Willner 1985). Anderson (1983), in a review of this subject, concluded . . .

Recent investigation of chronic antidepressant treatments using ligand binding, electrophysiological, and behavioral techniques have attempted to identify subgroups of receptors that might be affected uniquely and specifically by chronic antidepressant treatments. At the present time, however, the data produced by ligand binding experiments and electrophysiological experiments investigating serotonergic functioning do not fit together. In addition, interpretational problems and internal contradictions exist within each of the three bodies of data when straightforward hypotheses regarding a serotonergic role in antidepressant treatment are formulated.

To this summary it can be added that the available literature has focused on the effects of chronic administration of antidepressants and not on the effects of serotonin uptake inhibitors, which are distinct from other antidepressants. The relevant question is how do these specific anti-obsessional drugs differ from other antidepressants in their chronic effects?

There can be little intellectual solace in the results with *m*-CPP. Although early evidence implicated the 5-HT$_{1B}$ receptor as the major mediator of *m*-CPP's physiological effects in rodents, the absence of selective antagonists precludes closure on this issue. Certainly, on the basis of competitive binding studies, *m*-CPP has clear affinity for 5-HT$_{1C}$, 5-HT$_2$, and 5-HT$_{1A}$ sites as well. More bothersome, 5-HT$_{1B}$ sites are not detectable in human brain, although the 5-HT$_{1D}$ site found in man but not rodents may prove similar to the 5-HT$_{1B}$ receptor (neither have been cloned as yet). The affinity of *m*-CPP for the serotonin receptor subtypes in human brain has not been characterized. The point is not merely academic—the evolution of serotonergic function has been mediated not only by changes in receptor distribution but also by changes in the receptors themselves. Extrapolation from rodent receptor pharmacology to clinical response is therefore fraught with assumptions that need to be tested in human tissue.

With these caveats in mind, the mechanistic model for *m*-CPP's effects in

OCD patients could be built in two ways. The behavioural hyper-responsiveness to oral m-CPP could result from hypersensitive receptors—leading to increased serotonergic effects at a subpopulation of receptors which mediate OC symptoms. Acute treatment with serotonin uptake inhibitors might be expected to have similar behavioural effects. Chronic treatment with serotonin uptake inhibitors could lead to adaptive down-regulation of the receptor, decreased sensitivity to m-CPP, and decreased sensitivity to endogenous serotonin.

An alternative mechanism posits m-CPP as primarily decreasing serotonergic neurotransmission, either via autoreceptor effects (as demonstrated for 5-HT_{1B} receptors) or through direct antagonist effects at cortical 5-HT_2 receptors (suggested in recent studies of phosphoinositol hydrolysis). This model presumes a decrease in serotonergic neurotransmission in OCD patients, as suggested by the blunted prolactin response to fenfluramine. This decrease is exacerbated by m-CPP and corrected by serotonin uptake inhibitors.

Neither the platelet studies nor the preliminary reports of increased CSF 5-HIAA in OCD patients are particularly helpful in resolving these two models. Moreover, although the neuroendocrine responses to serotonin agonists suggest subsensitivity, this may be misleading. Behavioural and neuroendocrine responses may be mediated by different receptors in different terminal fields. In the rat, hypothalamic receptors are innervated by median raphe neurones and are largely 5-HT_2 and 5-HT_{1A}. The emerging story from neuro-imaging studies of OCD patients implicates the striatum in this disorder (Baxter *et al.* 1987). Serotonin receptors in striatum are 5-HT_{1B} (and 5-HT_{1D} in man) and 5-HT_2, with innervation from the dorsal raphe. So a report of a blunted prolactin response to fenfluramine or m-CPP in female OCD patients does not shed much light on the mechanism for the behavioural effects of m-CPP or serotonin re-uptake inhibitors.

Several pieces of the puzzle are missing. Post-mortem data on serotonergic receptors in those regions implicated in OCD psychopathology (striatum, orbital cortex, cingulate cortex) would be helpful for resolving the questions of subtypes and sensitivity. Studies of differences between the regional effects of long-term treatment with serotonin re-uptake inhibitors as opposed to other antidepressants would help to elucidate the key to anti-obsessional drug action. And further study of *behavioural* consequences of acute challenge with several serotonergic agonists and antagonists in OCD patients should help to put the m-CPP findings in perspective.

Conclusion

This paper reviews the accumulating evidence implicating serotonin in the treatment and the pathophysiology of OCD. Thus far, only serotonin uptake blockers have been shown to be anti-obsessional, but whether their effects reflect an increase or a decrease in central serotonergic function remains unclear. The role of serotonin in the pathophysiology of OCD remains speculative, but is strongly suggested by the increased behavioural response to *m*-CPP. Finally, it should be mentioned that serotonin may have a general role in the modulation of aggression or impulsivity, so that the results from studies of OCD could be understood in a larger context of investigations of several diagnostic categories varying on a dimension of impulsiveness. Although more studies are needed, the current data report high concentrations of CSF 5-HIAA in OCD patients (with low impulsiveness) and low concentrations of CSF 5-HIAA in violent criminals, arsonists, and suicidal patients (with high impulsiveness). This notion linking CSF 5-HIAA to impulsiveness is largely consistent with Soubrié's hypothesis (1986) that central serotonin function is inversely correlated with the release of suppressed behaviour.

Acknowledgement

Aspects of this chapter were published in Insel, T. R. *et al.*, in *The Neuropharmacology of Serotonin*, (ed. P. M. Whitaker-Azmitia and S. J. Peroutka), New York Academy of Sciences, in press.

References

Aloi, J. A., Insel, T. R., Mueller, E. A., and Murphy, D. L. (1984). Neuroendocrine and behavioural effects of m-chlorophenylpiperazine administration in rhesus monkeys. *Life Sciences*, **34**, 1325–31.

Ananth, J., Pecknold, J. C., van den Steen, N., and Engelsmann, F. (1981). Double-blind comparative study of clomipramine and amitriptyline in obsessive neurosis. *Progress in Neuro-psychopharmacology and Biological Psychiatry*, **5**, 257–62.

Anderson, J. L. (1983). Serotonin receptor changes after chronic antidepressant treatments. Ligand binding, electrophysiological, and behavioural studies. *Life Sciences*, **32**, 1791–1801.

Baxter, L. R., Phelps, M. E., Mazziotta, J. C., Guze, B. H., Schwartz, J. M., and Selin C. E. (1987). Local cerebral glucose metabolic rates in obsessive-compulsive disorder: a comparison with rates in unipolar depression and normal controls. *Archives of General Psychiatry*, **44**, 211–18.

Benkelfat, C., Murphy, D. L., Zohar, J., Hill, J. L., Grover, G., and Insel, T. R. (1989). Clomipramine in obsessive-compulsive disorder: further evidence for a serotonergic mechanism of action. *Archives of General Psychiatry*, **46**, 23–8.

Blier, P. and de Montigny, C. (1985). Short term lithium administration enhances serotonergic neurotransmission: electrophysiologic evidence in the rat CNS. *European Journal of Pharmacology*, **113**, 69–77.

Brown, G., Ebert, M., Goyer, P., Jimerson, D., Klein, W., Bunney, W., and Goodwin, F. (1982). Aggression, suicide, and serotonin: relationship to CSF amine metabolites. *American Journal of Psychiatry*, **139**, 741–6.

Charney, D. S., Goodman, W. K., Price, L. H., Woods, S. W., Rasmussen, S. A., and Heninger, G. R. (1988). Serotonin function in obsessive-compulsive disorder: a comparison of the effects of tryptophan and m-chlorophenylpiperazine in patients and healthy subjects. *Archives of General Psychiatry*, **45**, 177–85.

Delgado, P. L., Charney, D. S., Price, L. H., Goodman, W. K., Aghajanian, G. K., and Heninger, G. R. (1989). Behavioral effects of acute tryptophan depletion in psychiatric patients and healthy subjects. Society for Neuroscience 19th Annual Meeting, Phoenix, Arizona, Abstract Q-3.

de Montigny, C. and Aghajanian, G. K. (1978). Tricyclic antidepressants: long-term treatment increases responsivity of rat forebrain neurons to serotonin. *Science*, **202**, 1303–6.

de Montigny, C., Blier, P., and Chaput, Y. (1984). Electrophysiologically-identified serotonin receptors in the rat CNS. Effect of antidepressant treatment. *Neuropharmacology*, **23**, 1511–20.

de Veaugh-Geiss, J., Landau, P., and Katz, R. (1989). Treatment of obsessive-compulsive disorder with clomipramine. *Psychiatric Annals*, 19, 97–101.

Flament, M. F., Rapoport, J. L., Berg, C. J., Sceery, W., Kilts, C., Mellstrom, B., and Linnoila, M. (1985). Clomipramine treatment of childhood obsessive-compulsive disorder: a double-blind controlled study. *Archives of General Psychiatry*, **42**, 977–83.

Flament, M. F., Rapoport, J. L., Murphy, D. L., Berg, C. J., and Lake, C.R. (1987). Biochemical changes during clomipramine treatment of childhood obsessive-compulsive disorder. *Archives of General Psychiatry*, **44**, 219–25.

Foa, E. B., Steketee, G., Kozak, M. J., and Dugger, D. (1987). Effects of imipramine on depression and obsessive-compulsive symptoms. *Psychiatry Research*, **21**, 123–6.

Fontaine, R. and Chouinard, G. (1985). Fluoxetine in the treatment of obsessive-compulsive disorder. *Progress in Neuro-psychopharmacology and Biological Psychiatry*, **9**, 605–8.

Fontaine, R., Chouinard, G., and Iny, L. (1985). An open clinical trial of zimelidine in the treatment of obsessive-compulsive disorder. *Current Therapy Research*, **37**, 326–32.

Golden, R. N., Morris, J. E., and Sack, D. A. (1988). Combined lithium-tricyclic treatment of obsessive-compulsive disorder. *Biological Psychiatry*, **23**, 181–5.

Goodman, W. K., Price, L. H., Rasmussen, S. A., Delgado, P. L., Heninger, G. R., and Charney, D. S., (1989). Efficacy of fluvoxamine in obsessive-compulsive disorder: a double-blind comparison with placebo. *Archives of General Psychiatry*, **46**, 36–44.

Gorman, J. M., Leibowitz, M. R., Fyer, A. J., Davies, S. O., and Klein, D. F. (1985). Lactate infusions in obsessive-compulsive disorder. *American Journal of Psychiatry*, **142**, 864–66.

Hewlett, W. A., Vinogradov, S., Berman, S., Csernansky, J., and Agras, W. S. (1989). Fenfluramine stimulation of prolactin release in obsessive-compulsive disorder. *New York Academy of Sciences Neuropharmacology of Serotonin Conference*, Abstract 129.

Hollander, E., Fay, M., Cohen, B., Campeas, R., Gorman, J. M., and Liebowitz, M. R. (1988). Serotonergic and noradrenergic sensitivity in obsessive-compulsive disorder: behavioral findings. *American Journal of Psychiatry*, **145**, 1015–17.

Hollander, E., DeCaria, C., Gully, B., Nitescu, A., and Liebowitz, M. R. (1989). Serotonergic challenges in obsessive-compulsive disorder. *New York Academy of Sciences Neuropharmacology of Serotonin Conference*, Abstract 130.

Hytell, J. Overo, K. F., and Arnt, J. (1984). Biochemical effects and drug levels in rats after long-term treatment with the specific 5-HT uptake inhibitor citalopram. *Psychopharmacology*, **83**, 20–7.

Insel, T. R. and Zohar, J. (1987). Psychopharmacologic approaches to obsessive-compulsive disorder. In *Psychopharmacology: the third generation of progress*, (ed. H. Meltzer), pp. 1205–9. Raven Press, New York.

Insel, T. R., Murphy, D. L., Cohen, R. M., Alterman, I., Kilts, C., and Linnoila, M. (1983). Obsessive-compulsive disorder: a double-blind trial of clomipramine and clorgyline. *Archives of General Psychiatry*, **40**, 605–12.

Insel, T. R., Mueller, E. A., Gillin, J. C., Siever, L. J., and Murphy, D. L. (1984). Biological markers in obsessive-compulsive and affective disorders. *Journal of Psychiatric Research*, **18**, 407–23.

Insel, T. R., Mueller, E. A., Alterman, I., Linnoila, M., and Murphy, D. L. (1985). Obsessive-compulsive disorder and serotonin: Is there a connection? *Biological Psychiatry*, **20**, 1174–89.

Jenike, M. A. and Baer, L. (1988). Buspirone in obsessive-compulsive disorder: an open trial. *American Journal of Psychiatry*, **145**, 1285–6.

Kahn, R., Westenberg, H. G. M., and Jolles, J. (1984). Zimelidine treatment of obsessive-compulsive disorder. *Acta Psychiatrica Scandinavica*, **69**, 259–61.

Kahn, R. S., Asnis, G. M., Wetzler, S., van Praag, H. M., Kahn, R. S., and Strauman, T. (1988). Behavioral indications for serotonin receptor hypersensitivity in panic disorder. *Psychiatry Research*, **25**, 101–4.

Leonard, H., Swedo, S., Rapoport, J. L., Coffey, M., and Cheslow, D. (1988). Treatment of childhood obsessive compulsive disorder with clomipramine and desmethylimipramine: A double-blind crossover comparison. *Psychopharmacology Bulletin*, **24**, 93–5.

Lidberg, L., Tuck, J., Asberg, M., Scalia-Tomba, G., and Bertilsson, L. (1985). Homicide, suicide, and CSF 5-HIAA. *Acta Psychiatrica Scandinavica*. **71**, 230–6.

Linnoila, M., Virkkunen, M., Scheinin, M., Nuutila, A., Rimon, R., and Goodwin, F. K. (1983). Low cerebrospinal fluid 5-HIAA concentration differentiates impulsive from non-impulsive violent behaviour. *Life Sciences*, **33**, 2609–14.

McDougle, C. J., Goodman, W. K., Price, L. H., Delgado, P. L., Krystal, J. H., Charney, K. S., and Heninger, G. R. (1989). Addition of dopamine antagonists in fluvoxamine-refractory obsessive compulsive disorder. Society for Neuroscience 19th Annual Meeting, Phoenix, Arizona, Abstract Z-10.

Maj, J. and Lewandowska, A. (1980). Central serotoninmimetic action of phenylpiperazine. *Polish Journal of Pharmacology and Pharmacy*, **32**, 495–504.

Marks, I., Stern, R., Mawson, D. *et al.* (1980). Clomipramine and exposure for obsessive compulsive rituals. *British Journal of Psychiatry*, **136**, 1–25.

Mavissakalian, M., Turner, S., Michelson, L., and Jacob, R. (1985). *American Journal of Psychiatry*, **142**, 572–6.

Mennini, T., Poggasi, E., Caccia, S., Bendotti, C., Borsini, F., and Samanin, R. (1980). Adaptive changes in central serotonin receptors after long-term treatment in rats. In *Neurotransmitters and their receptors*, (ed. U. Z. Littauer, Y. Dudai, and I. Silman). Wiley, New York.

Montgomery, S. A. (1980). Clomipramine in obsessional neurosis: A placebo controlled trial. *Pharmacology and Medicine*, **1**, 189–92.

Mueller, E. A., Murphy, D. L., and Sunderland, T. (1985). Neuroendocrine effects of m-chlorophenylpiperazine, a serotonin agonist in humans. *Journal of Clinical Endocrinology and Metabolism*, **61**, 1179–84.

Murphy, D. L., Mueller, E. A., Hill, J. L., Tolliver, T. J., and Jacobsen, F. M. (1989). Comparative anxiogenic, neuroendocrine, and other physiologic effects of m-chlorophenylpiperazine given intravenously or orally to healthy volunteers. *Psychopharmacology*, **98**, 275–82.

Olpe, H. R. (1981). Differential effect of chlorimipramine and clorgyline on the sensitivity of cortical neurons to serotonin. *European Journal of Pharmacology*, **69**, 375–7.

Pato, M. T., Pigott, T. A., Hill, J.L., Grover, G., Bernstein, S. E., and Murphy, D. L. (1989). Clomipramine versus buspirone in OCD: a controlled trial. The 1989 Annual Meeting of the American Psychiatric Association, San Francisco, New Research Abstract 14.

Paul, S. M., Rehavi, M., Rice, K., Ittah, Y., and Skolnick, P. (1981). Does high affinity [³H]-imipramine binding label serotonin reuptake sites in brain and platelets? *Life Sciences*, **28**, 2753–60.

Pauls, D. L., Towbin, K. E., Lechman, J. F. *et al.* (1986). Gilles de la Tourette syndrome and obsessive-compulsive disorder: evidence supporting an etiological relationship. *Archives of General Psychiatry*, **43**, 1180–2.

Peroutka, S. J. and Snyder, S. H. (1980). Long-term antidepressant treatment decreases spiroperidol-labelled serotonin receptor binding. *Science*, **210**, 88–90.

Perse, T. L., Greist, J. H., Jefferson, J. W., Rosenfeld, R., and Dar, R. (1987). Fluvoxamine treatment of obsessive-compulsive disorder. *American Journal of Psychiatry*, **144**, 1543–48.

Pigott, T. A., Murphy, D. L., Pato, M. T., Hill, J. L., and Grover, G. (1989). Serotonin agonist and antagonist studies in patients with obsessive-compulsive disorder. *New York Academy of Science Neuropharmacology of Serotonin Conference*, Abstract 131.

Pigott, T. A., Pato, M. T., Bernstein, S. E., Grover, G. N., Hill, J. T., Tolliver, T. J., and Murphy, D. L. (1990). A controlled comparison of clomipramine and fluoxetine in the treatment of obsessive-compulsive disorder: behavioral and biological results. *Archives of General Psychiatry*, in press.

Prasad, A. (1985). A double blind study of imipramine versus zimelidine in treatment of obsessive compulsive neurosis. *Pharmacology and Biochemical Behavior*, **22**, 347–8.

Rasmussen, S. A. (1984). Lithium and tryptophan augmentation in clomipramine-resistant obsessive-compulsive disorder. *American Journal of Psychiatry*, **141**, 1283–5.

Rasmussen, S. A., Goodman, W. K., Woods, S. W., Heninger, G. R., and Charney, D. S. (1987). Effects of yohimbine in obsessive-compulsive disorder. *Psychopharmacology*, **93**, 308–13.

Ross, S. B. and Renyi, A. L. (1977). Inhibition of the neuronal uptake of 5-hydroxytryptamine and noradrenaline in rat brain by (Z) and (E)-3-(4-bromophenyl)-*N*,*N*-dimethyl-3-(3-pyridyl) allylamines and their secondary analogues. *Neuropharmacology*, **16**, 57–63.

Samanin, R., Mennini, T., and Ferraris, A. (1979). m-Chlorophenylpiperazine: a central serotonin agonist causing powerful anorexia in rats. *Naunyn-Schmiedeberg's Archives of Pharmacology*, **308**, 159–63.

Soubrié, P. (1986). Reconciling the role of central serotonin neurons in human and animal behavior. *Behavioral Brain Science*, **9**, 319–64.

Stern, R. S., Marks, I. M., Wright, J., and Luscombe, D. K. (1980). Clomipramine: plasma levels, side effects, and outcome in obsessive-compulsive neurosis. *Postgraduate Medical Journal*, **56**, 134–9.

Stolz, J. F., Marsden, C. A., and Middlemiss, D. N. (1983). Effect of chronic antidepressant treatment and subsequent withdrawal on [³H]-5-hydroxytryptamine and [³H]-spiperone binding in rat frontal cortex and serotonin receptor mediated behaviour. *Psychopharmacology*, **80**, 150–5.

Thoren, P., Asberg, M., Bertilsson, L., Mellstrom, B., Sjoqvist, F., and Traskman, L. (1980a). Clomipramine treatment of obsessive-compulsive disorder. II. Biochemical aspects. *Archives of General Psychiatry*, **37**, 1289–94.

Thoren, P., Asberg, M., Cronholm, B., Jornestedt, L., and Traskman, L. (1980*b*). Clomipramine treatment of obsessive-compulsive disorder. I. A controlled clinical trial. *Archives of General Psychiatry*, **37**, 1281–5.

Turner, S., Jacob, R., Beidel, D. C., and Himmelhoch, J. (1985). Fluoxetine treatment of obsessive–compulsive disorder. *Journal of Clinical Psychopharmacology*, **5**, 207–12.

Vetulani, J., Sansone, M., Bednarczyk, B., and Hano, J. (1982). Different effects of 3-chlorophenylpiperazine on locomotor activity and acquisition of conditioned avoidance response in different strains of mice. *Naunyn-Schmiedeberg's Archives of Pharmacology*, **319**, 271–4.

Virkkunen, M., Nuutila, A., Goodwin, F., and Linnoila, M. (1987). Cerebrospinal fluid monoamine metabolite levels in male arsonists. *Archives of General Psychiatry*, **44**, 241–7.

Volavka, J., Neziroglu, F., and Yaryaru-Tobias, J. A. (1985). Clomipramine and imipramine in obsessive-compulsive disorder. *Psychiatry Research*, **14**, 83–91.

Weizman, A., Carmi, M., Hermesh, H., Shahar, A., Apter, A., Tyano, S., and Rehavi, M. (1986). High-affinity imipramine binding and serotonin uptake in platelets of eight adolescent and ten adult obsessive-compulsive patients. *American Journal of Psychiatry*, **143**, 335–9.

Willner, P. (1985). Antidepressants and serotonergic neurotransmission: an integrative review. *Psychopharmacology*, **85**, 387–404.

Wozniak, K. M. (1984). Interaction between inhibitors of monoamine oxidase and amine re-uptake in rats. Ph.D. thesis, University of London.

Yaryura-Tobias, J. A. and Bhagavan, H. N. (1977). L-Tryptophan in obsessive-compulsive disorders. *American Journal of Psychiatry*, **134**, 1298–9.

Zohar, J. and Insel, T. R. (1987). Obsessive-compulsive disorder: psychobiological approaches to diagnosis, treatment, and pathophysiology. *Biological Psychiatry*, **22**, 667–87.

Zohar, J., Mueller, E. A., Insel, T. R., Zohar-Kadouch, R. C., and Murphy, D. L. (1987). Serotonergic responsivity in obsessive-compulsive disorder: comparison of patients and healthy controls. *Archives of General Psychiatry*, **44**, 946–51.

Zohar, J., Insel, T. R., Zohar-Kadouch, R. C., Hill, J. L., and Murphy, D.L. (1988). Serotonergic responsivity in obsessive-compulsive disorder: effects of chronic clomipramine treatment. *Archives of General Psychiatry*, **45**, 167–72.

Discussion

COPPEN: What is the course of obsessive-compulsive disorder? For how long do we need to give these drugs?

INSEL: OCD has a chronic course, whether treated or not. Patients who are treated with clomipramine need to remain on the drug. This has brought up an entirely new safety issue because previously antidepressants have been used for six months or a year. Nobody has asked what would be the physiological consequences of long-term administration, say for 15 years, of a tricyclic antidepressant. Yet the need for long-term administration seems clear. Pato *et al.* (1988) studied patients withdrawn in a double-blind fashion from clomipramine after six to 24 months of treatment. Seventeen out of 18 patients relapsed within the first seven weeks of withdrawal, and they all responded when they were restarted on the drug. Thus, although chronic, indefinite treatment of OCD with clomipramine raises serious questions, this is a very severe, disabling illness; untreated patients will continue to get worse, or at least fail to get better.

COPPEN: We face this issue with recurrent depression and bipolar illness; we require long-term management with lithium and other psychotropic medication.

What about the patients who do not respond?

INSEL: There is always a question about pharmacodynamic differences between individuals. Dr Linnoila and I found about a five-fold variation in individual plasma levels after the same oral dose of clomipramine (Insel *et al.* 1983). It is possible that a patient could be given what appeared to be a very high oral dose without getting therapeutic levels in plasma.

If someone has therapeutic levels but is not responding, there is some evidence that augmentation agents such as lithium, L-tryptophan, and even buspirone, may be useful. Also, although they may be equipotent, the various 5-HT re-uptake inhibitors are not identical in their effects. Some patients appear to respond better to one agent than another; someone who does not respond to clomipramine may respond to fluoxetine. We don't know why that happens.

LINNOILA: The average age of onset of OCD appears to be about eight or nine. We know nothing about the effects of administering these drugs throughout development. Because of the severity of the illness there is reason to suspect that the psychological development of these individuals is markedly hampered by OCD. Thus, it would be rational to start the therapy early, but treatment could be required for a long time.

Dr Insel, you mentioned that clomipramine administration has a long-lasting effect on platelet imipramine binding. Clomipramine differs from other antidepressants in its binding to the serotonin (5-hydroxytryptamine, 5-HT) uptake site in human platelets; it is an almost irreversible inhibitor. This was confirmed in rat brain and may explain the efficacy of clomipramine in OCD.

BELMAKER: Have you looked at fenfluramine or amphetamine as possible exacerbaters of OCD?

INSEL: As far as I know, fenfluramine has only been studied when given as a single oral dose, which has no effect. However, three hours after a single oral challenge of d-amphetamine (30 mg) 11 of 12 patients reported a remarkable decrease in symptoms. It was not strictly an anti-obsessional effect, but a striking effect on their ability to concentrate. This was not related simply to euphoria; some patients on amphetamine became quite dysphoric. One of our most severely affected patients began sobbing and saying that this was the first time she had mourned her father's death. She noticed two hours later that it was also the first time she had not had to wash her hands in that period of time. We monitored the ability of these patients to focus attention with a series of continuous performance tests. We found a nice relationship between the decrease of OCD symptoms and the increase in performance. This was exactly the opposite of what we had expected: we predicted that amphetamine would make OCD patients worse. We began treating patients for one week at a time with oral amphetamine. Invariably the patients felt they were much better, but their families complained that their symptoms had returned, sometimes with even greater severity. So we stopped the trial after three or four patients.

BRILEY: This reminds me of the effect of amphetamine on hyperkinetic children. Are there any other similarities between these disorders?

INSEL: In adults with OCD the male: female ratio is equal, but in children it is about 2:1 (Swedo *et al.* 1989). In hyperkinetic or attention deficit disorder this ratio is closer to 9:1, but at least the difference is in the same direction.

GUARDIOLA-LEMAITRE: Exacerbation of OCD has not been reported after long-term treatment with fenfluramine, but the studies were not designed to observe this kind of behaviour. In an international double-blind, placebo-controlled trial, 400 patients were treated with d-fenfluramine. No effects suggesting onset of OCD were reported (Guy-Grand *et al.* 1989).

MENDLEWICZ: How do you interpret the fact that the delay of action with clomipramine seems to be longer in OCD than in depression, although the doses are similar? Secondly, have there been prophylactic long-term studies of the efficacy of clomipramine in OCD?

INSEL: I am not sure why the time course is different, but this may be related partly to our rating instruments. In more recent studies with better instruments, such as the *Yale-Brown Obsessive-Compulsive Scale* (Y-BOCS), significant effects of the drug are evident as early as two weeks after the start of treatment. Previously our instruments were not very sensitive. Also, this patient group is loathe to report change of any sort. This subjective rigidity may contribute to the delayed time for drug response and it is probably why there is not much placebo response in OCD patients.

The CIBA-GEIGY study followed patients for a year after the double-blind trial which lasted 10 weeks. That study showed the persistence of improvement. I don't think there has been a longer study than that.

MURPHY: In the CIBA-GEIGY study (de Veaugh-Geiss *et al.* 1989) the effect of clomipramine was significant after two weeks, but it was nine or ten weeks at least before a plateau was reached in the majority of patients. This differs from the action of antidepressant drugs.

MELTZER: What percentage improvement is seen?

MURPHY: This trial used the observer-rated Y-BOCS scale. The total improvement was about 40 per cent.

COPPEN: What would the score be for the normal population?

MURPHY: It would be very low on this scale, unlike in the Maudsley inventory of OC symptoms, where, for example, groups of scientists show some modestly elevated scores.

COWEN: Acute tryptophan depletion did not worsen symptoms in untreated OCD patients, but has been reported to lead to a relapse of depression in depressed patients maintained on antidepressant drugs (Delgado *et al.* 1990). It would be interesting to see if a similar effect occurred in OCD patients who had responded to clomipramine.

INSEL: The tryptophan depletion test has been given to both depressed and OCD patients during the course of chronic treatment. Remarkably, depressed patients become significantly worse and OCD patients show no change in symptoms (D. Charney, personal communication).

YOUDIM: It is interesting that clorgyline had no effect on OCD. Clorgyline has different effects on 5-HT metabolism in different parts of the brain. One area where it has least effect is in the raphe, where the large component of the B form of monoamine oxidase (MAO-B) will continue to metabolize serotonin when MAO-A is selectively inhibited by clorgyline. Have you used another MAO inhibitor? Functionally you cannot increase serotonin activity with clorgyline alone in the rat. If you combine l-deprenyl with clorgyline the functional activity of serotonin is increased by inhibition of the MAO-B site and elevation of brain 5-HT (Green and Youdim 1975).

INSEL: That follows on from earlier remarks that sometimes 'dirty' drugs are better. In the original study of clorgyline versus clomipramine, we treated with tranylcypromine some of the patients who had a partial response to clorgyline or who could not tolerate clomipramine and had not responded to clorgyline. These were open trials, not a careful double-blind study, but tranylcypromine produced some of the best anti-obsessional results I have seen. It is a superb drug for a small group of patients. I don't know how to identify these patients, but the OCD patients who were not very improved on clorgyline seemed to respond better to tranylcypromine.

YOUDIM: In animal studies we also see a better response with tranylcypromine because this inhibitor inactivates both forms of MAO and causes a greater increase in brain serotonin than clorgyline.

MURPHY: In a cross-over study comparing clomipramine and fluoxetine in OCD, most patients who responded to one drug also responded to the other drug; both drugs were equally effective in an equal number of patients (Pigott et al. 1990).

YOUDIM: Did you try a combination of antidepressants? Was there a resistant group?

MURPHY: Yes, there was a resistant group. Dr Pigott is making a systematic comparison of several agents added to clomipramine in an attempt to obtain evidence for an additive effect under double-blind, controlled conditions. Our trial of buspirone versus clomipramine, to which Dr Insel referred, was a deliberate attempt to study a serotonergic agent which we expected to have no anti-OCD effects. Buspirone is an anti-anxiety agent and there are few parallels between OCD and the other anxiety disorders. Twenty OCD patients were randomly assigned to buspirone or clomipramine in a parallel double-blind study. We crossed the patients over afterwards. The buspirone dose averaged 60 mg per day, and we used a higher dose of clomipramine (238 mg per day) than is used with this drug as an antidepressant. We did not use placebos because we did not expect any greater effect of buspirone than in the earlier studies. However, on both the Y-BOCS and the NIH obsessive-compulsive scales at the end of six weeks we saw no difference between clomipramine and buspirone. In the cross-over phase, after 14 weeks, there was still no difference, although there were some interesting trends for patients on clomipramine to have lower Hamilton Depression scale scores.

DOOGAN: Dr Insel, in the light of your comments on increased impulse control and high concentrations of 5-hydroxyindoleacetic acid (5-HIAA) in cerebrospinal fluid (CSF), do you have any data on the suicide rate in these OCD patients?

INSEL: There have been some reports of increases in suicide ideation but a decreased likelihood that obsessional patients will commit the act. Gittleson (1966) described this in obsessional patients with major depression. These publications led psychiatrists to become too complacent about obsessional patients who had suicidal thoughts. These patients do commit suicide, but we have no clear statistics on the incidence.

DOOGAN: Are they depressed?

INSEL: No; they are usually desperate, rather than depressed. For example, one of our patients tried to throw himself through a window rather than touch a 'contaminated' door handle.

GOTTFRIES: Do people with OCD develop alcoholism to the same extent as panic anxiety patients?

INSEL: This has not been looked at carefully enough. Karno et al. (1988) reported an increased incidence of alcoholism (24 per cent), but their data are based on the Epidemiologic Catchment Area (ECA) survey and those identified as having OCD in this survey do not appear to be typical of a clinical population.

DEAKIN: If serotonin is involved in impulse control, and if OCD arises from serotonin deficiency, why don't patients with OCD have more generalized disturbances? They do not have a high suicide rate; they are not gamblers; they do not have eating disturbances; they do not vomit; they are far from aggressive. On the contrary, they are rather over-controlled, inhibited people.

LÓPEZ-IBOR: The question of impulse control and OCD is difficult because we do not know enough about the psychopathology of OCD and the impulsive disorders. The latter can be characterized from a clinical point of view by a lack of impulse control, and from the biological perspective by findings which suggest a deficiency in functional 5-HT. They share a therapeutic response to treatments which enhance 5-HT turnover (López-Ibor 1988). Alterations in 5-HT metabolism have been demonstrated in OCD (Insel *et al.* 1985; Zohar *et al.* 1987), which also responds partially to drugs that enhance 5-HT turnover. Impulsive individuals are not impulsive all of the time. They might be very controlled for a period (much like bulimic patients) and then let the impulse go wild. OCD patients sometimes lose control and become extremely violent or suicidal; they perpetrate the most violent and dramatic attempts of suicide possible, although most patients do not reach this stage. Hoehn-Saric and Barksdale (1983) found in a sample of OCD patients a childhood history of problems related to poor impulse control. A correlation between alterations in 5-HT metabolites and self-aggressive and hetero-aggressive behaviour, especially when the patients are violent, is often reported (Banki and Arato 1983; Asberg *et al.* 1984; Linnoila *et al.* 1984; López-Ibor *et al.* 1985).

Thus, a common link in the psychopathology of OCD and the group of impulsive disorders (the 'impulsivists', Lacey and Evans 1986), is poor impulse control, in the sense that new inner or outer experiences are not translated into adequate behaviour patterns. The experience is ignored or quickly abandoned in favour of an action — the impulse. In both types of disorder, as Janet (1903) wrote, 'the insignificant (substitutes) the significant'.

The improvement of OCD patients under psychopharmacological treatment is different from that obtained with similar drugs in depressed patients. OCD patients recognize that they are better long after an important change in their life style has been observed by their relatives and doctors. Although the obsessions continue, they dominate the patient less and less.

If the treatments fail we try to increase the serotonergic activity by adding 5-hydroxytryptophan (5-HTP) to the therapy. If that does not work psychiatric surgery may be indicated (López-Ibor and López-Ibor 1975).

COPPEN: Has anyone studied the effect of long-term lithium treatment on OCD? I think that lithium somehow affects the 5-HT system. This would have to be studied over several months.

LÓPEZ-IBOR: Based on the theory that affective patients are slightly obsessional and that prevention of depression may arise from an ability to modify obsessive traits of the pre-depressive personalities, Tellenbach (1983) published a study on this topic. However, this has not been replicated.

EVENDEN: How effective is simple behavioural therapy without drugs?

LÓPEZ-IBOR: Several studies have proved that using both is better than either alone.

INSEL: Behavioural therapy appears to be highly effective for OCD (Marks 1981). However, in behavioural therapy the non-responders are often those who drop out. Thus, it cannot be easily compared with drug treatment. More interesting is whether behavioural therapy may be altering the same neural substrate that these drugs alter. Nobody has studied whether behavioural therapy affects any of the serotonergic markers affected by the anti-obsessional drugs.

COWEN: Professor López-Ibor's description of the evolution of the effect of treatment in OCD was similar to the pattern of response seen with behavioural therapy.

LÓPEZ-IBOR: One patient's compulsion was to wash his hands if he touched something which had been touched by someone else. When I saw him playing table tennis and suggested he was improved he insisted that he was still very obsessed. A few days later, after playing table tennis he was watching others play. He claimed he still had his obsession. When I said 'But you are not washing your hands after touching the racket', he replied, 'Well, the match was so interesting that I wanted to stay here'.

MENDLEWICZ: I also experience this denial of improvement by OCD patients. I have problems with compliance because patients deny the benefit of the treatment for some time, despite improvement that is recognized by their families.

LÓPEZ-IBOR: One useful aspect of the Y-BOCS scale is that it measures the time devoted to the obsession and compulsion. This is one of the first things to change; the obsession and compulsion slowly begin to occupy less time.

MELTZER: Might the worsening of symptoms produced by metergoline in clomipramine-treated patients be a dopamine agonist effect, a kind of stereotypy? If it is not, I should like to consider a serotonergic mechanism. The typical tricyclic antidepressants are as effective serotonin uptake blockers as clomipramine, even if they are not as specific. Thus, although the clomipramine class of agents is identified by its specificity for serotonin uptake blockade, it is hard to attribute their efficacy in OCD to this mecahnism. Yet everything seems to point to serotonin as the basis for their action.

We consistently find that the hormonal response to both 5-HTP and MK 212 is blunted in our OCD patients, but we found no exacerbation with MK 212 (Bastani *et al*. 1990). With chronic fluoxetine treatment we saw dramatic potentiation of the cortisol and prolactin responses to both MK 212 and 5-HTP. We have not seen that with typical tricyclic antidepressants or with clomipramine. I hoped that clomipramine would show this effect because that would be some indication that in man these agents produce potentiation of serotonergic activity that is not seen with the typical drugs.

COWEN: Price *et al*. (1989) found that fluvoxamine enhanced the prolactin response to L-tryptophan to a much greater extent than amitriptyline. We also see a large enhancement of this response with clomipramine. Might the lack of enhancement of the MK 212 response be because clomipramine has some 5-HT_2 receptor-blocking effects that may offset the MK 212 neuroendocrine response? On the other hand, the L-tryptophan prolactin response, which is 5-HT_1-mediated, would not be affected by this mechanism.

MURPHY: Clomipramine does have potent 5-HT_2 antagonist effects, as do some of the other tricyclics. Fluvoxamine and fluoxetine do not.

MELTZER: We would want to look at some type of 5-HT receptor, which brings us back to busiprone. Markowitz *et al*. (1990) found that buspirone enhances the efficacy of fluoxetine in OCD patients. That is more evidence for a post-synaptic 5-HT_{1A} mechanism being important in OCD.

INSEL: There is still no clear picture of the difference between the actions of 5-HT uptake inhibitors and those of other tricyclic antidepressants.

PEROUTKA: The tricyclics are uptake or transporter antagonists. The selective agents do not interact with any other known receptor. In contrast, amitriptyline, imipramine, and clomipramine are essentially equipotent at the post-synaptic 5-HT_2 receptors and at the transporter.

FRAZER: There is evidence that chronic treatment with sertraline or fluoxetine blocks a response produced by $5\text{-}HT_2$ receptor activation. However, they do not down-regulate $5\text{-}HT_2$ receptors. Typical tricyclic antidepressants both down-regulate $5\text{-}HT_2$ receptors and block function. However, sertraline and fluoxetine still block 5-HT-mediated phosphoinositide turnover after chronic administration. So the functional effects of selective and non-selective uptake inhibitors are the same, although there is a difference in their $5\text{-}HT_2$ antagonist properties *in vitro*.

YOUDIM: There may be a threshold effect. In rats, monoamine oxidase inhibition and uptake inhibition show threshold effects; a certain degree of inhibition (85 per cent) is required before the functional increase of serotonin can occur (Green *et al.* 1977).

LINNOILA: Claude de Montigny claimed that he had evidence of differential effects on autoreceptors of the highly selective re-uptake inhibitors versus the classical tricyclic antidepressants.

MELTZER: He does postulate different mechanisms for the two classes, but it comes to the same thing in the end; they all potentiate serotonergic activity. The question is why there seems to be only one way to do this in OCD that leads to a partial therapeutic effect.

How many people have had a complete cessation of their OCD symptoms?

INSEL: None. One patient whom I treated in 1979 recently told me that he still had the symptoms although I had not seen him for five or six years and he had remained on his drugs throughout.

MELTZER: This is very different from the affective disorders and anxiety disorders.

DEAKIN: What about the association of OCD with Tourette's syndrome? There is an association with sociopathic behaviour. It seems that the obsessional symptoms in Tourette's syndrome are improved by 5-HT re-uptake blockers, but the movement disturbance is not.

INSEL: There also appears to be a genetic overlap; even those patients with Tourette's syndrome who do not have OC symptoms have an increased number of family members with OC symptoms or with OCD itself. The genetic vulnerability seems to be for both disorders. We still do not understand the relationship between them and how dopamine fits into OCD or how serotonin fits into Tourette's syndrome.

COPPEN: What is known about the genetics of OCD?

INSEL: There are several reports of identical twins that are concordant, but people often do not report the discordant twins. There are some dizygotic twins that are concordant. Torgersen (1983) found that of 12 pairs of twins none, dizygotic or monozygotic, was concordant. It appears that what is inherited may not be OCD *per se*, but some predisposition to obsessional characteristics, including a tendency to ritualize, introversion, self-doubt, and eccentric behaviours.

MURPHY: CIBA-GEIGY and the Federal Drug Administration reduced the maximum dose of clomipramine that could be prescribed in the USA to 250 mg per day because of a slightly higher incidence of seizures observed at higher doses. When we therefore reduced the dose for some patients from 300 mg to 250 mg, we encountered a recurrence of symptoms in at least one patient.

COPPEN: Wasn't there a correlation between plasma level and therapeutic effect?

INSEL: Yes, in the first study. Stern *et al.* (1980) also found a correlation, but Thoren (1980) showed an inverse relationship between the plasma level and improvement, and Flament *et al.* (1985) found no correlation at all.

MURPHY: Pato *et al.* (1990) systematically attempted to reduce the dosage of clomipramine in patients who had improved during long-term clomipramine treatment. They could reduce the average daily dose by approximately 100 mg from their initial treatment dose without encountering symptom recurrence. Individual dose reductions in the daily dose ranged from 50 to 100 mg.

COPPEN: Many clinicians become impatient; if something does not work immediately they increase the dose.

MURPHY: The patients had been receiving clomipramine for six months to six years.

MENDLEWICZ: What was the drop-out rate in the CIBA-GEIGY study?

INSEL: It was under 10 per cent. The earlier study had a much higher drop-out rate. Clomipramine has been approved in the United States as the first anti-obsessional drug.

LINNOILA: Regulation of these drugs remains a problem. The 250 mg upper limit recommended in the USA is totally arbitrary. There is no hard evidence that at higher doses there are more seizures. That is a very ineffective method of regulation which leaves drugs potentially ineffective for a significant proportion of patients, because plasma levels vary after a standard dose. Physicians need to know what the average plasma level is at the average dose in a large population sample. Then they could titrate the dose.

COPPEN: That is how we were going to regulate antidepressants 15 years ago.

CARLSSON: When the selective drugs and the less selective tricyclic antidepressants were compared and the selective ones were found to be more efficacious, did anybody study serotonin or serotonin uptake in platelets, or 5-HIAA in CSF?

MURPHY: Yes; clomipramine and fluoxetine reduce platelet serotonin content by 95 per cent, whereas desipramine reduces it by only 50 to 60 per cent (Pigott *et al.* 1990).

MELTZER: Inhibition of serotonin uptake by desipramine is surprisingly high, despite the belief that it is a selective noradrenaline uptake blocker.

CARLSSON: With therapeutic dosages there is so much blockade in the platelets that comparison of drugs may sometimes be difficult.

INSEL: Thoren *et al.* (1980) compared nortriptyline, placebo, and clomipramine in OCD patients, and there was no significant effect of nortriptyline on CSF 5-HIAA. As I mentioned earlier, the correlational data suggest that among the clomipramine patients it was those that had the decrease in CSF 5-HIAA that improved.

MURPHY: Table 18.4 shows an aggregate of findings from the literature on the relative changes in 5-HIAA and 3-methoxy-4-hydroxyphenylglycol (MHPG) after administration of agents with relatively selective 5-HT effects, such as clomipramine and fluvoxamine, and other drugs. For clomipramine and the other 5-HT-selective drugs, this ratio is about threefold higher than that found for nortriptyline, imipramine, and amitriptyline. Thus, there is evidence from patients that the preferential serotonergic effects observed in animal brain are greater than noradrenergic effects of these uptake inhibitors.

MELTZER: You almost have to hypothesize that changes in the noradrenaline system are having an effect opposite to the effect on the serotonergic system.

MURPHY: That is an interesting proposal.

LINNOILA: One can directly compare central serotonergic effects of most drugs using CSF 5-HIAA which does not permeate the blood–brain barrier. For MHPG, however, peripheral and central effects of the drug are mixed, if that ratio is used without correction for the peripheral production of MHPG.

TABLE 18.4.   *Differential effects of some 5-HT-selective uptake-inhibiting antidepressants and some non-selective antidepressants on monoamine metabolites in CSF*

Antidepressant		Percentage change		
		5-HIAA	MHPG	5-HIAA/MHPG
5-HT-selective agents				
Clomipramine		−48	−33	1.46
Zimelidine		−38	−20	1.95
Citalopram		−28	−11	2.55
Fluvoxamine		−46	(NS)	−
	Means	−40	−21	1.99
Other agents				
Nortriptyline		−20	−36	0.56
Imipramine		−35	−39	0.90
Amitriptyline		−36	−41	0.88
Clorgyline		−45	−87	0.52
	Means	−34	−51	0.73

Changes in homovanillic acid were negligible in all these studies. MHPG, 3-methoxy-4-hydroxyphenylglycol. Data from Major *et al.* (1979), Bertilsson and Asberg (1984), Bowden *et al.* (1985), Bjerkenstedt *et al.* (1985), and Martin *et al.* (1987).

References

Asberg, M., Edman, G., Rydin, E., Schalling, D., Traskman-Bendz, and Wagner, A. (1984). Biological correlates of suicidal behaviour. *Clinical Neuropharmacology*, **7**, 758–9.

Banki, C. M. and Arato, M. (1983). Amine metabolites and neuroendocrine responses related to depressions and suicide. *Journal of Affective Disorders*, **5**, 223–32.

Bastani, B., Nash, J. F., and Meltzer, H. Y. (1990). Prolactin and cortisol responses to MK-212, a serotonin agonist, in obsessive-compulsive disorder. *Archives of General Psychiatry*, **47**, 833–9.

Bertilsson, L. and Asberg, L. M. (1984). Amine metabolites in the cerebrospinal fluid as a measure of central neurotransmitter function: methodological aspects. *Advances in Biochemical Psychopharmacology*, **39**, 27–34.

Bjerkenstedt, L., Flyckt, L., Over, K. F., and Lingjaerde, O. (1985). Relationship between clinical effects, serum drug concentration and serotonin uptake inhibition in depressed patients treated with citalopram: a double-blind comparison of three dose levels. *European Journal of Pharmacology*, **28**, 553–7.

Bowden, C. L., Kowlow, S. H., Hanin, I., Maas, J. W., Davis, J. M., and Robins, E. (1985). Effects of amitriptyline and imipramine on brain amine neurotransmitter metabolites in cerebrospinal fluid. *Clinical Pharmacology and Therapeutics*, **37**, 316–24.

Delgado, P. L., Charney, D. S., Price, L. H., Aghajanian, G. K., Landis, H., and Heninger, G. R. (1990). Serotonin function and the mechanism of antidepressant actions: reversal of antidepressant induced remission by rapid depletion of plasma tryptophan. *Archives of General Psychiatry*, **47**, 411–18.

de Veaugh-Geiss, J., Landau, P., and Katz, R. (1989). Preliminary results from a multicenter trial of clomipramine in obsessive-compulsive disorder. *Psychopharmacology Bulletin*, **25**, 36–40.

Flament, M. F., Rapoport, J. L., Berg, C. J., Sceery, W., Kiltz, C., McUstrom, B., and Linnoila, M. (1985). Clomipramine treatment of childhood obsessive-compulsive disorder: a double-blind controlled study. *Archives of General Psychiatry*, **42**, 977–83.

Gittleson, N. (1966). The fate of obsession in depressive psychosis. *British Journal of Psychiatry*, **112**, 705–8.

Green, A. R. and Youdim, M. B. H. (1975). Effect of monoamine oxidase inhibition by clorgyline, deprenyl and tranylcypromine on 5-hydroxytryptamine concentration in rat brain and hyperactivity following subsequent tryptophan administration. *British Journal of Pharmacology*, **55**, 415–22.

Green A. R., Milchell, B. D., Tordoff, A. F., and Youdim, M. B. H. (1977). Evidence for dopamine deamination by both type A and type B monoamine oxidase in rat brain *in vivo* and for the degree of inhibition of enzyme necessary for increased functional activity of dopamine and 5-hydroxytryptamine. *British Journal of Pharmacology*, **60**, 343–9.

Guy-Grand, B., Apfelbaum M., Crepaldi, G., Gries, A., Lefebvre, P., and Turner, P. (1989). International trial of long-term Dexfenfluramine in obesity. *Lancet*, **ii**, 1142–4.

Hoehn-Saric, R. and Barksdale, V. C. (1983). Impulsiveness in obsessive-compulsive patients. *British Journal of Psychiatry*, **143**, 177–83.

Insel, T. R., Murphy, D. L., Cohen, R. M., Alterman, I., Kilts, C., and Linnoila, M. (1983). Obsessive-compulsive disorder. A double-blind trial of clomipramine and clorgyline. *Archives of General Psychiatry*, **40**, 605–12.

Insel, T., Mueller, E. A., and Alterman, I. (1985). Obsessive-compulsive disorder and serotonin: is there a connection? *Biological Psychiatry*, **20**, 1174–88.

Janet, P. (1903). *Les obsessions et la psychasthenie*, Alcan, Paris.

Karno, K., Golding, J. M., Sorenenson, S. B., and Burnam, M. A. (1988). The epidemiology of obsessive-compulsive disorder in five US communities. *Archives of General Psychiatry*, **45**, 1094–9.

Lacey, J. H. and Evans, C. D. H. (1986). The impulsivist: a multi-impulsive personality disorder. *British Journal of Addiction*, **81**, 641–9.

Linnoila, M., Virkkunen, M., Scheinin, M., Nuutila, A., Rimon, R., and Goodwin, F. K. (1984). Low cerebrospinal fluid 5-hydroxyindoleacetic acid concentration differentiates impulsive from non-impulsive violent behaviour. *Life Sciences*, **33**, 2609–14.

López-Ibor, Jr. J. J. (1988). The involvement of serotonin in psychiatric disorders and behaviour. *British Journal of Psychiatry*, **153**, Suppl. 3, 26–39.

López-Ibor, J. J. and López-Ibor, Jr. J. J. (1975). Selection criteria for patients who should undergo psychiatric surgery. In *Neurosurgical treatments in psychiatry, pain and epilepsy*, (ed. W. H. Sweet, S. Obrador, and J. G. Martin), pp. 151–62. University Park Press, Baltimore.

López-Ibor, Jr. J. J., Sáiz-Ruiz, J., and Perez de los Cobos, J. C. (1985). Biological correlations suicide and aggressivity in major depressions (with melancholia):

5-hydroxyindoleacetic acid and cortisol in cerebral spinal fluid, dexamethasone suppression test and therapeutic response to 5-hydroxytryptophan. *Neuropsychobiology*, **14**, 67–74.

López-Ibor, Jr. J. J., Sáiz-Ruiz, J., and Moral, L. (1988). The fenfluramine challenge test as an index of severity of the affective disorders. *Pharmacopsychiatry*, **26**, 252–62.

Major, L. F., Lake, C. R., Lipper, S., Lerner, P., and Murphy, D. L. (1979). The central noradrenergic system and affective response to MAO inhibitors. *Progess in Neuropsychopharmacology*, **3**, 535–42.

Markovitz, P. J., Stagno, S. J., and Calabrese, J. R. (1990). Buspirone augmentation of fluoxetine in obsessive-compulsive disorder. *American Journal of Psychiatry*, **147**, 798–800.

Marks, I. M. (1981). Review of behavioural psychotherapy: I. Obsessive-compulsive disorders. *American Journal of Psychiatry*, **138**, 584–92.

Martin, P. R., Adinoff, B., Bone, G. A. H., Stapleton, J. M., Eckardt, M. J., and Linnoila, M. (1987). Fluvoxamine treatment of alchoholic chronic organic brain syndrome. *Clinical Pharmacology and Therapeutics*, **41**, 211 (Abstract).

Pato, M. T., Zohar-Kadouch, R., Zohar, J., and Murphy, D. L. (1988). Return of symptoms after discontinuation of clomipramine in patients with obsessive-compulsive disorder. *American Journal of Psychiatry*, **145**, 1521–5.

Pato, M. T., Hill, J. L., and Murphy, D. L. (1990). A clomipramine dosage reduction study in the course of long-term treatment of obsessive-compulsive disorder patients. *Psychopharmacology Bulletin*, in press.

Pigott, T. A., Pato, M. T., Bernstein, S. E., Grover, G. N., Hill, J. L., Tolliver, T. J., and Murphy, D. L. (1990). A controlled comparison of clomipramine and fluoxetine in the treatment of obsessive-compulsive disorder: behavioural and biological results. *Archives of General Psychiatry*, **47**, 926–34.

Price, L. H., Charney, D. S., Delgado, P. L., Anderson, G. M., and Heninger, G. R. (1989). Effects of desipramine and fluvoxamine treatment on the prolactin response to tryptophan. *Archives of General Psychiatry*, **45**, 625–31.

Stern, R. S., Marks, I. M., and Mawson, D. (1980). Clomipramine and exposure for compulsive rituals: plasma levels, side effects and outcome. *British Journal of Psychiatry*, **136**, 161–6.

Swedo, S. E., Rapoport, J. L., Leonard, H., *et al.* (1989). Obsessive compulsive disorders in children and adolescents. *Archives of General Psychiatry*, **46**, 335–45.

Tellenbach, H. (1983). *Melancholie*, (4th edn.). Springer, Berlin.

Thoren, P., Asberg, M., Bertilsson, L., Melstrom, B., Sjoqvist, F., and Traskman, L. (1980). Clomipramine treatment of obsessive compulsive disorder: II. Biochemical aspects. *Archives of General Psychiatry*, **37**, 1289–95.

Torgersen, S. (1983). Genetic factors in anxiety disorders. *Archives of General Psychiatry*, **40**, 1085–9.

Zohar, J., Mueller, E. A., Insel, T. R., Zohar-Kadouch, R. C., and Murphy, D. L. (1987). Serotonergic responsivity in obsessive-compulsive disorder. *Archives of General Psychiatry*, **44**, 946–51.

19. Monoamines, glucose metabolism, and impulse control

Markku Linnoila and Matti Virkkunen

Many animal and human studies have explored biochemical concomitants of aggressive and self-destructive behaviours. A small number of these studies have used pharmacological manipulations to provoke or reduce such behaviours. A common factor in these investigations is central nervous system (CNS) serotonin (5-hydroxytryptamine, 5-HT); decreasing serotonergic functioning is conducive of aggressive and impulsive behaviours, increasing it reduces such behaviours.

Another factor associated with impulsive, violent offences in some humans is a tendency to become mildly hypoglycaemic after an oral glucose load. Such mild hypoglycaemia is a state associated with irritability and impulsivity.

This review develops the arguments that CNS serotonin metabolism may, to some extent, control glucose metabolism and that reduced central serotonin turnover may be causally linked to hypoglycaemic tendency in impulsive violent offenders and fire-setters.

Animal studies

Aggressive behaviour and serotonin metabolism

Italian investigators, studying isolation-induced fighting in male mice and mouse-killing behaviour in rats, observed an association between such behaviours and a low 5-hydroxyindoleacetic acid (5-HIAA) to serotonin ratio in whole brain homogenates obtained from the aggressive animals (Valzelli 1969, 1971). A low ratio is thought to reflect a low rate of serotonin turnover. Reduction of CNS serotonin by pharmacological or dietary means also leads to increased shock-induced fighting or mouse-killing behaviour in rats (Kantak *et al.* 1981; Katz 1980). Mouse-killing behaviour produced by depletion of serotonin by *p*-chlorophenylalanine can be reduced by the serotonin re-uptake inhibitor fluoxetine (Berzenyi *et al.* 1983). Olfactory bulbectomy, which in mice leads to increased intraspecies aggression, produces serotonin accumulation in the CNS. This accumulation could be indicative of reduced serotonin turnover; moreover, the time courses of the serotonin accumulation and the expression of the aggressive behaviour are parallel (Garris *et al.* 1984).

Both isolation- and olfactory bulbectomy-induced aggression can be reduced by serotonin receptor agonists. Serotonin$_{1A}$ (5-HT$_{1A}$) receptor agonists, such as 8-hydroxy-*N,N*-dipropyl-2-aminotetralin (8-OH-DPAT), are more potent than serotonin$_{1B}$ (5-HT$_{1B}$) receptor agonists in these animal models (Molina *et al.* 1986). Serotonin itself and serotonin receptor agonists show anatomical specificity in their suppression of mouse-killing behaviour in rats. Injections into the amygdala are particularly effective (Pucilowkski *et al.* 1985). The monoaminergic neurone systems interact extensively in the CNS, and a certain level of activity in all of them is necessary for the expression of complex behaviours. Thus, it is not surprising that putative noradrenergic and dopaminergic manipulations also affect mouse-killing behaviour (Kozak *et al.* 1984; Broderick *et al.* 1985). Soubrié (1986) suggested that serotonin serves as an inhibitor of the expression of various behaviours. Thus, reduced serotonin function might not lead to aggressive behaviours *per se*, but would serve a permissive role for expression of aggressive impulses. According to this model, serotonin depletion leads to a primary increase in impulsivity and the increase in aggressiveness is but one manifestation of the behavioural change (Soubrié 1986).

Studies on the Y chromosome

A series of studies at the University of Connecticut has produced evidence for an association between characteristics of the Y chromosome and an increase in intermale aggression in various inbred mouse strains (Selmanoff *et al.* 1977*a*; Maxson *et al.* 1979, 1982; Ginsburg *et al.* 1981). Although there is a relationship between the length of the Y chromosome and aggressiveness—a long Y chromosome is in certain strains associated with increased aggressiveness—interactions between the Y and other chromosomes are also important in controlling aggressive behaviour.

As yet, the role of genes on the Y chromosome in controlling serotonin turnover has not been studied. If both serotonin turnover and Y chromosome characteristics are important in controlling aggressiveness, or if both are associated with impulse control, correlations between these two variables should be found. Specifically, it could be postulated that in certain, particularly aggressive, mouse strains a long Y chromosome would be associated with reduced serotonin turnover in parts of the CNS that are important in controlling aggression or impulsivity.

Studies on glucose metabolism

Yamamoto *et al.* (1984*a,b,c*, 1985) have demonstrated that rats with suprachiasmatic nucleus (SCN) lesions exhibit hypoglycaemia during their active period. These rats show hyperinsulinemic and hypoglucagonemic responses to glucose and deoxyglucose challenges, respectively. Furthermore, they do not show reactive hyperglycaemia in response to central glucopenia produced by intracerebroventricular administration of deoxyglucose.

The suprachiasmatic nucleus projects to the ventromedial nucleus of the hypothalamus. This hypothalamic area together with the lateral hypothalamus, which is also connected to the SCN (Swanson and Cowan 1977; Kita *et al.* 1982), participates in the control of feeding and satiety, particularly with regard to carbohydrate intake. The SCN is thought to be the major endogenous circadian pacemaker in the CNS (Moore and Eichler 1972), and it receives a serotonergic input from the brainstem raphe nuclei (Palkovits *et al.* 1977). Thus, this nucleus provides an anatomical link between serotonin functions, regulation of circadian rhythms, such as the sleep-wake cycle, and regulation of glucose metabolism.

Serotonin is directly linked with CNS control of glucose metabolism by the work of Chaouloff and Jeanrenaud (1987), who demonstrated that intracerebroventricular administration of the serotonin$_{1A}$ receptor agonist 8-OH-DPAT produces hyperglycaemia in the rat.

Human studies: 5-hydroxyindoleacetic acid and homovanillic acid in cerebrospinal fluid

Depression

In 1971 van Praag and Korf discovered that concentrations of 5-hydroxyindoleacetic acid in the cerebrospinal fluid (CSF) of depressed patients after a probenecid load were bimodally distributed. Patients with low concentrations were characterized by a particularly severe form of illness which the authors called 'vital' depression.

In 1976, Asberg *et al.* reported an increased risk of violent suicide attempts among depressed patients with low CSF 5-HIAA concentrations. This finding has been replicated by many investigators (Roy-Byrne *et al.* 1983). The relationship is generally stronger between CSF 5-HIAA concentration and actual suicidal behaviour rather than ideation. Moreover, the relationship does not hold in patients with bipolar depression, who are at a high risk of committing suicide (Agren 1983; Berrettini *et al.* 1985).

Some authors reported a significantly lower mean concentration of homovanillic acid (HVA) rather than of 5-HIAA in their suicidal patients (Agren 1980; Montgomery and Montgomery 1982; Roy *et al.* 1986a). In a clinical and animal study, Agren *et al.* (1986) elucidated the nature of the relationship between the concentrations of 5-HIAA and HVA in CSF. Statistically, a sigmoid 'dose-response' relationship from 5-HIAA to HVA described the data better than a straight regression line. Together with the animal data, the results were interpreted to reflect serotonergic control of dopamine turnover in regions of the CNS controlling the concentration of HVA in lumbar CSF.

Personality disorders

Brown *et al.* (1979, 1982) found a negative correlation (−0.78) between CSF 5-HIAA concentration and an index of the severity and number of aggressive actions by young navy men and marines being evaluated for discharge from service because of a pattern of recurrent aggressive and impulsive behaviours. A similar correlation (−0.77) was found between CSF 5-HIAA and scores on the Minnesota Multiphasic Personality Inventory (MMPI) psychopathic deviate scale. Brown *et al.* (1986) described a negative correlation (−0.63) between the concentration of 5-HIAA in CSF and a history of aggressive behaviours in childhood in the same men. The relationships between the MMPI scores and CSF 5-HIAA, and aggressiveness during childhood and CSF 5-HIAA measured in young adulthood, suggest that low concentrations of 5-HIAA in CSF of these patients are an indicator of a trait rather than a state.

There is a noteworthy absence of research on CSF 5-HIAA in women with borderline personality disorder; very few such patients with notorious impulse control problems have been studied systematically.

Alcoholism

CSF 5-HIAA concentrations in alcoholics have been studied in Japan, the USA, and Hungary. Takahashi *et al.* (1974), investigating 30 alcoholics, found that only patients with severe withdrawal symptoms had lower 5-HIAA concentrations than controls. Major *et al.* (1977) reported a lower mean CSF HVA concentration in alcoholics during withdrawal than in controls. Ballenger *et al.* (1979) performed two lumbar punctures (LPs) on a group of alcoholics; the first within 48 hours of consumption of the last drink and the other after four weeks of supervised abstinence. The alcoholics in this study were young naval men (mean age 28.8 years). CSF 5-HIAA concentrations were significantly reduced from the first to the second LP. Furthermore, the average concentration in the second sample was significantly lower than the mean concentration of CSF 5-HIAA in controls with personality disorders. From their findings and results of previous animal research, the authors postulated that alcoholics as a group have a central serotonin deficit, and that alcohol functionally remedies such a deficit by releasing the transmitter.

Banki (1981), investigating female alcoholics in Hungary, made findings similar to those of Ballenger *et al.*; a negative correlation between the number of days of abstinence before the LP and the CSF 5-HIAA concentration. Branchey *et al.* (1984) found a low ratio of the plasma concentration of tryptophan to that of other neutral amino acids in a subgroup of alcoholics with histories of depressed mood and aggressive behaviour. This ratio is thought to regulate the rate of entry of tryptophan, the amino acid precursor of serotonin, into the brain. Because tryptophan hydroxylase, the rate-limiting enzyme in serotonin synthesis, is not saturated in the brain, the rate of entry of tryptophan may be the rate-limiting step in the synthesis of the transmitter. Thus, the patients studied by Branchey *et al.* may have low CNS serotonin turnover. This interpretation warrants some caution, however, because Hagenfelt *et al.* (1984) found very low correlations between precursor amino acid and neurotransmitter metabolite concentrations in human CSF.

More recently, Buydens-Branchey *et al.* (1989*a,b*) have increased the sample size, and emphasized that alcoholics with an early onset of alcohol abuse are most likely to have the low ratio of tryptophan: other amino acids in plasma. These patients were characterized as more likely to have been depressed, to have attempted suicide, and to have been imprisoned for physical violence. Moreover, they had alcoholic fathers significantly more often than did those who had a late onset of alcoholism.

Relatives of alcoholics

Rosenthal *et al.* (1980) investigated depressed relatives of alcoholics and found that they had a lower mean CSF 5-HIAA concentration than depressed patients without a family history of alcoholism. This study and the results of Buydens-Branchey *et al.* (1989*b*) raise an important issue because they suggest that low CSF 5-HIAA concentrations may not only be a trait but may also be a familial trait.

A familial trait of antisocial behaviours has been associated with 'type 2' or male-limited alcoholism (Cloninger *et al.* 1981). Roy *et al.* (1987) speculated that this subgroup of alcoholics, about 25 per cent of all male alcoholics, may be biochemically characterized by low CSF 5-HIAA concentrations. In agreement with this postulate, we found that of 54 alcohol-abusing violent offenders and impulsive fire-setters 35 had alcoholic fathers. In addition, these 35 had a significantly lower mean CSF 5-HIAA concentration than the group with non-alcoholic fathers (Linnoila *et al.* 1989).

Violent offenders

To further elucidate associations between specific behaviours and CNS serotonin metabolism we studied 36 violent offenders (Linnoila *et al.* 1983). The idea was to have two equally violent groups and classify them according to the impulsiveness of their behaviour. The hypothesis was that impulsive violent offenders would have a lower mean CSF 5-HIAA concentration than non-impulsive offenders, independent of violent behaviour *per se*. Patients with a clear premeditation of their crime were classified as non-impulsive while patients without established premeditation (attacking without provocation, without expectation of monetary gain, and not knowing the victim) were classified as impulsive. The source of the information was the police report on the crime for which they were convicted. Using this method, nine patients were classified as non-impulsive and 27 as impulsive.

Diagnoses were made according to criteria in the Diagnostic and Statistical Manual (DSM III) (American Psychiatric Association 1980) by a forensic research psychiatrist who was not blind to the criminal records of the patients. The impulsive patients had either intermittent explosive or antisocial personality disorder, whereas the non-impulsive patients had either paranoid or passive aggressive personality disorder. All patients fulfilled the criteria for alcohol abuse. Seventeen of the 25 impulsive patients had a past history of suicide attempts. The impulsive patients had a significantly lower mean CSF 5-HIAA concentration than the non-impulsive patients. Moreover, patients with a history of suicide attempts had the lowest mean CSF 5-HIAA. There was no difference in CSF free testosterone concentrations between the groups (Roy *et al.* 1986*b*).

Lidberg *et al.* (1984, 1985) and Selmanoff (1977) found a low CSF 5-HIAA concentration in murderers killing their children or lovers, but not in alcoholic murderers.

Arsonists

Impulsive fire-setters are thought to show relatively little interpersonal aggressive behaviour. Therefore, to investigate further whether low CSF 5-HIAA concentration is primarily associated with impulsiveness or aggressiveness we studied 20 impulsive arsonists (Virkkunen *et al.* 1987). Impulsivity in these patients was defined as a sudden uncontrollable urge to set a fire. Subjects setting fires for economic gain, such as insurance fraud, were excluded from the sample. The arsonists were compared to 20 age and sex-matched violent offenders and ten controls. The arsonists were found to have the lowest mean CSF 5-HIAA concentration, followed by the violent offenders, who had a lower concentration than the healthy volunteers. Interestingly, mean CSF HVA concentrations were practically identical in the three groups, but CSF 3-methoxy-4-hydroxyphenylglycol (MHPG) concentrations paralleled CSF 5-HIAA concentrations. Thus, low mean concentrations of both 5-HIAA and MHPG in CSF were more strongly associated with impulsivity than with violence in these samples of violent offenders and impulsive fire-setters.

Patients with frontal lobe lesions

Patients who have suffered brain damage to the frontotemporal regions often have uncontrollable bursts of anger and show 'emotional lability'. In one Dutch study (van Woerkom *et al.* 1977), 11 patients who had an LP within one to nine days of sustaining a frontotemporal brain insult had significantly lower CSF 5-HIAA concentrations than 30 patients with diffuse brain injuries of equal severity or ten non-specified controls.

Because the behavioural disturbances observed in some patients with frontotemporal lesions can be construed as indicative of impaired impulse control, further studies on CSF 5-HIAA concentration should be performed in this patient population. It would be particularly desirable to investigate patients who have a stable condition after the insult.

Healthy volunteers

Roy *et al.* (1988) found a negative correlation between acting out hostility and CSF 5-HIAA concentration in healthy volunteers. Individuals with low CSF 5-HIAA were more likely to rate themselves high on a standardized scale quantifying the pretence of hostility than those with high CSF 5-HIAA. Additionally, men had lower mean CSF 5-HIAA concentrations and higher mean hostility scores than women. Like the mouse Y chromosome experiments reviewed above, this finding emphasizes a potential role of the Y chromosome or androgens in controlling CNS serotonin metabolism.

Brewerton *et al.* (1988) found in a small number of healthy volunteers a significant seasonal variation in CSF 5-HIAA concentrations; in early spring the concentrations were on average 40 per cent lower than those in the late summer. If this finding is replicated, investigators should use season as a covariant in all studies concerning CSF 5-HIAA.

Treatments of violent behaviours in humans

Tryptophan and lithium have, in controlled studies, been shown to reduce violent incidents in aggressive schizophrenics and prisoners, respectively (Morand *et al.* 1983; Sherd *et al.* 1976). Propranolol, also in a controlled study, reduced assaultive behaviours in patients with organic brain disorders (Greendyke *et al.* 1986).

In uncontrolled clinical reports, propranolol, metoprolol, nadolol, and a combination of trazodone and tryptophan have been alleged to be useful for treatment of violent behaviours in patients with schizophrenia and mental retardation arising from various causes (Sorgi *et al.* 1986; Mattes 1985; O'Neil *et al.* 1986).

All these treatments have serotonergic effects; lithium and propranolol enhance pre-synaptic serotonergic functioning by different mechanisms (Hotta *et al.* 1986; Sprouse and Aghajanian 1986), and tryptophan is the precursor amino acid for serotonin synthesis.

Glucose metabolism

Depression

Glucose tolerance has been studied in depression for more than two decades. Patients with unipolar depression become hyperglycaemic and hyperinsulinemic after an oral or intravenous glucose load (Pryce 1958*a*,*b*). Patients with bipolar depression are not different from healthy people in this respect and differ significantly from patients with unipolar depression (Pryce 1958*b*).

Successful treatment of depression reverses the abnormal glucose tolerance (van Praag and Leijnse 1965). Furthermore, Heninger *et al.* (1975) found that in patients with psychotic unipolar depression suicidality was weakly, but significantly, associated with reduced disappearance of glucose and hyperinsulinemia. The difference between unipolar and bipolar depressives in oral glucose tolerance tests parallels the reported difference in the relationship between CSF 5-HIAA and suicidality in these diagnostic groups.

Violent offenders

Virkkunen and collaborators (Virkkunen and Huttunen 1982; Virkkunen 1982, 1983, 1986*a,b*) demonstrated that impulsive violent offenders have a tendency to become hypoglycaemic and hyperinsulinemic after an oral glucose load. Offenders with intermittent explosive personality disorder show a more rapid onset of, and recovery from, hypoglycaemia than patients with antisocial personality disorder. These time course differences parallel the characteristic time courses of disturbed behaviours in these two groups of patients.

Like the patients with low CSF 5-HIAA concentrations studied by Brown *et al.* (1979, 1982) the patients studied by Virkkunen who have clinically significant hypoglycaemic responses have life-long histories of aggressive, violent, and antisocial behaviours. They are also more likely to have fathers with histories of antisocial and criminal behaviours and low concentrations of 5-HIAA (Linnoila *et al.* 1989). Thus, both low CSF 5-HIAA concentrations and the tendency to become hypoglycaemic after an oral glucose load may be familial traits in impulsive patients with personality disorders.

Arsonists

In the study by Virkkunen *et al.* (1984), 11 out of 20 arsonists became mildly hypoglycaemic in the oral glucose tolerance test. They also had low CSF 5-HIAA concentrations but correlation between the two measures was not statistically significant. In a larger sample of 59 arsonists Virkkunen found mild hypoglycaemia during the oral glucose tolence test in 27 patients.

Healthy volunteers

Benton and Kumari (1982) studied 24 healthy male volunteers and found significant correlations between the degree of hypoglycaemia during an oral glucose tolerance test and the scores on two psychological tests of hostility and frustration tolerance administered during the glucose tolerance test. Subjects with low blood glucose concentrations showed more hostility and lower frustration tolerance.

Follow-up studies

We searched the Criminal Registry of Finland for repeat crimes in 58 violent offenders and fire-setters an average of about three years after they were released from prison. Thirteen had been sentenced for another violent offence. The recidivist offenders had significantly lower CSF 5-HIAA and HVA concentrations and blood glucose nadirs during the oral glucose tolerance test than the non-recidivists (Virkkunen *et al.* 1989*a*). Furthermore, in a discriminant function analysis a combination of blood glucose nadir and CSF 5-HIAA correctly classified 84.2 per cent of the subjects as recidivist or non-recidivist. Among the same subjects a history of suicide attempts was associated with low CSF 5-HIAA and MHPG concentrations and with the DSM-III diagnosis of dysthymia but not with a low blood glucose nadir (Virkkunen *et al.* 1989*b*).

Future directions

The strong associations between low CSF 5-HIAA and indices of reduced impulse control observed in a large number of human studies have led to surprisingly few studies of serotonergic intervention in impulsive, violent, and suicidal patients. More should be done to find treatments for these conditions.

The associations between CNS serotonin functioning and glucose metabolism should be explored further. The high incidence of violent behaviour, suicide, alcoholism, and adult onset of diabetes in certain populations may not be mere coincidence.

Finally, techniques of molecular biology should be applied to elucidate the putative control of serotonin functions by genes on the Y chromosome or by androgen responsive elements, and brain imaging should be used to explore the physiological CNS concomitants of low concentrations of 5-HIAA in CSF.

Acknowledgement

This review is an updated version of 'Monoamines, glucose metabolism and impulse control' by M. Linnoila, M. Virkkunen, A. Roy, and W. Z. Potter in *Violence and Suicidality: Perspective in Clinical and Psychobiological Research*, (ed. H. van Praag, R. Plutchik, and A. Apter), pp. 218–41. Brunner-Mazel, New York, 1990.

References

Agren, H. (1980). Symptom patterns in unipolar and bipolar depression correlating with monoamine metabolites in the cerebrospinal fluid. II. Suicide. *Psychiatry Research*, **3**, 225–36.

Agren, H. (1983). Life at risk: markers of suicidality in depression. *Psychiatric Developments*, **1**, 87–104.

Agren, H., Mefford, I. N., Rudorfer, M. V., Linnoila, M., and Potter, W. Z. (1986). Interacting neurotransmitter systems. A nonexperimental approach to the 5HIAA–HVA correlation in human CSF. *Journal of Psychiatric Research*, **20**, 175–93.

American Psychiatric Association (1980). *Diagnostic and statistical manual*, 3rd edn. American Psychiatric Association, Washington DC.

Asberg, M., Traskman, L., and Thoren, P. (1976). 5-HIAA in the cerebrospinal fluid—a biochemical suicide predictor? *Archives of General Psychiatry*, **33**, 1193–7.

Ballenger, J., Goodwin, F., Major, L., and Brown, G. (1979). Alcohol and central serotonin metabolism in man. *Archives of General Psychiatry*, **36**, 224–7.

Banki, C. (1981). Factors influencing monoamine metabolites and tryptophan in patients with alcohol dependence. *Journal of Neural Transmission*, **50**, 98–101.

Benton, D. and Kumari, N. (1982). Mild hypoglycemia and questionnaire measures of aggression. *Biological Psychology*, **14**, 129–35.

Berrettini, W. H., Nurnberger, J. I., Scheinin, M., Seppala, T., Linnoila, M., Simmons-Alling, S., and Gershon, E. (1985). Cerebrospinal fluid and plasma monoamines and their metabolites in euthymic bipolar patients. *Biological Psychiatry*, **20**, 257–69.

Berzenyi, P., Galateo, E., and Valzelli, L. (1983). Fluoxetine activity on muricidal aggression induced in rats by p-chlorophenylalanine. *Aggressive Behavior*, **9**, 333–8.

Branchey, L., Branchey, M., Shaw, S., and Lieber, C. S. (1984). Depression, suicide, and aggression in alcoholics and their relationship to plasma amino acids. *Psychiatry Research*, **12**, 219–26.

Brewerton, R. D., Berrettini, W. H., Nurnberger, J. I., and Linnoila, M. (1988). Analysis of seasonal fluctuations of CSF monoamine metabolites and neuropeptides in normal controls: findings with 5HIAA and HVA. *Psychiatry Research*, **23**, 257–65.

Broderick, P. A., Barr, G. A., Sharpless, N. S., and Bridger, W. H. (1985). Biogenic amine alterations in limbic brain regions of muricidal rats. *Research Communications in Chemical Pathology and Pharmacology*, **48**, 3–15.

Brown, G. L., Goodwin, F. K., Ballenger, J. C., Goyer, P. F., and Major, L. F. (1979). Aggression in humans correlates with cerebrospinal fluid metabolites. *Psychiatry Research*, **1**, 131–9.

Brown, G. L., Ebert, M. H., Goyer, D. C., Jimerson, D. C., Klein, W. J., Bunney, W. E., and Goodwin, F. K. (1982). Aggression, suicide and serotonin: relationship to CSF amine metabolites. *American Journal of Psychiatry*. **139**, 741–6.

Brown, G. L., Kline, W. J., Goyer, P. F., Minichiello, M. D., Kruesi, M. J. P., and Goodwin, F. K. (1986). Relationship of childhood characteristics to cerebrospinal fluid 5-hydroxyindoleacetic acid in aggressive adults. In *Biological psychiatry*, (ed. C. Chagass), pp. 177–9. Elsevier, New York.

Buydens-Branchey, L., Branchey, M., and Noumair, D. (1989a). Age of alcoholism onset. I. Relationship to psychopathology. *Archives of General Psychiatry*, **46**, 229–30.

Buydens-Branchey, L., Branchey, M., and Noumair, D. (1989b). Age of alcoholism onset. II. Relationship to susceptibility to serotonin precursor availability. *Archives of General Psychiatry*, **46**, 231–6.

Chaouloff, A. and Jeanrenaud, B. (1987). 5-HT $_{1A}$ and alpha-2 adrenergic receptors mediate the hyperglycemic and hypoinsulinemic effects of 8-hydroxy-2-(di-N-propylamino) tetralin in the conscious rat. *Journal of Pharmacology and Experimental Therapeutics*, **243**, 1159–66.

Cloninger, C., Bohman, M., and Sigvardsson, S. (1981). Inheritance of alcohol abuse: cross-fostering analysis of adopted men. *Archives of General Psychiatry*, **38**, 861–8.

Garris, D. R., Chamberlain, J. K., and DaVanzo, J. P. (1984). Histofluorescent identification of indoleamine-concentrating brain loci associated with intraspecies, reflexive biting and locomotor behavior in olfactory-bulbectomized mice. *Brain Research*, **294**, 385–9.

Ginsburg, B. E., Vigue, L. E., Larsom, W. A., and Maxson, S. C. (1981). Y-chromosome length in sublines of two mouse strains. *Behavioral Genetics*, **11**, 359–68.

Greendyke. R. M., Kanter, D. R., Schuster, D. B., Verstreate, S., and Wootton, J. (1986). Propranolol treatment of assaultive patients with organic brain disease. *Journal of Nervous and Mental Disorders*, **174**, 290–4.

Hagenfelt, L., Bjerkenstedt, G., Edman, G., Sedvall, G., and Wiesel F-A. (1984). Amino acids in plasma and CSF and monoamine metabolites in CSF: interrelationship in healthy subjects. *Journal of Neurochemistry*, **42**, 833–7.

Heninger, G. R., Mueller, P. S., and Davis, L. S. (1975). Depressive symptoms and the glucose tolerance test and insulin tolerance test. *Journal of Nervous and Mental Disorders*, **161**, 421–31.

Hotta, I., Yamawaki, S., and Segawa, T. (1986). Long-term lithium treatment causes serotonin receptor down-regulation via serotonergic presynapses in rat brain. *Neuropsychobiology*, **16**, 19–26.

Kantak, K. M., Hegstrand, L. R., and Eichelman, B. (1981). Facilitation of shock-induced fighting following intraventricular 5, 7-dihydroxytryptamine and 6-hydroxy-DOPA. *Psychopharmacology*, **74**, 157–60.

Katz, R. J. (1980). Role of serotonergic mechanisms in animal models of predation. *Progress in Neuro-Psychopharmacology and Biological Psychiatry*, **4**, 219–31.

Kita, H., Shibata, S., Oomura, Y., and Ohki, K. (1982). Excitatory effects of the suprachiasmatic nucleus on the ventromedial nucleus in the rat hypothalamic slice. *Brain Research*, **235**, 137–41.

Kozak, W., Valzelli, L., and Garattini, S. (1984). Anxiolytic activity on locus coeruleus-mediated suppression of muricidal aggression. *European Journal of Pharmacology*, **105**, 323–6.

Lidberg, L., Asberg, M., and Sundqvist-Stensman, U. B. (1984). 5-Hydroxyindole-acetic acid levels in attempted suicides who have killed their children. *Lancet*, **ii** 928.

Lidberg, L., Tuck, J. R., Asberg, M., Scalia-Tomba, G. P., and Bertilsson, L. (1985). Homicide, suicide and CSF 5-HIAA. *Acta Psychiatrica Scandinavica*, **71**, 230–6.

Linnoila, M., Virkkunen, M., Scheinin, M., Nuutila, A., Rimon, R., and Goodwin, F. K. (1983). Low cerebrospinal fluid 5-hydroxyindoleacetic acid concentration differentiates impulsive from nonimpulsive violent behavior. *Life Sciences*, **33**, 2609–14.

Linnoila, M., DeJong, J., and Virkkunen, M. (1989). Family history of alcoholism in violent offenders and impulsive fire setters. *Archives of General Psychiatry*, **46**, 613–16.

Major, L., Ballenger, J., Goodwin, F., and Brown, G. (1977). Cerebrospinal fluid homovanillic acid in male alcoholics: effect of disulfiram. *Biological Psychiatry*, **12**, 635–42.

Mattes, J. A. (1985). Metoprolol for intermittent explosive disorder. *American Journal of Psychiatry*, **142**, 1108–9.

Maxson, S. C., Ginsburg, B. E., and Trattner, A. (1979). Interaction of Y-chromosomal and autosomal gene(s) in the development of intermale aggression in mice. *Behavioral Genetics*, **9**, 219–369.

Maxson, S. C., Platt, T., Shrenker, P., and Tratner, A. (1982). The influence of the

Y-chromosome of Rb/1Bg mice on agonistic behaviors. *Aggressive Behavior*, **8** 285–91.

Molina, V. A., Gobaille, S., and Mandel, P. (1986). Effects of serotonin-mimetic drugs on mouse-killing behavior. *Aggressive Behavior*, **12**, 201–11.

Montgomery, S. and Montgomery, D. (1982). Pharmacological prevention of suicidal behavior. *Journal of Affective Disorders*, **4**, 291–8.

Moore, R. Y. and Eichler, V. B. (1972). Loss of a circadian adrenal corticosterone rhythm following suprachiasmatic lesions in the rat. *Brain Research*, **42**, 201–6.

Morand, C., Young, S. N., and Ervin, F. R. (1983). Clinical response of aggressive schizophrenics to oral tryptophan. *Biological Psychiatry*, **18**, 575–8.

O'Neil, M., Page, N., Adkins, W. N., and Eichelman, B. (1986). Tryptophan-trazodone treatment of aggressive behaviour. *Lancet*, **ii**, 859–60.

Palkovits, M., Saavedra, J. M., Jacobovits, D. M., Kizer, J. S., Zaborsky, L., and Brownstein, M. J. (1977). Serotonergic innervation of the forebrain: effect of lesions on serotonin and tryptophan hydroxylase levels. *Brain Research*, **130**, 121–34.

Pryce, I. G. (1958*a*). The relationship between glucose tolerance, body weight, and clinical state in melancholia. *Journal of Mental Science*, **104**, 1079–92.

Pryce, I. G. (1958*b*). Melancholia, glucose tolerance, and body weight. *Journal of Mental Science*, **104**, 421–7.

Pucilowski, O., Plaznik, A., and Kostowski, W. (1985). Aggressive behavior inhibition by serotonin and quipazine injected into the amygdala in the rat. *Behavioral and Neurological Biology*, **43**, 58–68.

Rosenthal, N., Davenport, Y., Cowdry, R., Webster, M., and Goodwin, F. (1980). Monoamine metabolites in cerebrospinal fluid of depressive subgroups. *Psychiatry Research*, **2**, 113–19.

Roy, A., Agren, H., Pickar, D., Linnoila, M., Doran, A. R., Cutler, N. R., and Paul, S. (1986*a*). Reduced CSF concentrations of homovanillic acid and homovanillic acid to 5-hydroxyindoleacetic acid ratios in depressed patients: relationship to suicidal behavior and dexamethasone nonsuppression. *American Journal of Psychiatry*, **143**, 1539–45.

Roy, A., Virkkunen, M., Guthrie, S., Poland, R., and Linnoila, M. (1986*b*). Monoamines, glucose metabolism and aggressive behaviors. *Psychopharmacology Bulletin*, **22**, 661–5.

Roy, A., Virkkunen, M., and Linnoila, M. (1987). Reduced central serotonin turnover in a subgroup of alcoholics? *Progress in Neuro-Psychopharmacology and Biological Psychiatry*, **11**, 173–7.

Roy, A., Adinoff, B., and Linnoila, M. (1988). Acting out hostility in normal volunteers: negative correlation with CSF 5HIAA levels. *Psychiatry Research*, **24**, 187–94.

Roy-Byrne, P., Post, R. M., Rubinow, D. R., Linnoila, M., Savard, R., and Davis, D. (1983). CSF 5HIAA and personal and family history of suicide in affectively ill patients: a negative study. *Psychiatry Research*, **10**, 263–74.

Selmanoff, M. K., Goldman, B. D., Maxson, S. C., and Ginsburg, B. E. (1977*a*). Correlated effects of the Y-chromosome of mice on developmental changes in testosterone levels and intermale aggression. *Life Sciences*, **20**, 359–66.

Selmanoff, M. K., Abreu, E., Goldman, B. D., and Ginsburg, B. E. (1977*b*). Manipulation of aggressive behavior in adult DBA/2/Bg and c57BL/10/Bg male mice implanted with testosterone in silastic tubing. *Hormones and Behavior*, **8**, 377–90.

Sherd, M. H., Marini, J. L., Bridges, C. I., and Wagner, E. (1976). The effect of lithium on impulsive aggressive behavior in man. *American Journal of Psychiatry*, **133**, 1409–13.

Soubrié, P. (1986). Reconciling the role of central serotonin neurons in human and animal behavior. *Behavioral Brain Science*, **9**, 319–64.

Sorgi, P. J., Ratey, J. J., and Polakoff, S. (1986). β-adrenergic blockers for the control of aggressive behaviors in patients with chronic schizophrenia. *American Journal of Psychiatry*, **143**, 775–6.

Sprouse, J. S. and Aghajanian, G. K. (1986). (−)-Propranolol blocks the inhibition of serotonergic dorsal raphe cell firing by 5-HT 1A selective agonists. *European Journal of Pharmacology*, **128**, 295–8.

Swanson, L. W. and Cowan, W. M. (1977). The efferent projections of the suprachiasmatic nucleus of the hypothalamus. *Journal of Comprehensive Neurology*, **160**, 1–12.

Takahashi, S., Yamane, H., Kondo, H., and Tani, N. (1974). CSF monoamine metabolites in alcoholism, a comparative study with depression. *Folia Psychiatrica and Neurologica Japanica*, **28**, 347–54.

Valzelli, L. (1969). Aggressive behaviour induced by isolation. In *Excerpta Medica*, (ed. S. Garattini and E. B. Sigg), pp. 70–6. Amsterdam.

Valzelli, L. (1971). Further aspects of the exploratory behavior in aggressive mice. *Psychopharmacologia*, **19**, 91–4.

van Praag, H. M. and Korf, J. (1971). Endogenous depressions with and without disturbances in the 5-hydroxytryptamine metabolism: a biochemical classification. *Psychopharmacology*, **19**, 148–52.

van Praag, H. M. and Leijnse, B. (1965). Depression, glucose tolerance, peripheral glucose uptake and their alterations under the influence of anti-depressive drugs of the hydrazine type. *Psychopharmacologia*, **8**, 67–78.

van Woerkom, T. C. A. M., Teelken, A. W., and Minderhoud, J. M. (1977). Difference in neurotransmitter metabolism in frontotemporal-lobe contusion and diffuse cerebral contusion. *Lancet*, **i**, 812–13.

Virkkunen, M. (1982). Reactive hypoglycemic tendency among habitually violent offenders. *Neuropsychobiology*, **8**, 35–40.

Virkkunen, M. (1983). Insulin secretion during the glucose tolerance test in antisocial personality. *British Journal of Psychiatry*, **142**, 598–604.

Virkkunen, M. (1984). Reactive hypoglycemic tendency among arsonists. *Acta Psychiatrica Scandinavica*, **69**, 445–52.

Virkkunen, M. (1986a). Insulin secretion during the glucose tolerance test among habitually violent and impulsive offenders. *Aggressive Behavior*, **12**, 303–10.

Virkkunen, M. (1986b). Reactive hypoglycemic tendency among habitually violent offenders. *Nutrition Review*, Suppl., 94–103.

Virkkunen, M. and Huttunen, M. O. (1982). Evidence for abnormal glucose tolerance test among violent offenders. *Neuropsychobiology*, **8**, 30–4.

Virkkunen, M., Nuutila, A., Goodwin, F. K., and Linnoila, M. (1987). CSF monoamine metabolites in male arsonists. *Archives of General Psychiatry*, **44**, 241–7.

Virkkunen, M., DeJong, J., Bartko, J., Goodwin, F. K., and Linnoila, M. (1989a). Relationship of psychobiological variables to recidivism in violent offenders and impulsive fire setters: a follow up study. *Archives of General Psychiatry*, **46**, 600–3.

Virkkunen, M., DeJong, J., Bartko, J., and Linnoila, M. (1989b). Psychobiological concomitants of history of suicide attempts among violent offenders and impulsive fire setters. *Archives of General Psychiatry*, **46**, 604–6.

Yamamoto, H., Nagai, K., and Nakagava, H. (1984*a*). Bilateral lesions of the suprachiasmatic nucleus enhance glucose tolerance in rats. *Biomedical Research*, **5**, 47–54.

Yamamoto, H., Nagai, K., and Nakagava, H. (1984*b*). Role of the suprachiasmatic nucleus in glucose homeostasis. *Biomedical Research*, **5**, 55–60.

Yamamoto, H., Nagai, K., and Nakagava, H. (1984*c*). Bilateral lesions of the SCN abolish lipolytic and hyperphagic responses to 2DG. *Physiology and Behavior*, **32**, 1017–20.

Yamamoto, H., Nagai, K., and Nakagava, H. (1984*d*). Additional evidence that the suprachiasmatic nucleus is the center for regulation of insulin secretion and glucose homeostasis. *Brain Research*, **304**, 237–41.

Yamamoto, H., Nagai, K., and Nakagava, H. (1985). Lesions involving the suprachiasmatic nucleus eliminate the glucagon response to intracranial injection of 2-deoxy-D-glucose. *Endocrinology*, **117**, 468–73.

Discussion

SANDLER: I would be the first to agree with you that many factors are involved in aggression. Some years ago, we measured phenylacetic acid, the major metabolite of phenylethylamine, in aggressive psychopaths and found an increase of both free and conjugated compound (Sandler *et al.* 1978). Yu *et al.* (1984) were not able to confirm this finding, however. When we studied a population of vervet monkeys in St. Kitts (Elsworth *et al.* 1985), we found that the alpha male, the leader of the pack, consistently had higher amounts of free and conjugated phenylacetic acid than the non-dominant males.

I feel uneasy about the studies on 5-hydroxyindoleacetic acid (5-HIAA) in cerebrospinal fluid (CSF) from alcoholics. Alcoholics who are supposedly abstinent may be drinking in secret. When 5-HIAA is measured, only a little alcohol is required to cause a shift from the oxidative to the reductive metabolite pathway, with a consequent increase in 5-hydroxytryptophol at the expense of 5-HIAA. In patients with carcinoid tumours, who have large amounts of 5-HIAA in their urine, a small glass of sherry will convert most of that 5-HIAA into 5-hydroxytryptophol. If one is measuring 5-HIAA, this may result in a negative test for carcinoid.

LINNOILA: In the large number, about 300, of alcoholics on my research ward during the past six years, and in about 50 controls from the same ward, there is no mean difference in the CSF 5-HIAA levels after a minimum of four weeks sober on a supervised ward. Every time patients return to the ward they blow into a breathalyser, and we also monitor urinary alcohol output and liver enzymes. It is known that patients are discharged if they fail the tests. On the other hand, if we look at the early onset aggressive male alcoholics, a difference begins to emerge. With Theodore George and Dennis Murphy, we were surprised to find that 90 per cent of early onset alcoholics get 'high' on *m*-chlorophenylpiperazine (*m*-CPP), whereas only one late onset alcoholic and two controls showed this response, which suggests that this is a subgroup-related phenomenon.

I am aware of your phenylacetic acid studies. Dr Farouk Karoum would say that all phenylacetic acid is produced in the periphery via decarboxylation of phenylalanine. I am not competent to judge that issue.

I find it intriguing that, as Tom Insel elegantly stated, in impulsivity we may have a dimension that in certain respects cuts across diagnostic categories. I did not expect the finding that verbal acting of hostility by healthy volunteers correlates, for both sexes, negatively with CSF 5-HIAA. We used the Brown–Goodwin aggression scale for 100 alcoholics from my ward. Those who rated the patients did not know the subgrouping or the biochemistries. Even in this group of relatively non-aggressive alcoholics we find a reasonably robust negative correlation.

We are not the only people finding these low levels of CSF 5-HIAA. For example, in the literature on unipolar depression, 16 of 19 studies reported that individuals with low 5-HIAA make more suicide attempts.

SANDLER: I am not sure that it matters whether what we study is a peripheral phenomenon or not; it is a marker of *something* going on and, as long as it helps to distinguish one clinical group from another, it does not make any difference if the finding is an empirical one.

You did not mention the drugs that Duphar call serenics. Olivier and his colleagues (see Olivier and Mos 1986) developed these drugs using rats who had just given birth as a model of aggression. The current reference compound in this group, eltoprazine, is probably a 5-HT$_{1A}$ agonist. Apart from reversing aggressivity, it appears to abolish sexual drive altogether, at least in males.

LINNOILA: Infusion of 5-HT$_{1A}$ agonists, such as 8-hydroxy-N,N-dipropyl-2-aminotetralin (8-OH-DPAT), into the central nucleus or the amygdala is an effective anti-aggressive measure. The central nucleus is also intimately involved in the circuits which control the heart rate in fight/flight responses. Thus the circuitry makes some sense.

DEAKIN: I like the finding that aggressive and sociopathic individuals have low CSF 5-HIAA. Their problem could be that they lack an effective 5-HT (serotonin) punishment system. Sociopathic individuals are very poor at aversive conditioning, for example. Is their problem a lack of anxiety? Can you separate a lack of anxiety from impulsiveness?

You postulate a direct relationship between depleted 5-HT and hypoglycaemia. Could you test that in primates by lesioning raphe and showing that you get hyperglycaemic nadirs after glucose tolerance tests?

LINNOILA: The anxiety issue is complex. In a study of 60 violent offenders from Helsinki we had volunteers on the same ward, thus dealing with the possible artefact of isolation from society. The offenders excreted significantly less cortisol. We are looking at CSF corticotropin-releasing hormone (CRH) concentrations in these people. Because there are links between serotonin and noradrenaline and CRH and several other peptides, the relationships are not easy to decypher. Anxiety and lack of impulse control are not necessarily exactly the same phenomenon, but they may be linked.

It is difficult to selectively lesion the suprachiasmatic nucleus (SCN) in rats. H. Yamamoto *et al.* obtained clear-cut pure SCN lesions in only three of 20 rats. We have had similar experience. 5,7-Dihydroxytryptamine applied directly on the dorsal raphe or intracerebroventricularly does not cause significant depletion of the serotonin in the SCN. 5-HT$_{1A}$ agonists applied centrally produced hypoglycaemia, as expected. This makes me apprehensive in interpreting much of the literature about 5-HT and food intake. We know that there are feedback loops from plasma glucose to the brain. Even more baffling is the fact that in the satiated rat 5-HT$_{1A}$ agonists increase food intake whereas at the same time they increase blood glucose. We are doing the appropriate studies to evaluate these phenomena but we are not as far advanced as we would like to be.

GUARDIOLA-LEMAITRE: Pinealectomy is one way to induce a decrease in insulin, an increase in glucogen levels, and hyperglycaemia. Injection of melatonin restores the insulin level. In rats with diabetes induced by alloxan there is a diminution of melatonin, but no study has shown whether melatonin is able to restore the level of insulin.

LINNOILA: The effects of pinealectomy are interesting because there is a relatively high density of melatonin receptors on the SCN. There is undoubtedly cross-talk between the pineal and the SCN. In the rat, pinealectomy also produces quite severe hypertension, and the brainstem serotonin systems are involved in the maintenance of blood pressure. So it is a difficult situation for us to interpret.

Based on physical activity monitors, we have evidence that impulsive violent offenders show more disrupted sleep than healthy volunteers, if one takes increased activity during the night as an indication of disrupted sleep. Thus, the hypothesis of circadian rhythm disturbance in impulsive violent offenders seems to be supported. Melatonin rhythms should be studied in these patients in future.

Steven Paul found that just micrograms of alloxan given intracerebroventricularly destroys the glucostat in the hypothalamus. Thus, alloxan has effects on the central nervous system beyond acting at the pancreas. We used streptozotocin injections to produce experimental diabetes. After reasonably good glucose control by administration of insulin to the rat, the changes in monoamines are primarily noradrenergic, not serotonergic.

COPPEN: What happens to women who have low 5-HIAA?

LINNOILA: There are no good studies of CSF 5-HIAA in women with borderline personality disorder. In studies with fenfluramine and *m*-CPP the different responsiveness between aggressive psychopaths and normal individuals was found only in males, not females. In the *m*-CPP studies we have only about 10 women alcoholics, but none of these has shown the subjective response that the male alcoholics show. The biochemistry of women with borderline personality disorder is unknown, and may not be similar to that of the aggressive sociopathic male.

COPPEN: An important social manifestation of poor impulse control and aggression is in motor accidents. In the UK there are more motor accidents involving young men; the risk decreases after age 30. Have you studied this area?

LINNOILA: My doctoral thesis was on drinking and driving. The so-called accident proneness literature is confusing, but it is clear that young males under the influence of alcohol are at much higher risk than middle-aged males with the same blood alcohol concentration. We don't know why that is.

COPPEN: I imagine that your group of impulsive individuals has a high motor accident rate.

LINNOILA: They do have some motor accidents, but these are extremely impulsive individuals who tend to get into trouble at a young age, and in Finland they have less access to cars than they would in the United States, for example. In the new series we found that CSF 5-HIAA or blood glucose levels do not predict non-violent crime. They may predict violent crime.

OXENKRUG: Do low concentrations of CSF 5-HIAA reflect slow degradation of serotonin or low serotonin synthesis?

LINNOILA: We do not know what physiological feature low CSF 5-HIAA concentrations reflect. In human post-mortem studies on 5-HIAA in various parts of the brain and in the lumbar CSF, the best correlation, surprisingly, is between concentrations in the frontal cortex and in lumbar CSF. We need to be able to measure directly serotonin turnover in living human brain, and many of us are working towards that using positron emission tomography or single-photon emission computed tomography.

Contrary to the findings of G. Sedvall from Sweden in humans, in a large-scale study of rhesus monkeys we find high heritability of CSF 5-HIAA and homovanillic acid (HVA). This suggests that some of the CSF monoamine metabolites could be valid phenotypic markers that might be used to select individuals for further studies.

GLOVER: The groups where you found low CSF 5-HIAA are fairly similar to groups where low platelet monoamine oxidase (MAO) activity has been found. Oreland *et al.* (1984) have some evidence for a correlation between CSF 5-HIAA concentrations and platelet MAO activity. Have you looked at this?

LINNOILA: We have not measured platelet MAO activity, being fairly discouraged by the large-scale studies in Sweden, where the correlations are only of the order of 0.2–0.3.

GLOVER: It might be higher in extreme populations.

LINNOILA: That could be true. In these challenge studies we quickly reach the limit of blood available for the assays. Studying platelet MAO has not been high on the priority list.

GLOVER: What are the social implications of your data? You seem to suggest that you can predict who is going to commit further violent crime.

LINNOILA: I don't think I can predict that with the kind of accuracy that law courts would require. A better idea would be to find something early on so that one could prevent further violence by appropriate manipulations.

CARLSSON: How about treatment? The animal experiments and these results in humans provide a strong connection between aggression and low serotonin. You mentioned that fluoxetine has been tried in rodents. Have any trials been done in humans, for example of fluoxetine or buspirone in violent men?

LINNOILA: The control studies, few as they are, suggest that in prison conditions lithium has remarkably good efficacy, tryptophan is reasonable effective, and there is a questionable but statistically significant efficacy for high dose β-blockers, although there the mechanism of action is unclear. I am particularly interested in the results of application of 8-OH-DPAT in specific areas of the brain, because although there are some caveats, for example about dyskinesias, drugs such as buspirone are relatively free of side-effects. Controlled studies should be used. The best results I have had with buspirone are in women with borderline personality disorder, where in doses of 40–60 mg it seems to stabilize the situation. But in these patients we do not yet have evidence of serotonergic involvement.

GOTTFRIES: In humans there are stable, good correlations between concentrations of HVA and 5-HIAA in CSF. You show that the 5-HIAA is reduced whereas HVA is unchanged in impulsive individuals. Have you studied the ratio of 5-HIAA to HVA? That could explain more than the concentration of 5-HIAA alone.

LINNOILA: We find the same correlations, of the order of 0.6–0.8, depending on the samples, despite the fact that in some of the materials there is no difference. I always use the correlation to test the legitimacy of my data unless I have a specific reason not to expect the correlation. We have only seen a lack of correlation between 5-HIAA and HVA in non-responding depressives. There may be some kind of decoupling between the systems in these patients.

By using the ratio of 5-HIAA to HVA you theoretically remove the contribution of the acid transport system to the data. But I found that looking at that ratio in these materials did not add much to the existing data. There is also a penalty in that we have the variability of two assays, not one, even though we run it in the same chromatogram. The ratio is not valid when you evaluate a 5-HT re-uptake inhibitor or neuroleptic, because then you begin to directly manipulate one or the other metabolite.

PALFREYMAN: The killer rat model is very sensitive to manipulation of the GABA system. If you damage or remove the olfactory bulbs in non-killer animals you transform them into killer animals (Mandel *et al.* 1979). Is that relevant to the violent situation with which you deal? Is there any explanation of how the serotonergic system could impact on that aggressive behaviour?

LINNOILA: Attack latency seems to be very sensitive to serotonergic manipulation; manipulations thought to reduce serotonin function reduce attack latency. A study of predative behaviour in minks also showed that attack latency was affected by serotonergic manipulations.

Mouse-killing behaviour in rats is difficult to interpret because it is natural for the rat to protect its own habitat. But again the attack latency is affected. The olfactory bulbectomy model is questionable because the rat slowly gnaws the mouse to death. This is very different from the decisive attack by the intact rat, which usually involves a bite to the neck that kills the mouse immediately.

MELTZER: We reported that the 5-hydroxytryptophan-induced increase in cortisol was most elevated in people who made violent suicides (Meltzer *et al.* 1984). We subsequently showed that that response was negatively correlated with CSF 5-HIAA (Koyama *et al.* 1987). More recently, we found with Mann *et al.* (1986) that there were increased numbers of 5-HT$_2$ receptors only in patients who made violent suicides (Arora and Meltzer 1989). Non-violent suicides in that group had increased 5-HT$_{1A}$ receptors compared to normal controls. There was a trend for them also to differ from the violent suicides (Matsubara and Meltzer 1990). In animal models, one can up-regulate cortical 5-HT$_2$ receptors by decreasing seroto-nergic activity via reserpine (Stockmeier and Kellar 1986).

INSEL: How do you define non-violent suicides?

MELTZER: The non-violent suicides were drug overdoses, and the violent ones were mostly gunshots to the chest and some plunges from buildings. In our control group we separated people who died from car crashes from those who died of natural causes. We did not find any relationships to either the receptors or 5-HIAA. Nor did we find any difference in frontal cortical 5-HIAA levels between the violent and non-violent suicides.

DEAKIN: There is contradictory evidence on 5-HIAA in CSF for people who commit suicide. Arato *et al.* (1988) found an increase in CSF 5-HIAA in a large number of suicides sampled post-mortem in Budapest. Gjerris *et al.* (1987) found increased 5-HT concentrations in CSF from depressives.

LINNOILA: On the other hand, decreases in CSF 5-HIAA were reported in people who attempted suicide in Hungary. Both in Hungary, where there is a very high suicide rate, and Spain, where there is a very low suicide rate, low CSF 5-HIAA correlates with suicide attempts. Cultural factors probably can be excluded, and the vast majority of the 5-HIAA studies in depressed suicides are positive. All the studies on bipolar depressives are negative. We don't know what is the biochemical component of suicidal behaviour in bipolar patients, and yet these people are at a high risk of attempting or completing suicide.

LÓPEZ-IBOR: We had two patients with very low concentrations of CSF 5-HIAA in a group of non-suicidal patients. Both these patients died during suicide attempts about one year after the study (López-Ibor *et al.* 1985).

DEAKIN: Post-mortem brain studies of suicide victims are even more contradictory. Most studies do not find reduction of 5-HT metabolites. Two studies reported increases of 5-HIAA in the hippocampus of suicide victims.

LINNOILA: There are certainly discrepancies, but most brain studies suggest that in certain parts of the brain there are reductions in 5-HT. Marie Asberg and Lil Traskman told me that the Karolinska Institute ethics committee has ordered that a lumbar puncture should be performed if a unipolar depressed patient is admitted who has previously attempted suicide. This is because, unless they take special measures, about 30 per cent of their low 5-HIAA group attempt to kill themselves within a year of discharge, even though they are discharged without significant symptoms of depression. In the high 5-HIAA group the risk is around 1–2 per cent. In five years about 70 per cent of our melancholic patients with low 5-HIAA made significant suicide attempts, as opposed to 5 per cent of those with high CSF 5-HIAA. Thus, there does seem to be some predictive value in these studies.

COPPEN: Great attention should be paid to the follow-up of any patient who has attempted suicide, whatever the 5-HIAA level. The high risk of repetition is well documented.

LÓPEZ-IBOR: How stable are these impulsive and aggressive patients?

LINNOILA: Our trait studies suggest they are relatively stable, although the problem tends to escalate; in their early teens they tend to get into fights and the highest risk that they will kill someone is between the ages of 18 and 25. The situation may be more complex in the unipolar depressives; there is some recovery in the CSF 5-HIAA when unipolar depressive patients recover clinically. When they get depressed CSF 5-HIAA may be decreased again, perhaps suggesting that a sort of trait-state interplay occurs. I think the personality disorder patients are more stable over time.

MELTZER: How close is the concept of impulsivity to that of the sensation-seeking subject reported by Dennis Murphy and others to have low platelet MAO activity? Have you used the Zuckerman sensation scale and does it correlate with your measures of impulsivity?

LINNOILA: We used the TPQ, which did not correlate with any biochemical variable that we measured. The longitudinal aggression history with the fairly well-standardized Brown–Goodwin interview was the only clinical variable which correlated. We have not done the direct study with the Zuckerman scale.

The pathological gamblers that Alec Roy and I studied fulfilled DSM-III criteria, did not have sociopathy, but had lost a tremendous amount of money in gambling. They clearly had a different kind of impulse control disorder, which was fairly stable over time. In CSF, plasma, and urine we found indices for noradrenergic dysregulation, and these gamblers fit more closely to the characteristics that Zuckerman described in the sensation-seeking model.

DEAKIN: Why are these impulsive people not depressed with this deficiency of 5-HT?

LINNOILA: Most of them would fulfil criteria for dysthymia. They have a chronic low-level dysphoria, which is one reason, I believe, that they start to drink. Many of them say that the drinking gives them a good feeling. However, when they continue drinking they lose the effect. Some of the animal studies on ethanol effects on serotonin metabolism suggest that initially there is increased release, but that chronically there is a depletion.

DEAKIN: The other factor that may be important is that, whereas they lack a 5-HT anxiety system, they have an intact reward system, which is catecholamine mediated. Someone with depression has an inactive reward-detecting system.

INSEL: Is there any evidence that 5-HIAA has biological effects?

LINNOILA: No, but pharmacological studies with 5-HIAA were done a long time ago.

SANDLER: Its equivalent in plants, indoleacetic acid, is extremely important as the major auxin.

MELTZER: There are many suggestions in the literature that CSF 5-HIAA is not a good measure of neuronal activity and that it reflects mainly interneuronal catabolism. Yet it seems to have these striking and robust correlations with behaviour.

LINNOILA: That is why I hope that we shall soon be able to measure directly serotonin turnover in brain.

MELTZER: I should like to see a replication of your results in the normal volunteers. That is what makes this story so fascinating. The relationship with CSF 5-HIAA seems to hold across the whole spectrum of human aggression, if one takes this verbal hostility in volunteers as a measure of aggression.

LINNOILA: We are trying to replicate those findings. The study of oral glucose tolerance tests in healthy volunteers shows a similar association—the lower the blood glucose, even within the normal range, the more impulsive and aggressive the volunteers are during the double-blind test, according to standardized rating scales.

LÓPEZ-IBOR: Oreland *et al.* (1981) also found correlations between low 5-HIAA concentrations and hostility traits in the Rorschach Psychodiagnostic Test.

References

Arato, M., Falus, A., Sotonyi, P., Somogyi, E., Tothfalusi, L., Magyer, K., *et al.* (1988). Postmortem neurochemical investigation of suicide. In *Current issues of suicidology*, (ed H. J. Moller, A. Schmidtke, and R. Weiz). Springer-Verlag, Amsterdam.

Arora, R. C. and Meltzer, H. Y. (1989). Serotonergic measures in the brains of suicide victims: 5-HT$_2$ binding sites in the frontal cortex of suicide victims and control subjects. *American Journal of Psychiatry*, **146**, 730–6.

Elsworth, J. D., Redmond, D. E. Jr., Ruthven, C. R. J., and Sandler, M. (1985). Phenylacetic acid production in dominant and non-dominant vervet monkeys. *Life Sciences*, **37**, 1727–30.

Gjerris, A., Sorensen, A. S., Rafaelsen, O. J., Wederlin, L., Alling, G., and Linnoila, M. (1987). 5-HT and 5-HIAA in cerebrospinal fluid in depression. *Journal of Affective Disorders*, **12**, 13–22.

Koyama, T., Lowy, M. T., and Meltzer, H. Y. (1987). 5-Hydroxytryptophan-induced cortisol response and CSF 5-HIAA. *American Journal of Psychiatry*, **144**, 334–7.

López-Ibor, Jr. J. J., Sáiz-Ruiz, J., and Pérez de los Cobos, J. C. (1985). Biological correlations of suicide and aggressivity in major depressions (with melancholia): 5-hydroxyindoleacetic acid and cortisol in cerebral spinal fluid, dexamethasone suppression test and therapeutic response to 5-hydroxytryptophan. *Neuropsychobiology*, **14**, 67–74.

Mandel, P., Ciesielski, L., Maitre, M., Simler, S., Mack, G., and Kempf, E. (1979). Involvement of central gaba-ergic systems in convulsions and aggressive behavior. In *GABA—biochemistry and CNS function*, (ed. P. Mandel, and F. V. DeFeudis), pp. 475–92. Plenum Press, New York.

278 *M. Linnoila and M. Virkkunen*

Mann, J. J., Stanley, M., McBride, P. A., and McEwen, B. S. (1986). Increased serotonin₂ and β-adrenergic receptor binding in the frontal cortices of suicide victims. *Archives of General Psychiatry*, **43**, 954–9.

Matsubara, S. and Meltzer, H. Y. (1990). Serotonergic measures in suicide brain. II. 5-HT$_{1A}$ binding sites in frontal cortex of suicide victims. *Neuropsychopharmacology*, in press.

Meltzer, H. Y., Perline, R., Tricou, B. J., Lowy, M. T., and Robertson, A. (1984). Effect of 5-hydroxytryptophan on serum cortisol levels in major affective disorders. II. Relation to suicide, psychosis and depressive symptoms. *Archives of General Psychiatry*, **41**, 379–87.

Olivier, B. and Mos, J. (1986). Serenics and aggression. *Stress Medicine*, **2**, 197–209.

Oreland, L., Wiberg, A., Asberg, M., Träksman, L., Sjostrand, L., Thoren, P., *et al.* (1981). Platelet MAO activity and monoamine metabolism in CSF in depressed and suicidal patients and in healthy controls. *Psychiatry Research*, **4**, 21–9.

Oreland, L., Von Knorring, L., and Schalling, D. (1984). Connections between monoamine oxidase, temperament and disease. In *Proceedings of the Ninth International Congress of Pharmacology*, (ed. W. Patton, J. Mitchell, and P. Turner), pp. 193–202. Macmillan, London.

Sandler, M., Ruthven, C. R. J., Goodwin, B. L., Field, H., and Matthews, R. (1978). Phenylethylamine overproduction in aggressive psychopaths. *Lancet*, **ii**, 1269–70.

Stockmeier, C. A. and Kellar, K. J. (1986). In vivo regulation of the serotonin-2 receptor in rat brain. *Life Sciences*, **38**, 117–27.

Yu, P. H., Davis, B. A., Bowen, R. D., Wormith, S., Addington, D., and Boulton, A. A. (1984). The catabolism of trace amines in some psychiatric disorders. In *Neurobiology of the trace amines. Analytical, physiological, pharmacological, behavioral, and clinical aspects*, (ed. A. A. Boulton, G. G. Baker, W. G. Dewhurst, and M. Sandler), pp. 475–86. Humana, Clifton.

20. 5-Hydroxytryptamine in the control of feeding and its possible implications for appetite disturbance

G. Curzon

Introduction

It is hardly surprising that numerous influences impinge on such an important activity as feeding. Many sensory, metabolic, endocrine, and neurochemical inputs are involved and have been discussed in detail (Brewerton *et al*. 1990; Leibowitz *et al*. 1990; Morley and Blundell 1988). This article focuses on the relationships between 5-hydroxytryptamine (5-HT, serotonin) and feeding and describes both neurochemical and pharmacological findings. Neurochemical research has centred on the effects of feeding on brain 5-HT metabolism in laboratory animals, but its effects on the availability of 5-HT to receptors were only reported recently. Pharmacological research has shown that serotonergic drugs influence appetite. Thus the 5-HT system is relevant to appetite disorders and their treatment.

Taken together, these results imply (but do not prove) that effects of feeding or starvation on 5-HT function may be involved in the control of appetite. They lead to tentative hypotheses on how appetite disorder could arise through disturbances of these effects. Testing such hypotheses demands work on central 5-HT function in humans with appetite disorders. Relevant data are at present limited, apart from some potentially important neuroendocrine findings.

In common with most areas of research on brain 5-HT, work on its relationships with feeding is now being stimulated by the revelation of increasing numbers of 5-HT receptor types and of drugs acting selectively at them, and by the use of methods for monitoring transmitters in the living brain.

Neurochemical findings

Neurochemical research on 5-HT and feeding has been stimulated by evidence that both rat (Carlsson and Lindqvist 1978) and human (Gillman *et al.* 1981) brain tryptophan hydroxylases are normally only about half-saturated with substrate which means that synthesis of 5-HT in the brain depends on the availability to the brain of dietary tryptophan. However, it seems unlikely that 5-HT function throughout the brain is at the mercy of acute changes of dietary tryptophan content. On the contrary, there is evidence that brain 5-HT synthesis is *normally* well protected against the dietary tryptophan deficiency that *might* be assumed to occur during limited periods of starvation or after non-protein meals.

In rats, food deprivation for 24 hours can *increase* brain tryptophan because plasma unesterified fatty acids increase and displace tryptophan bound to plasma albumin, making it more available to the brain (Knott and Curzon 1972; Fuenmayor and Garcia 1984; Chaouloff *et al.* 1986). Similarly, a large high carbohydrate, low protein (and therefore low tryptophan) meal can increase brain tryptophan because the resultant insulin secretion decreases plasma levels of large neutral amino acids which compete with tryptophan for transport to the brain (Fernstrom and Wurtman 1973; Sarna *et al.* 1984). However, it has been argued (Curzon 1985) that although the *presence* of these amino acids in plasma has a major influence on brain tryptophan concentration, normal effects of diet on their levels probably have little effect in most subjects. A number of findings are in agreement (Ashley *et al.* 1985; Scriver *et al.* 1985; Fernstrom *et al.* 1987; Peters and Harper 1987*a*,*b*). Nevertheless, *extremes* of meal composition and size can affect brain tryptophan concentration and hence 5-HT synthesis (Moller 1985; Yokogoshi and Wurtman 1986).

Most of the above papers concern work on moderate numbers of subjects over short periods. As values obviously range more widely within larger groups or during longer periods, it is conceivable that brain tryptophan and 5-HT concentrations in some subjects or at some times respond readily to dietary influence.

We know little about the effects of normal feeding patterns on the availability of 5-HT to receptors in the human brain. Schwartz *et al.* (1989*a*) used *in vivo* brain dialysis and reported that feeding, or even the sight or smell of food (Schwartz *et al.* 1989*b*), increases extracellular 5-HT in the lateral hypothalamus of the rat. They suggest that these changes could mediate meal termination, which seems reasonable because injection of 5-HT into the hypothalamus suppresses feeding (reviewed in Leibowitz *et al.* 1990).

Pharmacological findings: effects of serotonergic drugs on feeding

The literature about effects on feeding of inhibitors of 5-HT synthesis, precursors of 5-HT, and 5-HT releasers, such as fenfluramine, has been reviewed comprehensively (Blundell 1977; Brewerton *et al.* 1990; Rowland and Carlton 1986; Sugrue 1987) and will not be described in detail. Recent work on the effects of drugs with selectivity for particular 5-HT receptor types will be discussed more fully.

5-HT$_{1A}$ agonists

Agonists for 5-HT$_{1A}$ receptors, such as 8-hydroxy-*N,N*-dipropyl-2-aminotetralin (8-OH-DPAT) (Dourish *et al.* 1985; Bendotti and Samanin 1987), buspirone, ipsapirone (Dourish *et al.* 1986*a*), gepirone (Gilbert and Dourish 1987), and LY 165163 (Hutson *et al.* 1987), increase food intake by free-feeding rats but not by food-deprived rats. As non-selective, indirect 5-HT agonists (e.g. fenfluramine and 5-hydroxytryptophan, 5-HTP) decrease feeding, and the 5-HT synthesis inhibitor *p*-chlorophenylalanine (*p*-CPA) increases it (Rowland and Carlton 1986; Blundell 1977), 8-OH-DPAT was suggested to cause hyperphagia by activating pre-synaptic 5-HT$_{1A}$ receptors so that 5-HT release from terminals is decreased (Dourish *et al.* 1986*a*). The absence of 8-OH-DPAT- and LY 165163-induced hyperphagia after depletion of 5-HT by *p*-CPA (Hutson *et al.* 1987; Dourish *et al.* 1986*b*) is consistent with this mechanism.

Pre-synaptic 5-HT$_{1A}$ receptors are not detectable on 5-HT terminals (Middlemiss 1984) but occur densely on 5-HT cell bodies in the raphe nuclei (Verge *et al.* 1985). The hyperphagic mechanism proposed by Dourish *et al.* (1986*a*) was confirmed by the demonstration that injecting 8-OH-DPAT into the raphe increases feeding (Hutson *et al.* 1986) and decreases synthesis of 5-HT and its release at terminals (Hutson *et al.* 1989). 8-OH-DPAT has high affinity for 5-HT$_{1A}$ sites and lower affinity for 5-HT$_{1B}$, 5-HT$_{1C}$, 5-HT$_{1D}$, and 5-HT$_2$ sites (Hoyer 1988), and for α_2-adrenergic sites (Middlemiss 1987). The effects of antagonists on 8-OH-DPAT hyperphagia agree with its mediation by 5-HT$_{1A}$ sites (Hutson *et al.* 1988*a*).

It is unlikely that the hyperphagia occurs as part of a general activation of motor and consummatory behaviour because systemic (Dourish *et al.* 1985) or raphe (Hutson *et al.* 1986) injection at low dosage increased feeding significantly even though locomotor effects were, at most, marginal. However, as raphe lesions can enhance dopamine-dependent stereotypical gnawing (Costall and Naylor 1974), the proposal that 8-OH-DPAT increases feeding by this mechanism (Montgomery *et al.* 1988, Chaouloff *et al.* 1988) is worth considering. Nevertheless, animals given 8-OH-DPAT and a choice between food pellets and wood blocks, chose to eat the food (Dourish *et al.* 1985), and the drug increased intakes of both pelleted and finely powdered food (G. S. Sarna, P. Whitton, G. Curzon, and P. D. Leathwood, unpublished) and of a liquid diet (Dourish *et al.* 1988). However, any behaviour with a motor component may be influenced by dopaminergic activity and Muscat *et al.* (1989) reported that dopamine receptor antagonists prevent 8-OH-DPAT-induced feeding.

5-HT$_{1B}$ and 5-HT$_{1C}$ agonists

That hyperphagia arises from decreased 5-HT at post-synaptic sites when 5-HT$_{1A}$ agonists are given implies involvement of post-synaptic 5-HT receptors. In the rat, 5-HT$_{1B}$ receptors are implicated because the 5-HT$_{1B}$ agonist RU 24969 has the opposite effect, causing hypophagia (Kennett *et al.* 1987*a*). Also, 1-(3-chlorophenyl)piperazine (*m*-CPP) and 1-[3-(trifluoromethyl)-phenyl]piperazine (TFMPP), which have substantial affinity for 5-HT$_{1B}$, 5-HT$_{1C}$, and 5-HT$_2$ sites (Hoyer 1988), cause hypophagia in both normally fed and food-deprived rats (Kennett *et al.* 1987*a*; Samanin *et al.* 1979).

As *m*-CPP and TFMPP also cause hypoactivity which is mediated by central 5-HT$_{1C}$ receptors (Kennett and Curzon 1988*a*), we suspected that they induce hypophagia at similar sites. Preliminary results in the hypoactivity study were supportive and when *m*-CPP and TFMPP were given under conditions more appropriate to the study of hypophagia, that is after food deprivation (Kennett and Curzon 1988*b*), the effects of antagonists indicated that *m*-CPP (and possibly TFMPP) causes hypophagia by stimulating 5-HT$_{1C}$ receptors, although 5-HT$_{1B}$ receptors also seemed necessary for the response. RU 24969, however, acted solely by activating 5-HT$_{1B}$ receptors, and as it was effective after *p*-CPA treatment (Kennett *et al.* 1987*a*) the receptors are not the pre-synaptic sites described by Middlemiss (1985) but are post-synaptic. (−)-Pindolol behaved anomalously; unlike other 5-HT$_{1B}$ antagonists, it blocked hypophagia induced by RU 24969 but not *m*-CPP.

If *m*-CPP and TFMPP cause hypophagia by acting partly on a 5-HT$_{1B}$-dependent mechanism and partly on a separate 5-HT$_{1C}$-dependent mechanism, blocking only one receptor subtype would only partially reverse the hypophagias. However, both mianserin, which has an affinity for 5-HT$_{1C}$ sites 2.8 log units greater than it has for 5-HT$_{1B}$ sites, and (±)-cyanopindolol, which has an affinity for 5-HT$_{1B}$ sites 4.1 log units greater than it has for 5-HT$_{1C}$ sites, completely reversed *m*-CPP- and TFMPP-induced hypophagia (Kennett and Curzon 1988*b*). These results suggest that activation of 5-HT$_{1C}$ receptors leads to activation of 5-HT$_{1B}$ receptors in a common hypophagic pathway and that *m*-CPP and TFMPP at the doses used have little direct effect on 5-HT$_{1B}$ receptors, an interpretation which is consistent with their higher affinities for 5-HT$_{1C}$ than for 5-HT$_{1B}$ sites (Hoyer 1988).

Evidence that *m*-CPP and TFMPP cause hypolocomotion (Kennett and Curzon 1988*a*), hypophagia (Kennett and Curzon 1988*b*), and anxiety (Kennett *et al.* 1989; Whitton and Curzon 1990) by action at 5-HT$_{1C}$ receptors now indicates that these sites may mediate behaviour. However, most antagonists with high affinity for 5-HT$_{1C}$ sites also bind strongly to 5-HT$_2$ sites (Hoyer 1988), and activation of either site induces phosphoinositide hydrolysis (Conn and Sanders-Bush 1987). Indeed, some reports suggest involvement of 5-HT$_2$ receptors in the hypophagia. Thus, the 5-HT releaser fenfluramine was thought to cause hypophagia by activating 5-HT$_2$ sites because its effect was blocked by the 5-HT$_2$ antagonist ketanserin (Hewson *et al.* 1988). This interpretation was later disputed (Neill and Cooper 1989), but the facts that hypophagia induced by 1-(2,5-dimethoxy-4-iodophenyl)-2-aminopropane (DOI) is blocked by LY 53857 and 1-naphthylpiperazine (Schechter and Simansky 1988) and that TFMPP-induced hypophagia is blocked by ketanserin and ritanserin (Klodzinska and Chojnacka-Wojcik 1990) were taken as evidence of the involvement of 5-HT$_2$ sites.

These disagreements may reflect experimental differences and the use of *in vitro* affinity constants to predict which receptors the antagonists are likely to block *in vivo*. *In vitro* values do not necessarily indicate *in vivo* potencies. We therefore determined the *in vivo* potencies in rats of nine drugs against both *m*-CPP-induced hypophagia and an authentic 5-HT$_2$ receptor-mediated behaviour, head shakes induced by 5-HTP (Kennett and Curzon 1991). The results were highly consistent with *m*-CPP inducing hypophagia by activating 5-HT$_{1C}$ receptors, as ID$_{50}$ values for inhibition of the hypophagia correlated significantly ($p < 0.01$) with their affinities (Hoyer 1988) for 5-HT$_{1C}$ but not for 5-HT$_2$, 5-HT$_{1A}$, or 5-HT$_{1B}$ receptors, whereas the ID$_{50}$ values for inhibition of the head shakes correlated significantly ($p < 0.02$) with affinities for 5-HT$_2$ but not for the other 5-HT receptors. Furthermore, the ratios of ID$_{50}$(hypophagia) to ID$_{50}$(head shakes) correlated highly significantly ($p < 0.001$) with the ratios of the affinities of the drugs for 5-HT$_2$ receptors to their affinities for 5-HT$_{1C}$ receptors.

The drug-induced hypophagias studied are not merely secondary to other behavioural effects. Thus, hypophagia induced by RU 24969 is not secondary to its hyperlocomotor effect, as haloperidol (Kennett *et al.* 1987*a*; Green *et al.* 1984; Tricklebank *et al.* 1986) and (+)-pindolol (Tricklebank *et al.* 1986) block this but not the hypophagia (Kennett *et al.* 1987*a*), whereas metergoline blocks the hypophagia (Kennett *et al.* 1987*a*; Kennett and Curzon 1986*b*) but potentiates the hyperlocomotion (Green *et al.* 1984; Tricklebank *et al.* 1986). Infusion of RU 24969 into the hypothalamus caused only hypophagia (Hutson *et al.* 1988*b*). Similarly, *m*-CPP (and TFMPP) probably causes hypophagia, hypolocomotion, and anxiety by three separate mechanisms; chronic pre-treatment with chlordiazepoxide prevented only the anxiety (Kennett *et al.* 1989), cyanopindolol prevented only the hypophagia (Kennett and Curzon 1988*b*), and injection of TFMPP into the paraventricular nucleus caused hypophagia but not hypoactivity (Hutson *et al.* 1988*b*). The 5-HT$_{1B}$ and 5-HT$_{1C}$ agonists do not seem to cause hypophagia via drug-induced malaise as the antiemetic drug trimethobenzamide prevented the hypophagic response of rats to acetyl salicylate (a known emetic in man and dogs) but not the hypophagia induced by RU 24969, *m*-CPP, and TFMPP (Kennett and Curzon 1988*c*).

Whereas the 5-HT$_{1C}$ antagonists mianserin, 1-naphthylpiperazine, cyproheptadine, and mesulergine opposed both *m*-CPP-induced hypophagia and hypoactivity, they increased feeding (but not activity) when given alone

(Kennett and Curzon 1988a,b) to normally fed rats but not when given to food-deprived rats. Therefore, hyperphagia produced by the antagonists may be rate dependent or caused by effects on appetite rather than satiety. These findings may explain contradictory reports about the effect of cyproheptadine on the intake of food by rats (Baxter et al. 1970; Ghosh and Parvathy 1973).

The above studies on 5-HT$_1$ agonists suggest that in the rat activation of 5-HT$_{1A}$ autoreceptors on cell bodies of 5-HT neurones decreases 5-HT release at terminals, with resultant hyperphagia. Terminals in the paraventricular, ventromedial, and suprachiasmatic nuclei of the medial hypothalamus are important for appetite control. Increasing serotonergic function in the paraventricular nucleus by infusion of either 5-HT or the 5-HT releaser norfenfluramine causes hypophagia, probably by inhibiting α_2-noradrenergic stimulation of feeding (Leibowitz et al. 1990). Our results indicate that 5-HT receptors of the 5-HT$_{1B}$ and 5-HT$_{1C}$ types are involved. They do not exclude roles of 5-HT in feeding at other central sites, for example the lateral hypothalamus (McClelland et al. 1990), or at extracerebral sites (Rowland and Carlton 1986). They do, however, reveal ways in which serotonergic drugs can affect feeding and suggest how 5-HT could mediate both normal and abnormal feeding mechanisms.

5-HT in appetite disorders

Food intake in humans depends on specifically human factors such as the desire to conform to accepted indices of attractiveness or success. It is also likely to involve central mechanisms that are held in common with other mammals. Therefore, relationships between 5-HT and feeding in animals suggest how disturbances of feeding might develop in humans.

Anorexia nervosa

General aspects of anorexia nervosa have been described by Ploog and Pirke (1987). Chronic abnormalities of food intake both here and in other disorders of appetite can lead to gross metabolic disturbances and it can be difficult to distinguish those which could have a role in maintaining the feeding disorder from those which do not. The greater incidence of anorexia nervosa in women is of special interest with regard to 5-HT because animal experiments suggest that serotonergic activity is greater in females (reviewed in Haleem et al. 1990).

Increased release of 5-HT in the paraventricular nucleus of the hypothalamus has been proposed as a cause of the disorder (Morley et al. 1986). One way this might develop is by slimming, in some subjects, leading to excessive activity of the mechanisms that normally protect the brain against tryptophan deficiency in starvation. Thus, abnormally large starvation-induced increases of plasma free tryptophan and brain tryptophan could occur (Knott and

Curzon 1972), resulting in increased 5-HT synthesis, increased release of 5-HT in the hypothalamus, and suppression of appetite (Shor-Posner *et al.* 1986). These tryptophan changes can be enhanced by stress (Curzon and Knott 1975; Knott *et al.* 1977), a suggested causal factor in anorexia nervosa (reviewed in Donohoe 1984). Although the route from plasma tryptophan changes to altered 5-HT release normally tends to be a 'negative cascade', with less marked consequences at successive stages (Yuwiler *et al.* 1977), the magnitude of these consequences could vary considerably between subjects. This is not improbable as factors that might be relevant to central 5-HT function and appetite control show considerable inter-subject variation in humans; for example, plasma amino acid concentrations (Scriver *et al.* 1985) and magnitudes of effects of serotonergic drugs on feeding (Silverstone and Goodall 1986). However, the evidence does not suggest increased net brain 5-HT synthesis in anorexia nervosa (reviewed in Brewerton *et al.* 1990). Although this seems to go against the hypothesis, more data on factors that influence brain 5-HT synthesis during the development of anorexia nervosa could be of interest; information on the initial effects of slimming regimes might be particularly useful.

Abnormalities occurring specifically at points closer to the hypothalamic outflow of the cascade could also be implicated in anorexia nervosa; for example, the release of hypothalamic 5-HT to receptors on food presentation, intake (Schwartz 1989*a,b*), or even on thinking about food, might be particularly large. Alternatively, 5-HT release might be normal but post-synaptic responsiveness to it enhanced. It is relevant that dieting may increase the sensitivity of hypothalamic 5-HT receptors specifically in women because it increased prolactin release on tryptophan loading in them but not in men (Goodwin *et al.* 1987). On the other hand, prolactin release on giving either tryptophan or *m*-CPP to women with anorexia nervosa is reported to be low (Brewerton *et al.* 1990).

However, the results of Goodwin *et al.* (1987) suggest a mechanism by which dieting-induced anorexia could develop. It is relevant that female rats are more vulnerable than males to 5-HT-dependent hypophagia; fenfluramine (Rowland 1986), RU 24969, and *m*-CPP (D. J. Haleem, A. M. C. Barnfield, G. A. Kennett and G. Curzon, unpublished work) are more hypophagic in females than in males. The high incidence of anorexia nervosa in women might therefore result from their greater tendency to submit to drastic dieting regimes combined with a sex-dependent higher responsiveness of 5-HT-mediated anorectic mechanisms which could be particularly marked in vulnerable subjects.

In our rat experiments, we also found that a single two-hour restraint stress caused hypophagia over the next 24 hours in both males and females, but that after daily restraint for five days (Kennett *et al.* 1986; Haleem *et al.* 1988) food intake returned to normal in the males but not the females. The hypophagia was not explicable as a response to stress-induced gastric lesions

(Donohoe *et al.* 1987). It is intriguing that plasma corticosterone rose more in female rats than in males after both stress (Haleem *et al.* 1988) and injection of the 5-HT$_{1A}$ agonist 8-OH-DPAT into the paraventricular nucleus (Haleem *et al.* 1989) because injection of 5-HT$_{1B}$ and 5-HT$_{1C}$ agonists (but not 8-OH-DPAT) into the same nucleus causes hypophagia (Hutson *et al.* 1988*b*). Also, levels of corticotropin-releasing hormone (CRH) and cortisol in cerebrospinal fluid (CSF) and plasma cortisol are raised in underweight anorectic women. This probably arises from a defect at or above the hypothalamus, causing CRH to be hypersecreted (Kaye *et al.* 1987). This activation of the hypothalamo-pituitary-adrenal axis could cause hypophagia because intraventricular CRH decreased feeding (Britton *et al.* 1982) and the impaired food intake of repeatedly stressed female rats was opposed by the inhibitor of corticosterone synthesis, metyrapone (Haleem *et al.* 1988).

Anorexia nervosa has been treated with drugs that alter serotonergic transmission for over a decade, but without striking success (reviewed in Brewerton *et al.* 1990). This may partly reflect heterogeneity of the populations studied; Halmi *et al.* (1986) reported that the 5-HT receptor blocker cyproheptadine (previously used with largely disappointing results) was beneficial to non-bulimic anorexics but harmful to bulimic anorexics.

Little is known yet about the utility of 5-HT$_{1A}$ agonists in human anorexic disorders, although in rats hypophagia over 24 hours after a two-hour stress was partly prevented if the 5-HT$_{1A}$ agonists 8-OH-DPAT, buspirone, and ipsapirone were injected two hours after the termination of stress (Dourish *et al.* 1987). Cyproheptadine given in the same way, or daily injection for two weeks of the tricyclic antidepressants desipramine and sertraline, did not decrease the hypophagia, although the latter two drugs and the 5-HT$_{1A}$ agonists all opposed the locomotor deficit of rats placed in an open field on the day after restraint, a property which is an indicator of antidepressant properties of the drugs (Kennett *et al.* 1987*c*).

How relevant are these findings to the control of feeding in humans? The 5-HT$_{1A}$ agonists buspirone and gepirone have been used as anxiolytics and (more recently) as antidepressants (Cott *et al.* 1988). Secondary effects on appetite are therefore possible, both in anxiety or depression and in anorexia nervosa where the symptoms overlap considerably with those of depression (Brambilla *et al.* 1985). However, it is interesting that two patients on gepirone experienced a craving for chocolate (Amsterdam *et al.* 1987) because carbohydrate intake is selectively increased in rats given 8-OH-DPAT (G. S. Sarna, P. Whitton, G. Curzon, and P. D. Leathwood, unpublished). On the other hand, the hyperphagic effects of 5-HT$_{1A}$ agonists arise from a decrease in 5-HT release (Dourish *et al.* 1986*a*; Hutson *et al.* 1986, 1989) which seems unlikely when the antidepressant effects of the agonists become manifest because these probably result from a subsequent *increase* of 5-HT release through autoreceptor desensitization (Kennett *et al.* 1987*b*; Beer *et al.* 1990).

Bulimic disorders

It is obvious that obesity is a frequent result of bulimia (an abnormal craving for food). Bulimia nervosa (weight control by binge eating followed by self-induced vomiting) has similarities with both ordinary bulimia and anorexia nervosa. Although bulimia nervosa is psychopathologically similar to anorexia nervosa in so far as both involve great interest in food and a dread of obesity (Russell 1985), they are characterized by opposite disturbances of appetite. However, subjects can be bulimic at one time and anorexic at another, which is hard to explain except in terms of an instability of the mechanisms controlling appetite.

The data on 5-HT metabolism in bulimia do not point to abnormal availability of tryptophan for brain 5-HT synthesis; the ratio of plasma tryptophan to other large neutral amino acids was normal in normal weight bulimics (Lydiard *et al.* 1988), and there is no evidence of abnormal concentrations of CSF 5-HIAA. A defect in hypothalamic 5-HT function is suggested by the markedly low prolactin response to *m*-CPP (Brewerton *et al.* 1990). This can be contrasted with the elevated hypothalamic response to tryptophan seen in normal dieting women (Goodwin *et al.* 1987). The results of Brewerton *et al.* are consistent with increased appetite and thus might explain bingeing in bulimia. Only bulimics who became satiated and stopped bingeing and vomiting had increased ratios of plasma tryptophan to large neutral amino acids after bingeing. If this caused increased 5-HT release to receptors, it could counteract the postulated hypothalamic defect (Kaye *et al.* 1988). A similar defect might play a part in the seasonal changes in appetite that occur in exaggerated form in seasonal affective disorder. This illness is characterized by regular winter depressions that are usually associated with carbohydrate craving (Rosenthal *et al.* 1984, 1988). It is therefore interesting that in a post-mortem study on subjects who had died without neurological or psychiatric illness Carlsson *et al.* (1980) found that hypothalamic 5-HT values were at their lowest in winter.

These findings imply that drugs which increase serotonergic transmission should be beneficial in bulimia nervosa. For example, acute fenfluramine treatment decreased bingeing (Robinson *et al.* 1984). The neurotoxicity of this drug in the rat shown by Appel *et al.* (1989) but not by Schaechter and Wurtman (1989) has raised questions about its use. However, these studies involved much higher doses than those found to be effective appetite suppressants in man. The selective 5-HT re-uptake inhibitor fluoxetine is an obvious candidate drug for bulimia (Fuller and Wong 1989).

It is not clear whether 5-HT_{1B} agonists could be used to control bingeing because evidence is largely against the presence of 5-HT_{1B} sites in human brain (Hoyer *et al.* 1986). 5-HT_{1D} sites are distributed in man in a similar manner to 5-HT_{1B} sites in rats and may be their functional equivalents (Waeber *et al.* 1988). If this is so, then 5-HT_{1D} agonists able to penetrate the blood–brain barrier could be effective. Whether 5-HT$_{1C}$ agonists are useful is not known, but in humans the agonist *m*-CPP is anxiogenic (Charney *et al.* 1987) and causes migraine in some subjects (Brewerton *et al.* 1988). Hypophagic doses of *m*-CPP in rats also induce anxiety-like behaviour (Kennett *et al.* 1989; Kennett and Curzon 1990). Despite these problems, new drugs with selectivity for 5-HT receptor subtypes might have advantages in the treatment of bulimia over the unselective or poorly selective compounds, such as fenfluramine, fluoxetine, and cyproheptadine, that are used at present.

The craving for food in bulimia without self-induced vomiting could, as in bulimia nervosa, result from defective hypothalamic 5-HT function. There is some evidence of this as the normal increase of plasma prolactin after an insulin tolerance test was impaired or absent in obese subjects (Bernini *et al.* 1989). This defect is not simply caused by obesity because it was still present in some obese patients on attainment of normal body weight after jejuno-ileal bypass (Kopelman *et al.* 1980). The suggested hypothalamic disorder may result from insufficient 5-HT release rather than a defect in post-synaptic responsiveness as the 5-HT releaser fenfluramine enhanced the prolactin responses to insulin of obese subjects but not of normal ones (Bernini *et al.* 1989). The Osborne-Mendel rat may be a useful animal model; it is genetically prone to obesity and has a lower rate of synthesis and lower concentrations of 5-HT in brain than the Sprague-Dawley strain (Weekley *et al.* 1982).

Obesity is often associated with excessive snacking between meals and normal calorie intake in main meals. Wurtman *et al.* (1987) found that obese carbohydrate-selective snackers (group 1) showed a greater decrease in snacking than obese non-selective snackers (group 2) when given d-fenfluramine over three months. During meals, group 1 showed smaller but significant decreases in intake and group 2 were not affected. However, the evidence that fenfluramine selectively decreases intake of carbohydrate snacks is not persuasive because group 1 ate very few protein snacks. Thus, the relative effects of the drug on protein and carbohydrate intake were not determined for group 1. Moreover, the decreases in both carbohydrate and protein snacks by group 2 over the three-month period were similar.

5-HT and macronutrient selection

The above study on obesity (Wurtman *et al.* 1987) was derived from earlier work in which it was proposed that 5-HT influenced carbohydrate/protein macronutrient choice (Wurtman and Wurtman 1979). The hypothesis was that carbohydrate consumption increased synthesis and release of 5-HT in the brain, resulting in decreased appetite. Fenfluramine (which releases 5-HT) was postulated to decrease hunger for carbohydrates by simulating the effect of carbohydrate intake.

It seems unlikely that this mechanism influences choice by normal subjects in the absence of drug treatments (Curzon 1988*b*; Peters and Harper

1987*a,b*). Furthermore, the data of Wurtman *et al.* (1987) suggest that whereas carbohydrate snackers are particularly sensitive to fenfluramine, the resultant hypophagia is not carbohydrate selective. On the other hand, many results are consistent with increased serotonergic activity causing selective carbohydrate hypophagia in a carbohydrate/protein choice (Blundell and Hill 1987; Li and Anderson 1984; Shor-Posner *et al.* 1986; White *et al.* 1988). Decreased serotonergic activity had the opposite effect; the 5-HT receptor antagonists metergoline (Stallone and Nicolaidies 1989) and 8-OH-DPAT (G. S. Sarna, P. Whitton, G. Curzon, and P. D. Leathwood, unpublished) selectively increased carbohydrate intake.

There are various problems in interpreting choice experiments (Blundell 1983), and carbohydrate/protein choice may depend on sensory clues rather than on diet composition (Booth 1987). Fernstrom (1988) questioned the biological role of a specific mechanism for carbohydrate intake because: (1) spontaneous carbohydrate intake is not tightly controlled; (2) calorie and protein intake but not carbohydrate intake is maintained when bar-pressing is required for food delivery; and (3) there is no known nutritional advantage in specific control of carbohydrate intake.

Other data suggest that 5-HT is probably a determinant of both food intake and macronutrient choice but the nature of the choice depends on circumstances in a way that is not yet understood. Thus, when rats deprived of food for 24 hours were given a carbohydrate/protein choice, intakes were decreased indiscriminately by RU 24969 and *m*-CPP (G. S. Sarna, P. Whitton, G. Curzon, and P. D. Leathwood, unpublished) whereas in rats given access for eight hours to a fat/protein/carbohydrate choice with the fat component having twice the calorific value of either of the other diets, Orthen-Gambill and Kanarek (1982) found that fenfluramine selectively decreased fat and protein intake. However, in a similar study on rats deprived of food for two hours, Shor-Posner *et al.* (1986) found that fenfluramine selectively decreased (and cyproheptadine selectively increased) fat and carbohydrate intake. When Orthen-Gambill and Kanarek (1982) used three equicalorific diets fenfluramine selectively decreased the fat intake. Similar findings were obtained when only peripheral 5-HT receptors were activated, that is, when 5-HT was given intraperitoneally (Kanarek and Dushkin 1988).

Summary

This chapter describes relationships between 5-HT and feeding. Synthesis of 5-HT in the brain depends on dietary sources of tryptophan but effective mechanisms protect the brain against acute deficiencies in the tryptophan supply. Drugs that decrease and increase 5-HT-dependent responses increase and decrease feeding respectively. Thus, in the rat 5-HT$_{1A}$ agonists activate autoreceptors on cell bodies of 5-HT neurones to decrease 5-HT release and cause hyperphagia. 5-HT_{1B} and 5-HT_{1C} agonists cause hypophagia. Receptors in the paraventricular nucleus and other hypothalamic sites are involved.

These and other findings are discussed in relation to human appetite control. Anorexia nervosa and bulimia could result from disturbed 5-HT synthesis and release, or from abnormal responsiveness of hypothalamic 5-HT receptors which mediate appetite. Neuroendocrinological findings suggest that bulimia may involve defective activation of these receptors. The observations that dieting increased the sensitivity of hypothalamic 5-HT receptors in normal women but not in men and that female rats are more vulnerable to hypophagic effects of stress or 5-HT agonists may be relevant to the greater incidence of anorexia nervosa in women.

The reported effects of serotonergic drugs on appetite disorders are consistent with the above findings. For example, the 5-HT antagonist cyproheptadine was beneficial in anorexia but exacerbated bulimia, whereas the 5-HT releaser fenfluramine was useful in bulimic obesity, especially in subjects with carbohydrate craving. These and other serotonergic drugs also have various effects on macronutrient choice.

References

Amsterdam, J. D., Berwish, N., Potter, L., and Rickels, K. (1987). Open trial of gepirone in the treatment of major depressive disorder. *Current Therapeutic Research*, **41**, 185–93.

Appel, N. M., Contrera, J. F., and De Souza, E. B. (1989). Fenfluramine selectively and differentially decreases the density of serotonergic nerve terminals in rat brain: evidence from immunocytochemical studies. *Journal of Pharmacology and Experimental Therapeutics*, **249**, 928–43.

Ashley, D. V. M., Liardon, R., and Leathwood, P. D. (1985). Breakfast meal composition influences plasma tryptophan to large neutral amino acid ratios of healthy lean young men. *Journal of Neural Transmission*, **63**, 271–83.

Baxter, M. J., Miller, A. A., and Soroko, F. E. (1970). The effect of cyproheptadine on food consumption in the fasted rat. *British Journal of Pharmacology*, **39**, 229–30.

Beer, M., Kennett, G. A., and Curzon, G. (1990). A single dose of 8-OH-DPAT reduces raphe binding of [³H]-8-OH-DPAT and increases the effect of raphe stimulation on 5-HT metabolism. *European Journal of Pharmacology*, **178**, 179–87.

Bendotti, C. and Samanin, R. (1987). The role of putative 5-HT_{1A} and 5-HT_{1B} receptors in the control of feeding in rats. *Life Sciences*, **41**, 635–42.

Bernini, G. P., Argenio, G. F., Vivaldi, M. S., DelCorso, C., Sgro, M., Franchi, F., and Luisi, M. (1989). Effects of fenfluramine and ritanserin on prolactin response to insulin-induced hypoglycemia in obese patients: evidence for failure of the serotoninergic system. *Hormone Research*, **31**, 133–7.

Blundell, J. E. (1977). Is there a role for serotonin (5-hydroxytryptamine) in feeding? *International Journal of Obesity*, **1**, 15–42.

Blundell, J. E. (1983). Problems and processes underlying the control of food selection and nutrient intake. In *Nutrition and the brain*, Vol. 6, (ed. R. J. Wurtman and J. J. Wurtman), pp. 163–221. Raven, New York.

Blundell, J. E. and Hill, A. J. (1987). Influence of tryptophan on appetite and food selection in man. In *Amino acids in health and disease: new perspectives*, (ed. S. Kaufman), pp. 403–19. Alan R. Liss, New York.

Booth, D. A. (1987). Central dietary 'feedback onto nutrient selection': not even a scientific hypothesis. *Appetite*, **8**, 195–201.

Brambilla, F., Cavagnini, F., Invitti, C., Poterzio, F., Lampertillo, M., Sali, L., *et al.* (1985). Neuroendocrine and psychopathological measures in anorexia nervosa, resemblances to primary affective disorders. *Psychiatric Research*, **16**, 165–76.

Brewerton, T. D., Murphy, D. L., Mueller, E. A., and Jimerson, D. C. (1988). Induction of headaches by the serotonin agonist m-chlorophenylpiperazine. *Clinical Pharmacology and Therapeutics*, **43**, 605–9.

Brewerton, T. D., Brandt, H. A., Lesem, M. D., Murphy, D. L., and Jimerson, D. C. (1990). Serotonin in eating disorders. In *Serotonin in major psychiatric disorders*, (ed. E. F. Coccaro and D. L. Murphy), pp. 153–84. American Psychiatric Press, Washington.

Britton, D. R., Koob, G. F., Rivier, J., and Vale, W. (1982). Intraventricular corticotrophin-releasing factor enhances behavioural effects of novelty. *Life Sciences*, **31**, 363–7.

Carlsson, A. and Lindqvist, M. (1978). Dependence of 5-HT and catecholamine synthesis on concentrations of precursor amino acids in rat brain. *Naunyn-Schmiedeberg's Archives of Pharmacology*, **303**, 157–64.

Carlsson, A., Svennerholm, L., and Winblad, B. (1980). Seasonal and circadian monoamine variations in human brains examined post mortem. *Acta Psychiatrica Scandinavica*, **61**, Suppl. 280, 75–85.

Chaouloff, F., Kennett, G. A., Serrurrier, B., Merino, D., and Curzon, G. (1986). Amino acid analysis demonstrates that increased plasma free tryptophan causes the increase of brain tryptophan during exercise in the rat. *Journal of Neurochemistry*, **46**, 1647–50.

Chaouloff, F., Serrurrier, B., Merino, D., Laude, D., and Elghozi, J. L. (1988). Feeding responses to a high dose of 8-OH-DPAT in young and adult rats: influence of food texture. *European Journal of Pharmacology*, **151**, 267–73.

Charney, D. S., Woods, S. W., Goodman, W. K., and Heninger, G. R. (1987). Serotonin function in anxiety: II. Effects of the serotonin agonist MCPP in panic disorder patients and healthy subjects. *Psychopharmacology*, **92**, 14–21.

Costall, B. and Naylor, R. J. (1974). Stereotyped and circling behaviour induced by dopaminergic agonists after lesions of the midbrain raphe nuclei. *European Journal of Pharmacology*, **29**, 206-22.

Conn, F. J. and Sanders-Bush, E. (1987). Relative efficacies of piperazines at the phosphoinositide hydrolysis-linked serotonergic (5-HT$_2$ and 5-HT$_{1C}$) receptors. *Journal of Pharmacology and Experimental Therapeutics*, **242**, 552–7.

Cott, J. M., Kurtz, N. M., Robinson, D. S., Lancaster, S. P., and Copp, J. E. (1988). A 5-HT$_{1A}$ ligand with both antidepressant and anxiolytic properties. *Psychopharmacology Bulletin*, **24**, 164–7.

Curzon, G. (1985). Effects of food intake on brain transmitter amine precursors and amine synthesis. In *Psychopharmacology and food*, (ed. M. Sandler and T. Silverstone), pp. 59–70. Oxford University Press.

Curzon, G. (1988*a*). Serotonergic mechanisms of depression. *Clinical Neuropharmacology*, **11**, S11–S20.

Curzon, G. (1988*b*). Feeding, stress, exercise and the supply of tryptophan to the brain. In *Amino acid availability and brain function in health and disease*. (ed. G. Huether), pp. 39–59. Springer, Berlin.

Curzon, G. and Knott, P. J. (1975). Rapid effects of environmental disturbance on rat plasma unesterified fatty acid and tryptophan concentrations and their prevention by antilipolytic drugs. *British Journal of Pharmacology*, **54**, 389–96.

Donohoe, T. P. (1984). Stress-induced anorexia: implications for anorexia nervosa. *Life Sciences*, **34**, 203–18.

Donohoe, T. P., Kennett, G. A., and Curzon, G. (1987). Immobilisation stress-induced anorexia is not due to gastric ulceration. *Life Sciences*, **40**, 467–72.

Dourish, C. T., Hutson, P. H., and Curzon, G. (1985). Low doses of the putative serotonin agonist 8-Hydroxy-2-(di-n-propylamino) tetralin (8-OH-DPAT) elicit feeding in the rat. *Psychopharmacology*, **86**, 197–204.

Dourish, C. T., Hutson, P. H., Kennett, G. A., and Curzon, G. (1986*a*). 8-OH-DPAT induced hyperphagia: its neural basis and possible therapeutic relevance. *Appetite*, **7**, Suppl., 127–40.

Dourish, C. T., Hutson, P. H., and Curzon, G. (1986*b*). Parachlorophenylalanine prevents feeding induced by the serotonin agonist 8-hydroxy-2-(di-n-propylamino) tetralin (8-OH-DPAT). *Psychopharmacology*, **89**, 467–71.

Dourish, C. T., Kennett, G. A., and Curzon, G. (1987). The 5-HT$_{1A}$ agonists 8-OH-DPAT, buspirone and ipsapirone attenuate stress-induced anorexia in rats. *Journal of Psychopharmacology*, **1**, 23–30.

Dourish, C. T., Clark, M. L., and Iversen, S. D. (1988). 8-OH-DPAT elicits feeding and not chewing: evidence from liquid diet studies and a diet choice test. *Psychopharmacology*, **95**, 185–8.

Fernstrom, J. D. (1988). Carbohydrate ingestion and brain serotonin synthesis: relevance to a putative control loop for regulating carbohydrate ingestion and effects of aspartate consumption. *Appetite*, **11**, Suppl., 35–41.

Fernstrom, J. D. and Wurtman, R. J. (1973). Brain serotonin content: physiological regulation by plasma neutral amino acids. *Science*, **178**, 414–16.

Fernstrom, J. D., Fernstrom, M. H., and Grubb, P. E. (1987). Twenty-four hour variations in rat blood and brain levels of the aromatic and branched-chain amino acids: chronic effects of dietary protein content. *Metabolism*, **36**, 643-50.

Fuenmayor, L. D. and Garcia, S. (1984). The effect of fasting on 5-hydroxytryptamine metabolism in brain regions of the albino rat. *British Journal of Pharmacology*, **83**, 357–62.

Fuller, R. W. and Wong, D. T. (1989). Fluoxetine: a serotonergic appetite suppressant drug. *Drug Development Research*. **17**, 1–15.

Ghosh, M. N. and Parvathy, S. (1973). The effect of cyproheptadine on water and food intake and on body weight in the fasted adult and weanling rat. *British Journal of Pharmacology*, **48**, 328–9.

Gilbert, F. and Dourish, C. T. (1987). Effects of the novel anxiolytics gepirone, buspirone and ipsapirone on free feeding and on feeding induced by 8-OH-DPAT. *Psychopharmacology*, **93**, 349–52.

Gillman, P. K., Bartlett, J. R., Bridges, P. K., Hunt, A., Patel, A. J., Kantamaneni, B. D., and Curzon, G. (1981). Indolic substances in plasma, cerebrospinal fluid and frontal cortex of human subjects infused with saline or tryptophan. *Journal of Neurochemistry*, **37**, 410–17.

Goodwin, G. M., Fairburn, C. G., and Cowen, P. J. (1987). Dieting changes serotonergic function in women not men: implications for the aetiology of anorexia nervosa? *Psychological Medicine*, **17**, 839–42.

Green, A. R., Guy, A. P., and Gardner, C. R. (1984). The behavioural effects of RU 24969, a suggested 5-HT receptor agonist in rodents, and the effect on the behaviour of treatment with antidepressants. *Neuropharmacology*, **23**, 655–61.

Haleem, D. J., Kennett, G. A., and Curzon, G. (1988). Adaptation of female rats to stress: shift to male pattern by inhibition of corticosterone synthesis. *Brain Research*, **458**, 339–47.

Haleem, D. J., Kennett, G. A., and Curzon, G. (1990). Hippocampal 5-hydroxytryptamine synthesis is greater in female rats than in males and more decreased by the 5-HT$_{1A}$ agonist 8-OH-DPAT. *Journal of Neural Transmission*, **79**, 93–101.

Haleem, D. J., Kennett, G. A., Whitton, P. S., and Curzon, G. (1989). 8-OH-DPAT increases corticosterone but not other 5-HT$_{1A}$ receptor-dependent responses more in females. *European Journal of Pharmacology*, **164**, 435–43.

Halmi, K. A., Eckert, E., La Du, T. J., and Cohen, J. (1986). Anorexia nervosa. Treatment efficacy of cyproheptadine and amitriptyline. *Archives of General Psychiatry*, **43**, 177–81.

Hewson, G., Leighton, G. E., Hill, R. G., and Hughes, J. (1988). Ketanserin antagonises the anorectic effect of DL-fenfluramine in the rat. *European Journal of Pharmacology*, **145**, 227–30.

Hoyer, D. (1988). Functional correlates of serotonin 5-HT$_1$ recognition sites. *Journal of Receptor Research*, **8**, 59–81.

Hoyer, D., Pazos, A., Probst, A., and Palacios, J. M. (1986). Serotonin receptors in the human brain. I. Characterization and autoradiographic localization of 5-HT$_{1A}$ recognition sites. Apparent absence of 5-HT$_{1B}$ recognition sites. *Brain Research*, **376**, 85–96.

Hutson, P. H., Dourish, C. T. and Curzon, G. (1986). Neurochemical and behavioural evidence for mediation of the hyperphagic action of 8-OH-DPAT by 5-HT cell body autoreceptors. *European Journal of Pharmacology*, **129**, 347–52.

Hutson, P. H., Donohoe, T. P., and Curzon, G. (1987). Neurochemical and behavioural evidence for an agonist action of 1-[2-(4-aminophenyl)-4-(3-trifluoro-methylphenyl)piperazine at central 5-HT receptors. *European Journal of Pharmacology*, **138**, 215–23.

Hutson, P. H., Dourish, C. T. and Curzon, G. (1988a). Evidence that the hyperphagic response to 8-OH-DPAT is mediated by 5-HT$_{1A}$ receptors. *European Journal of Pharmacology*, **150**, 361–6.

Hutson, P. H., Donohoe, T. P. and Curzon, G. (1988b). Infusion of the 5-hydroxytryptamine agonists RU 24969 and TFMPP into the paraventricular nucleus of the hypothalamus causes hypophagia. *Psychopharmacology*, **95**, 550–2.

Hutson, P. H., Sarna, G. S., O'Connell, M. T., and Curzon, G. (1989). Hippocampal 5-HT synthesis and release in vivo is decreased by infusion of 8-OH-DPAT into the nucleus raphe dorsalis. *Neuroscience Letters*, **100**, 276–80.

Kanarek, R. B. and Dushkin, H. (1988). Peripheral serotonin administration selectively reduces fat intake in rats. *Pharmacology Biochemistry and Behaviour*, **31**, 113–22.

Kaye, W. H., Gwirtsman, H. E., George, D. T., Ebert, M. H., Jimerson, D. C., Tomai, T. P., *et al.* (1987). Elevated cerebrospinal fluid levels of immunoreactive corticotrophin-releasing hormone in anorexia nervosa: relation to state of nutrition, adrenal function and intensity of depression. *Journal of Clinical Endocrinology and Metabolism*, **64**, 203–8.

Kaye, W. H., Gwirtsman, H. E., Brewerton, T. D., George, D. T., and Wurtman, R. J. (1988). Bingeing behaviour and plasma amino acid: a possible involvement of brain serotonin in bulimia nervosa. *Psychiatry Research*, **23**, 31–43.

Kennett, G. A. and Curzon, G. (1988a). Evidence that mCPP may have behavioural effects mediated by 5-HT$_{1C}$ receptors. *British Journal of Pharmacology*, **94**, 137-47.

Kennett, G. A. and Curzon, G. (1988b). Evidence that hypophagia induced by mCPP and TFMPP requires 5-HT$_{1C}$ and 5-HT$_{1B}$ receptors: hypophagia induced by RU 24969 only requires 5-HT$_{1B}$ receptors. *Psychopharmacology*, **96**, 93–100.

Kennett, G. A. and Curzon, G. (1988c). The antiemetic drug trimethobenzamide prevents hypophagia due to acetyl salicylate but not to 5-HT$_{1B}$ or 5-HT$_{1C}$ agonists. *Psychopharmacology*, **96**, 101–3.

Kennett, G. A. and Curzon, G. (1991). Potencies of antagonists against 5-HT$_2$-mediated head shakes and mCPP-induced hypophagia indicate that 5-HT$_{1C}$ receptors mediate the latter effect. *British Journal of Pharmacology*, in press.

Kennett, G. A., Chaouloff, F., Marcou, M., and Curzon, G. (1986). Female rats are more vulnerable than males in an animal model of depression: the possible role of serotonin. *Brain Research*, **382**, 416–21.

Kennett, G. A., Dourish, C. T., and Curzon, G. (1987a). 5-HT$_{1B}$ agonists induce anorexia at a postsynaptic site. *European Journal of Pharmacology*, **141**, 429–35.

Kennett, G. A., Marcou, M., Dourish, C. T., and Curzon, G. (1987b). Single administration of 5-HT$_{1A}$ agonists decreases 5-HT presynaptic but not postsynaptic receptor-mediated responses: relationship to antidepressant-like action. *European Journal of Pharmacology*, **138**, 53–60.

Kennett, G. A., Dourish, C. T., and Curzon, G. (1987c). Antidepressant-like action of 5-HT$_{1A}$ agonists and conventional antidepressants in an animal model of depression. *European Journal of Pharmacology*, **134**, 265–74.

Kennett, G. A., Whitton, P., Shah, K., and Curzon, G. (1989). Anxiogenic-like effects of mCPP and TFMPP in animal models are opposed by 5-HT$_{1C}$ receptor antagonists. *European Journal of Pharmacology*, **164**, 445–54.

Klodzinska, A. and Chojnacka-Wojcik, E. (1990). Anorexia induced by m-trifluoro-methylphenylpiperazine (TFMPP) in rats. *Polish Journal of Pharmacology and Pharmacy*, **42**, 13–18.

Knott, P. J. and Curzon, G. (1972). Free tryptophan in plasma and brain tryptophan metabolism. *Nature*, **239**, 452-3.

Knott, P. J., Hutson, P. H., and Curzon, G. (1977). Fatty acid and tryptophan changes on disturbing groups of rats and caging them singly. *Pharmacology Biochemistry and Behaviour*, **7**, 245–52.

Kopelman, P. G., Pilkington, T. R. E., Jeffcoate, S. L., and White, N. (1980). Persistence of defective hypothalamic control of prolactin secretion in some obese women after weight reduction. *British Medical Journal*, **ii**, 358–9.

Li, E. T. S. and Anderson, G. H. (1984). 5-Hydroxytryptamine: a modulator of food composition but not quantity? *Life Sciences*, **34**, 2453–60.

Leibowitz, S. F., Shor-Posner, G., and Weiss, G. F. (1990). Serotonin in medial hypothalamic nuclei controls circadian patterns of macronutrient intake. In *Serotonin: from cell biology to pharmacology and therapeutics*, (ed. R. Paoletti and P. M. Vanhoutte), pp. 203–11. Kluwer, Amsterdam.

Lydiard, R. B., Brady, K. T., O'Neill, P. M., Schlesier-Carter, B., Hamilton, S., Rogers, Q., and Ballenger, J. C. (1988). Precursor amino acid concentrations in normal weight bulimics and normal controls. *Progress in Neuropsychopharmacology and Biological Psychiatry*, **12**, 893–8.

McClelland, R. C., Sarfaty, T., Hernandez, L., and Hoebel, B. G. (1990). The serotonergic appetite suppressant, d-FEN decreases self-stimulation at a feeding site in the lateral hypothalamus. *Pharmacology Biochemistry and Behaviour*, in press.

Middlemiss, D. N. (1984). 8-Hydroxy-2-(di-n-propylamino) tetralin is devoid of activity at the 5-hydroxytryptamine autoreceptor in rat brain. Implications for the proposed link between the autoreceptor and the [^{3}H]5-HT recognition site. *Naunyn-Schmiedeberg's Archives of Pharmacology*, **327**, 18–22.

Middlemiss, D. N. (1985). The putative 5-HT$_1$ receptor agonist RU 24969 inhibits the efflux of 5-hydroxytryptamine from rat frontal cortex slices by stimulation of the 5-HT autoreceptor. *Journal of Pharmacy and Pharmacology*, **37**, 434–7.

Middlemiss, D. N. (1987). Lack of effect of the putative 5-HT$_{1A}$ receptor agonist, 8-OH-DPAT on 5-HT release in vitro. In *Brain 5-HT$_{1A}$ receptors: behavioural and neurochemical pharmacology*, (ed. C. T. Dourish, S. Ahlenius, and P. H. Hutson), pp. 82–93. Ellis Horwood, Chichester.

Moller, S. E. (1985). Effect of various oral protein doses on plasma neutral amino acid levels. *Journal of Neural Transmission*, **61**, 183–91.

Montgomery, A. M. J., Willner, P., and Muscat, R. (1988). Behavioural specificity of 8-OH-DPAT induced feeding. *Psychopharmacology*, **94**, 110–14.

Morley, J. E. and Blundell, J. E. (1988). The neurobiological basis of eating disorders: some formulations. *Biological Psychiatry*, **23**, 53–78.

Morley, J. E., Levine, A. S., and Willenburg, M. L., (1986). Stress-induced feeding disorders. In *Pharmacology of eating disorders: theoretical and clinical developments*, (ed. M. V. Carruba and J. E. Blundell), pp. 71–99. Raven, New York.

Muscat, R., Montgomery, A. M. J., and Willner, P. (1989). Blockade of 8-OH-DPAT-induced feeding by dopamine antagonists. *Psychopharmacology*, **99**, 402–8.

Neill, J. C. and Cooper, S. J. (1989). Evidence that d-fenfluramine anorexia is mediated by 5-HT$_1$ receptors. *Psychopharmacology*, **97**, 213-18.

Orthen-Gambill, N. and Kanarek, R. B. (1982). Differential effects of amphetamine and fenfluramine on dietary self selection in rats. *Pharmacology Biochemistry and Behaviour*, **16**, 303–9.

Peters, J. C. and Harper, A. E. (1987*a*). A skeptical view of the role of central serotonin in the selection and intake of protein. *Appetite*, **8**, 206–10.

Peters, J. C. and Harper, A. E. (1987*b*). Acute effects of dietary proteins on food intake, tissue amino acids and brain serotonin. *American Journal of Physiology*, **252**, R902–14.

Ploog, D. W. and Pirke, K. M. (1987). Psychobiology of anorexia nervosa. *Psychological Medicine*, **17**, 843–59.

Rosenthal, N. E., Sack, D. A., Gillin, J. C., Lewy, A. J., Goodwin, J. C., Davenport, Y., *et al.* (1984). Seasonal affective disorder: a description of the syndrome and preliminary findings with light therapy. *Archives of General Psychiatry*, **41**, 72–80.

Rosenthal, J. I., Genhart, M., Sack, D. A., Skwerer, R. G., and Wehr, T. A. (1988). Seasonal affective disorder: relevance for treatment and research of bulimia. In *Psychobiology of bulimia*, (ed. J. I. Hudson and H. G. Pope). American Psychiatric Association, Washington.

Robinson, P. H., Checkley, S. A., and Russell, G. F. M. (1984). Suppression of eating by fenfluramine in patients with bulimia nervosa. *British Journal of Psychiatry*, **146**, 169–74.

Rowland, N. E. (1986). Effect of continuous infusions of dexfenfluramine on food intake, body weight and brain amines in rats. *Life Sciences*, **39**, 2581–6.

Rowland, N. E. and Carlton, J. (1986). Neurobiology of an anorectic drug: fenfluramine. *Progress in Neurobiology*, **27**, 13–62.

Russell, G. F. M. (1985). Bulimia revisited. *International Journal of Eating Disorders*, **4**, 681–92.

Sarna, G. S., Kantameneni, B. D., and Curzon, G. (1984). Variables influencing the effect of a meal on brain tryptophan. *Journal of Neurochemistry*, **44**, 1575–80.

Samanin, R., Mennini, T., Ferraris, A., Bendotti, C., Borsini, F., and Garattini, S. (1979). m-Chlorophenylpiperazine: a central agonist causing powerful anorexia in rats. *Naunyn-Schmiedeberg's Archives of Pharmacology*, **308**, 159–63.

Schaechter, J. D. and Wurtman, R. J. (1989). Effects of chronic D-fenfluramine administration on rat hypothalamic serotonin levels and release. *Life Sciences*, **44**, 265–71.

Schechter, L. E. and Simansky, K. J. (1988). 1-(2,5-Dimethoxy-4-iodophenyl)-2-aminopropane (DOI) exerts an anorexic action that is blocked by 5-HT$_2$ antagonists in rats. *Psychopharmacology*, **94**, 342–6.

Scriver, C. R., Gregory, D. M., Sovetts, D., and Tissenbaum, G. (1985). Normal plasma free amino acid values in adults: the influence of some common physiological variables. *Metabolism*, **34**, 868–73.

Schwartz, D. H., McClane, S., Hernandez, L., and Hoebel, B. G. (1989a). Feeding increases extracellular serotonin in the lateral hypothalamus of the rat as measured by microdialysis. *Brain Research*, **479**, 349–54.

Schwartz, D. H., Hernandez, L., and Hoebel, B. G. (1989b). Serotonin release in the medial and lateral hypothalamus during feeding and its anticipation. *Society for Neuroscience Abstracts*.

Silverstone, T. and Goodall, E. (1986). Serotonergic mechanisms in human feeding: the pharmacological evidence. *Appetite*, Suppl. 7, 85–97.

Shor-Posner, G., Grinker, J. A., Marinescu, C., Brown, O., and Leibowitz, S. F. (1986). Hypothalamic serotonin in the control of meal patterns and macronutrient selection. *Brain Research Bulletin*, **17**, 663–71.

Stallone, D. and Nicolaidis, S. (1989). Increased food intake and carbohydrate preference in the rat following treatment with the serotonin antagonist metergoline. *Neuroscience Letters*, **102**, 319–24.

Sugrue, M. F. (1987). Neuropharmacology of drugs affecting food intake. *Pharmacology and Therapeutics*, **32**, 145–82.

Tricklebank, M. D., Middlemiss, D. M., and Neill, J. (1986). Pharmacological analysis of the behavioural and thermoregulatory effects of the putative 5-HT$_1$ receptor agonist RU 24969 in the rat. *Neuropharmacology*, **25**, 877–86.

Verge, D., Duval, G., Patey, A., Gozlan, S., Mestikawy, E. L., and Hamon, M. (1985). Presynaptic 5-HT autoreceptors on serotonergic cell bodies and/or dendrites but not terminals are of the 5-HT$_{1A}$ subtype. *European Journal of Pharmacology*, **113**, 463–4.

Waeber, C., Dieth, M. M., Hoyer, D., Probst, A. and Palacios, J. M. (1988). Visualization of a novel serotonin recognition site (5-HT$_{1D}$) in the human brain by autoradiography. *Neuroscience Letters*, **88**, 11–16.

Weekley, L. B., Maher, R. W., and Kimbrough, T. D. (1982). Alterations of tryptophan metabolism in a rat strain (Osborne-Mendel) predisposed to obesity. *Comparative Biochemistry and Physiology*, **72A**, 747–52.

White, P. J., Cybulski, K. A., Primus, R., Johnson, D. F., Collier, G. H., and Wagner, G. L. (1988). Changes in macronutrient selection as a function of dietary tryptophan. *Physiology and Behaviour*, **43**, 73–7.

Whitton, P. and Curzon, G. (1990). Anxiogenic-like effect of infusing 1-(3-chlorophenyl)piperazine (mCPP) into the hippocampus. *Psychopharmacology*, **100**, 138–40.

Wurtman, J. J. and Wurtman, R. J. (1979). Drugs that enhance central serotonergic transmission diminish elective carbohydrate consumption by rats. *Life Sciences*, **24**, 895–904.

Wurtman, J., Wurtman, R., Reynolds, S., Tsay, R., and Chew, B. (1987). Fenfluramine suppresses snack intake among carbohydrate cravers but not among non-carbohydrate cravers. *International Journal of Eating Disorders*, **6**, 687–99.

Yokogoshi, H. and Wurtman, R. J. (1986). Meal composition and plasma amino acid ratios: effect of various proteins or carbohydrates and of various protein concentrations. *Metabolism*, **35**, 837–42.

Yuwiler, A., Oldendorf, W. H., Geller, E., and Braun, L. (1977). Effect of albumin binding and amino acid competition on tryptophan uptake into brain. *Journal of Neurochemistry*, **27**, 1015–23.

Discussion

PEROUTKA: 5-HT$_{1B}$ sites are also the autoreceptors on the terminal. Agonists decrease the release of 5-hydroxytryptamine (5-HT, serotonin) and other transmitters. How does that fit with the concept that increasing 5-HT activity is important?

CURZON: We went down to very low doses of RU 24969 because we thought that perhaps it might then activate terminal 5-HT$_{1B}$ sites, therefore decreasing 5-HT release and causing hyperphagia rather than hypophagia. We didn't find this. Although much emphasis has been placed on terminal 5-HT$_{1B}$ sites, most 5-HT$_{1B}$ sites in the rat are post-synaptic; when a 5-HT neurotoxin is given most of the 5-HT$_{1B}$ sites remain. One wonders, however, if any behavioural responses to activation of those terminal autoreceptors are known.

CARLSSON: We cannot say that 5-HT$_{1A}$ agonists are only autoreceptor agonists. They do have post-synaptic actions; you saw that when you detected the motor syndrome at higher doses. The clinical antidepressant action of 5-HT uptake inhibitors is most probably an agonist response. The 5-HT$_{1A}$ agonists have a similar effect. Thus, some, presumably important, 5-HT$_{1A}$ effects are post-synaptic, but are not manifest in this appetite control system. Is it possible that the post-synaptic 5-HT$_{1A}$ receptor responsiveness in this system is weak, perhaps even absent, and that other post-synaptic subtypes operate here?

We have a somewhat analogous problem in sexual behaviour. 5-Hydroxytryptophan (5-HTP) is inhibitory and the 5-HT$_{1A}$ agonists are the strongest available stimulants of sexual behaviour in male rats. This discrepancy could arise from an almost exclusive activity of the 5-HT$_{1A}$ agonists on the autoreceptors. The alternative explanation is that even a compound such as 8-hydroxy-*N*,*N*-dipropyl-2-aminotetralin (8-OH-DPAT) may be a partial agonist. If so, it could sometimes be an antagonist, for example in systems controlling sexual activity in the male rat, and perhaps also in appetite control.

CURZON: Although the increase of sexual activity fits well with earlier work on the effects of serotonergic drugs in male rats, 8-OH-DPAT has an opposing action in females (Ahlenius *et al.* 1989). Another problem is how to explain the antidepressant effects of 5-HT$_{1A}$ agonists in terms of autoreceptor activation decreasing 5-HT release when many findings suggest that antidepressant effects are associated with increased 5-HT availability to post-synaptic receptors. One explanation is that 5-HT$_{1A}$ agonists readily down-regulate the raphe cell body 5-HT$_{1A}$ autoreceptors so that they no longer damp down 5-HT release. This is indicated by our behavioural work in the rat in which a 5-HT$_{1A}$ agonist caused hyperphagia by activating the raphe sites so that 5-HT release was decreased, but the drug no longer was hyperphagic when given again on the next day (Kennett *et al.* 1987). We also found that a large single dose of the 5-HT$_{1A}$ agonist 8-OH-DPAT given 24 h previously decreased raphe 5-HT$_{1A}$ binding sites and increased the effect of electrical stimulation of the raphe on 5-HT metabolism in the frontal cortex (Beer *et al.* 1990). This suggests that 5-HT$_{1A}$ agonists may have antidepressant effects by down-regulating cell body 5-HT$_{1A}$ sites so that 5-HT release on firing is enhanced. These results also imply that the hyperphagic and antidepressant actions of 5-HT$_{1A}$ agonists would not be expected to occur together.

CARLSSON: But the 5-HT uptake inhibitors in man have appetite-reducing actions.

CURZON: Presumably they increase 5-HT release to hypothalamic sites at which 5-HT suppresses appetite. Also, antidepressant drugs may well alter feeding by other mechanisms that are secondary to changes of mood. Using drugs that are selective for receptor subtypes one can tease out mechanisms involved in feeding. But with antidepressant drugs which increase 5-HT release to numerous 5-HT receptors and may also have other effects, it becomes much more complicated.

COPPEN: That amitriptyline causes weight gain is well established. The increase correlates well with the clinical response. However, drugs such as fluoxetine also provide improvement. Thus, this weight increase cannot be ascribed entirely to the improvement in mood. On the other hand, amitriptyline seems to have little effect in anorexia.

In our patients on long-term amitriptyline the weight increase seems to continue even after the patient has recovered. I think that it is more marked in females than males. What is the mechanism for this amitriptyline-induced weight increase?

COWEN: Might the fact that certain tricyclics cause weight gain relate to their ability to block 5-HT$_{2/1C}$ receptors, which amitriptyline does potently? Mianserin is well known to cause weight gain and is a potent 5-HT$_{1C}$ receptor antagonist. Lithium, which can also cause weight gain, would be expected to lower 5-HT$_{2/1C}$ transmission through its effect on the phosphoinositide system which acts as a second messenger at 5-HT$_{2/1C}$ receptors.

CURZON: Those observations are completely consistent with the effects of mianserin described in my paper. They also agree with work by Dourish *et al.* (1989) that shows that metergoline, methiothepin, mesulergine, mianserin, and methysergide increase feeding in satiated rats.

MELTZER: What is known about the weight gain associated with buspirone-type drugs and any changes over time, when some desensitization of the somatodendritic autoreceptor might develop? I am not aware that changes in weight/appetite have been important clinically with these agents.

CURZON: I do not have any clinical information, but the lack of effect on appetite would agree well with our work on the desensitization of the cell body 5-HT$_{1A}$ sites.

ROBINSON: In the comprehensive safety review of buspirone, involving about 3500 patients, significant weight changes were not seen, even in patients ($n = 264$) treated with anxiolytic doses of buspirone continuously for one year.

MENDLEWICZ: Was this done on depressed patients?

ROBINSON: No, that is being done now.

CURZON: I look at 5-HT$_{1A}$ agonists as tools for studying mechanisms that are important for appetite. I do not see them as useful treatments in appetite disorders as I would not expect them to have any long-term effects on feeding.

CARLSSON: We did a 10-day treatment study with an analogue of 8-OH-DPAT that has the same pharmacological profile (unpublished work). In rats we saw a slight but significant retardation of the weight gain. The acute effects might differ from the chronic ones.

The species differences are very large, even between mice and rats. Whereas 5-HTP causes the classical 5-HT motor syndrome in both mouse and rat, 8-OH-DPAT only does so in the rat; it has almost no effect in the mouse. 8-OH-DPAT stimulates sexual behaviour in the male rat; in the male mouse 8-OH-DPAT inhibits sexual behaviour and 5-HTP stimulates it (Svensson *et al.* 1987).

MAÎTRE: In chronic toxicity studies with 5-HT uptake inhibitors in dogs a similar retardation of weight gain is seen after an initial decrease in weight. This effect persists over several months and is more pronounced in females than in males.

INSEL: Do the receptors which have been cloned have promoter elements for oestrogen in the non-coding region? That would be relatively simple to investigate.

PEROUTKA: The 5-HT_{1A}, 5-HT_{1C}, and the 5-HT_2 receptors have been cloned but, to my knowledge, oestrogen-related effects have not been studied.

GUARDIOLA-LEMAITRE: With fenfluramine, also, female rats are more sensitive than males (Rowland and Carlton 1988). Did you try to discover the abnormality or modification of the subtype of 5-HT receptors in obese animals or after inducing eating disorders?

CURZON: Most of our work has been on 200–250 g male Sprague-Dawley rats. We have not looked at obese animals. It is difficult to think of a good animal model for feeding disorders. We are all exposed to dietary stimuli yet only a small proportion of the population become severely bulimic or anorexic. Are there useful animal models of bulima or anorexia nervosa?

GUARDIOLA-LEMAITRE: There are many ways to induce obesity, such as stress, cafeteria diet, tail pinching, etc. There is also a more physiological model—the ageing animal. In particular, Sprague-Dawley rats become obese in old age.

CURZON: It may be relevant that 5-HT turnover is less in the obese Osborne-Mendel rat than in other strains (Weekley *et al.* 1982). It might be interesting to investigate the effects in these animals of serotonergic drugs on feeding and on extraneuronal 5-HT in the hypothalamus using *in vivo* dialysis.

MURPHY: Another possible model for eating disorders is the fawn-hooded rat strain (Wang *et al.* 1988; Aulakh *et al.* 1988a). These rats show growth retardation over time and are subsensitive to *m*-CPP and 8-OH-DPAT, both in eating behaviour responses and neuroendocrine responses. This strain might provide an interesting model for molecular genetic studies.

PALFREYMAN: Under the right circumstances benzodiazepines will increase feeding. This is most pronounced under high-light conditions when the animals are fed a normal diet but are stressed. Could part of the effect with the anxiolytic 5-HT_{1A} partial agonists arise from a similar anti-anxiety response? Could you explore that idea by changing the novelty or stress-associated component of the feeding in some way?

CURZON: That seems reasonable and worth pursuing. For the benzodiazepines decreased 5-HT release might be involved. We know that this occurs in the hippocampus (Pei *et al.* 1989). Perhaps a similar effect decreases 5-HT release in the hypothalamus and hence increases feeding.

PEROUTKA: Was there a correlation between agonist activity and the effect on feeding? Did 8-OH-DPAT increase feeding more than buspirone? Could you separate partial from full agonists?

CURZON: We have looked at the hyperphagic effects of six 5-HT$_{1A}$ agonists. We have not compared them systematically, but 8-OH-DPAT had a greater hyperphagic effect than buspirone and gepirone.

PEROUTKA: These agonists decrease core temperature to varying degrees. Is the hyperphagic effect secondary to altered metabolic activity?

MURPHY: 8-OH-DPAT at doses between 0.1 and 0.5 mg kg^{-1} produced parallel increases in temperature and food intake. *m*-CPP at doses of 1 to 5 mg kg^{-1} produced the opposite effect; parallel decreases in temperature and food intake (Aulakh *et al.* 1988*b*; Wozniak *et al.* 1989).

CURZON: How would one show whether there was a causal connection?

MURPHY: One would use antagonists, I suppose.

CARLSSON: If one studied the dose-response, the autoreceptor activation would be the same for both 8-OH-DPAT and buspirone. The rate of synthesis of 5-HT would be reduced to the same extent by both. However, there is a great difference in the expression of the 5-HT motor syndrome; it is very weak for buspirone.

CURZON: We did not study the 5-HT motor syndrome with buspirone but we used another 5-HT$_{1A}$ agonist, LY 165163, which causes hyperphagia but not the motor syndrome. It also inhibits components of the 5-HT syndrome induced by 5-methoxy-*N*,*N*-dimethyltryptamine which require dopamine (DA) as well as 5-HT. We ascribed this effect to blockade of dopamine receptors; neurochemical data agree as LY 165163 also increases dopamine synthesis (Donohoe *et al.* 1987).

EVENDEN: We tested the interaction between 8-OH-DPAT and raclopride. The 8-OH-DPAT-induced 5-HT syndrome is much enhanced by this DA$_2$ antagonist. Dopamine agonists also block many of the effects of 8-OH-DPAT (Renyi, personal communication). This is certainly not consistent with the ideas that you are putting forward at the moment.

The effects of 8-OH-DPAT on feeding when liquid diets are used instead of solid food are different. In my hands, the active dose of 8-OH-DPAT for increasing drinking of liquid diet is about 100 times less than the active dose for increasing feeding from a solid diet.

CURZON: There has been controversy about whether 5-HT$_{1A}$ agonists directly affect feeding, or are effective because they increase gnawing. Some people were unable to show hyperphagic effects with liquid diets. But in our first experiments with 8-OH-DPAT we had bits of wood in the cage and measured both feeding and gnawing. There was very little effect on gnawing. Also, we have found that the hyperphagic effect is similar whether we use a pelleted or finely powdered diet. I did not know that the dose-response curve was different with liquid diets. The hyperphagia must be with very low doses.

EVENDEN: The optimal dose is 0.01 mg kg^{-1}, that is towards the lower end of the range at which you have observed gnawing. If the dose is increased to one at which the food hyperphagia is observed, there is no increase in drinking. In fact, there is a reduction in drinking.

CURZON: This might, at least partly, explain why some groups (Dourish *et al.* 1988*a*,*b*; Neill and Cooper 1988) but not others (Fletcher 1987; Montgomery *et al.* 1988) found that 8-OH-DPAT increased intake of a liquid diet.

References

Ahlenius, S., Larsson, K., and Fernandez-Guasti (1989). Evidence for the involvement of central 5-HT$_{1A}$ receptors in the mediation of lordosis behaviour in the female rat. *Psychopharmacology*, **98**, 440–4.

Aulakh, C. S., Wozniak, K. M., Hill, J. L., Devane, C. L., Tolliver, T. J., and Murphy, D. L. (1988*a*). Differential neuroendocrine responses to the 5-HT agonist m-chlorophenylpiperazine in Fawn-Hooded rats relative to Wistar and Sprague-Dawley rats. *Neuroendocrinology*, **48**, 401–6.

Aulakh, C. S., Wozniak, K. M., Haas, M., Hill, J. L., Zohar, J., and Murphy, D. L. (1988*b*). Food intake, neuroendocrine and temperature effects of 8-OH-DPAT in the rat. *European Journal of Pharmacology*, **146**, 253–9.

Beer, M., Kennett, G. A., and Curzon, G. (1990). A single dose of 8-OH-DPAT reduces raphe binding of [^{3}H]8-OH-DPAT and increases the effect of raphe stimulation on 5-HT metabolism. *European Journal of Pharmacology*, **178**, 179–87.

Donohoe, T. P., Hutson, P. H., and Curzon, G. (1987). Blockade of dopamine receptors explains the lack of 5-HT stereotypy on treatment with the putative 5-HT$_{1A}$ agonist LY 165163. *Psychopharmacology*, **93**, 82–6.

Dourish, C. T., Cooper, S. J., Gilbert, F., Coughlan, J., and Iversen, S. D. (1988*a*). The 5-HT$_{1A}$ agonist 8-OH-DPAT increases consumption of palatable wet mash and liquid diets in the rat. *Psychopharmacology*, **94**, 58–63.

Dourish, C. T., Clark, M. L., and Iversen, S. D. (1988*b*). 8-OH-DPAT elicits feeding and not chewing: evidence from liquid diet studies and a diet choice test. *Psychopharmacology*, **95**, 185–8.

Dourish, C. T., Clark, M. L., Fletcher, A., and Iversen, S. D. (1989). Evidence that blockade of post-synaptic 5-HT receptors elicits feeding in satiated rats. *Psychopharmacology*, **97**, 54–8.

Fletcher, P. J. (1987). 8-OH-DPAT elicits gnawing and eating of solid but not liquid foods. *Psychopharmacology*, **92**, 192–5.

Kennett, G. A., Marcou, M., Dourish, C. T., and Curzon, G. (1987). Single administration of 5-HT$_{1A}$ agonists decreases 5-HT$_{1A}$ presynaptic but not postsynaptic receptor-mediated responses: relationship to antidepressant-like action. *European Journal of Pharmacology*, **138**, 53–60.

Montgomery, A. M. J., Willner, P., and Muscat, R. (1988). Behavioural specificity of 8-OH-DPAT induced feeding. *Psychopharmacology*, **94**, 110–14.

Neill, J. C. and Cooper, S. J. (1988). Evidence for serotonergic modulation of sucrose sham-feeding in the gastric-fistulated rat. *Physiology and Behaviour*, **44**, 453–9.

Pei, Q., Zetterstrom, T., and Fillenz, M. (1989). Both systemic and local administration of benzodiazepine agonists inhibit the *in vivo* release of 5-HT from ventral hippocampus. *Neuropharmacology*, **28**, 1061–6.

Rowland, N. E. and Carlton, J. (1988). Dexfenfluramine: effects on food intake in various animal models. *Clinical Neuropharmacology*, **11**, Suppl. 1, S33–S50.

Svensson, K., Larsson, K., Ahlenius, S., Arvidson, L. E., and Carlsson, A. (1987). Evidence for a facilitatory role of central 5-HT in male mouse sexual behaviour. In *Brain 5-HT$_{1A}$ receptors* (ed. C. T. Dourish, S. Ahlenius, and P. H. Hutson), pp. 199–210. Ellis Horwood, Chichester.

Wang, P., Aulakh, C. S., Hill, J. L., and Murphy, D. L. (1988). Fawn-hooded rats are subsensitive to the food intake suppressant effects of 5-HT agonists. *Psychopharmacology*, **94**, 558–62.

Weekley, L. B., Maher, R. W., and Kimbrough, T. D. (1982). Alterations of tryptophan metabolism in a rat strain (Osborne-Mendel) predisposed to obesity. *Comparative Biochemistry and Physiology*, **72A**, 747–52.

Wozniak, K. M., Aulakh, C. S., Hill, J. L., and Murphy, D. L. (1989). Hyperthermia induced by *m*-CPP in the rat and its modification by antidepressant treatments. *Psychopharmacology*, **97**, 269–74.

21. d-Fenfluramine and animal models of eating disorders

B. Guardiola-Lemaitre

Introduction

Pharmacological studies on food intake or body weight have traditionally used normal, young lean rats which are starved or fed a bland and balanced diet of laboratory chow, or rats that are genetically obese or diabetic. However, many parameters, such as food regimen, age, physiological state, and environmental stresses or stimuli, and life events influence the development of eating disorders and consequently of obesity. Experimental models must reproduce these parameters to give an indication of the effect of a drug in human eating disorders. This is illustrated by some preclinical data obtained with the serotonergic drug d-fenfluramine. The models used to investigate this drug can be classified (Table 21.1) as studying: (1) the motivation to eat; (2) the structure of eating behaviour; and (3) the hedonic value of food and choice of macronutrients. In addition, some of the animal models induce overeating or trigger food intake.

d-Fenfluramine acts by inhibition of the re-uptake of 5-hydroxytryptamine (5-HT, serotonin) and by releasing 5-HT from nerve terminals (Garattini *et al.* 1988). It has been marketed in Europe since 1985 and is used in the treatment of different forms of obesity; its efficacy has been confirmed by a double-blind, placebo-controlled, multicentre trial involving 800 patients (Guy-Grand *et al.* 1989). Comparison between d-fenfluramine and amphetamine (or d-amphetamine) at equianorectic doses enhances our understanding of the relative involvement of 5-HT and the catecholamines in the mechanism of eating disorders.

Motivation to eat

A motivation to eat may be induced not only by hunger and food deprivation but also by desire for food or for what it represents—reward and compensation. The motivation to eat can be measured by the use of the food-rewarded runway behaviour test. Rats are put behind a gate at one end of an alley and food is presented at the other end. The rats are trained to run to the food when the gate is opened. The motivation to obtain food is intensified in those

TABLE 21.1. *Comparison of equianoretic doses of d-fenfluramine and amphetamine on eating parameters*

Eating parameters	d-Fenfluramine (0.3–1.5 mg kg^{-1})	Amphetamine	Reference
Motivation to eat			
Food reward runway behaviour			
—starting speed	↓ *	→	Thurbly and Samanin 1981
—running speed	↓ *	→	Thurbly and Samanin 1981
Self-stimulation (reward)	↓	↑	Hoebel 1988 *et al.*
Hoarding behaviour	↓ *	→	Fantino *et al.* 1988
Structure of eating			
Food intake—calorific intake	↓ *	↓	Garattini 1986
Initiation of meal	normal	delayed	Blundell and Latham 1980
Eating rate	↓ *	↑	Blundell and Latham 1980
Meal duration	↓	↓	Blundell and Latham 1980
General pattern of eating	conserved	modified	Blundell and Latham 1980
Hedonic value of food			
Cafeteria	↓ ↓	↓ or →	Blundell and Hill 1985
Dessert test	↓ ↓ *	↓ or →	Borsini *et al.* 1985
Reward	↓	↑	Hoebel *et al.* 1988
Food choice			
Carbohydrates	↓	→	Hirsch *et al.* 1982
Induction of food intake			
Tail-pinching	↓ *	→	Antelman *et al.* 1981
Muscimol injection	↓ *	→	Garattini 1986
2-Deoxyglucose injection	↓	↓	Carruba *et al.* 1985
Insulin hypoglycaemia	↓	→	Carruba *et al.* 1985

*, antagonized by metergoline; ↓ , decreased; ↑ , increased; →, unchanged.

animals whose body weight has been decreased by 20 per cent. Measurements of the starting speed, the running speed, the delay before eating, and the amount of food eaten allow us to explore different components of the feeding process (Thurbly and Samanin 1981).

When rats are starved and their body weight decreases, they actively and compulsively hoard food in certain experimental conditions. The amount of food hoarded is positively correlated to the body weight deficit induced by the low calorie diet (Fantino and Cabanac 1980). In these models, rats treated with d-fenfluramine at low doses (0.3–0.6 mg kg⁻¹) behave like fed animals. Thus d-fenfluramine affects the parameters which reflect the motivation to approach, to hoard, and to acquire food. The effect of d-fenfluramine is antagonized by metergoline. On the other hand, amphetamine is less active or inactive in these models.

Stimulation-induced feeding responses and self-stimulation are modulated by physiological signals that control an animal's appetite and body weight. An animal will be self-stimulated at a lower rate immediately after it has eaten, if it is overweight, or if it is given an anorectic dose of insulin. d-Fenfluramine (1.5 mg kg⁻¹) inhibits lateral hypothalamus (LH) self-stimulation but not stimulation-escape. It also causes release of serotonin in the LH, as shown by microdialysis (Hoebel *et al.* 1988). Under the same conditions, amphetamine increases LH self-stimulation.

Structure of eating behaviour

Acute food deprivation is a reliable and easy way to stimulate appetite for a large meal in most laboratory animals. This is the most widely used paradigm in the screening of drugs for anorectic actions. d-Fenfluramine (< 1.2 mg kg⁻¹) is as effective as amphetamine in reducing the food intake of rats after food deprivation (Garattini 1986). However, this parameter has been criticized as irrelevant for normal free feeding and for overeating syndromes or disorders. The organization of the eating sequence includes initiation, maintenance, and termination of the feeding process (Blundell and Latham 1980). The eating behaviour of rats is represented by a sequence of activities in which episodes (bouts) of eating are interspersed with bouts of non-eating. In animals, the study of the microstructure of eating includes measuring total food intake, amount of time spent eating, latency (time elapsed before onset of eating), number of eating bouts, food intake during bouts, duration of bouts, and eating rate. This is recorded with a video-camera. Fenfluramine and amphetamine gave rise to quite distinctive readjustments in the structure of feeding behaviour. Amphetamine anorexia is characterized by a long initial delay and a rapid eating rate. These effects are antagonized by the dopamine receptor antagonist, pimozide. Fenfluramine activity is characterized by a marked slowing of the rate of eating, this effect being countered by the serotonin receptor antagonist, metergoline (Blundell and Latham 1980).

Hedonic value of food and choice of macronutrients

Consumption of food can be dominated by the sensory aspects of the diet, such as the taste of food (e.g., sweet versus salt), the aspect (e.g., liquid versus solid), or the composition (carbohydrates, proteins, lipids). One way to stimulate food consumption in rats is to give them free access to diverse, palatable, high-energy food, such as is available in a modern human diet (sugar, chocolate, rice, corn flakes). Under these conditions, some rats will become hyperphagic and subsequently obese (20 per cent overweight). This is the 'cafeteria' or 'supermarket' diet model (Sclafani and Springer 1976). Another model is the 'dessert test'. Undeprived rats are offered a sweet dessert once a day (sucrose solutions, sweetened drinks). After several days, the day-to-day intakes are stable and provide a baseline against which drug effects can be evaluated (Borsini *et al* 1985).

In both these tests, d-fenfluramine is very active in reducing food intake, this effect being countered by metergoline in the 'dessert test'. Amphetamine is not, or only weakly, active.

Carbohydrate consumption has been shown to be related to serotonin synthesis (via competition of amino acids with tryptophan for uptake into the brain) (Wurtman 1988). Animal models have been developed in which rats can select food from two dishes containing isocalorific diets, one low (5 per cent) and one high (45 per cent) in protein. Low doses of d-fenfluramine selectively reduce consumption of the low protein diet, thereby also reducing carbohydrate intake by a greater proportion than protein intake. In contrast d-amphetamine decreased protein and carbohydrate consumption proportionately (Hirsch *et al.* 1982).

Induction of food intake

Stressful circumstances are able to produce either anorexia or hyperphagia, depending upon the characteristics of an individual and the environmental conditions. In rats, restraint stress gives rise to a period of anorexia (see Curzon, this volume). Hyperphagia can be induced experimentally in animals by quite different means, for example stress, such as mild, non-painful pinching of tails, triggers transient hyperphagia in some rats when food is available (Antelman and Caggiula 1978). d-Fenfluramine, quipazine, *m*-chlorophenylpiperazine, and fluoxetine inhibit this stress-induced overeating. Compounds acting on the catecholaminergic pathways are poorly active or inactive in this model (Antelman *et al.* 1981; Garattini 1986).

Infusions of physiological or pharmacological agents such as insulin or 2-deoxyglucose induce so-called glucoprivic feeding. This overeating is blocked by d-fenfluramine as well as by other serotonergic drugs such as quipazine or fluoxetine, whereas amphetamine, acting through the dopaminergic system, antagonizes the hyperphagia induced by 2-deoxyglucose, but not that induced by insulin (Carruba *et al.* 1985). Muscimol, a GABAergic agonist, also induces feeding when injected into the dorsal raphe nucleus and this is blocked by d-fenfluramine. This action of d-fenfluramine is prevented by metergoline (Garattini 1986).

Conclusion

This paper is based on the recognition that human eating disorders involve more than abnormal calorie intake. If animal models are to be of any value in highlighting the possible therapeutic action of a drug, it seems appropriate to consider more than the mere ingestion of food. Aspects of feeding which precede, accompany, follow, or otherwise support, ingestion must also be considered.

d-Fenfluramine, a serotonergic drug acting both by inhibition of 5-HT uptake and by release of 5-HT, acts differently on the eating parameters compared to amphetamine. d-Fenfluramine decreases the motivation to eat, the eating rate, and the meal duration, but leaves unchanged the general pattern of eating. Hedonic values of food and carbohydrate consumption are decreased after d-fenfluramine administration, but protein consumption is spared. Stress-induced overeating is also countered by d-fenfluramine. On the other hand, amphetamine, which also decreases the total food intake, modifies the general pattern of eating. Amphetamine is poorly active on hedonic values of food and inactive on food selection. It does not counter the overfeeding induced by stress, insulin or muscimol injection. This information, taken together with the fact that metergoline antagonizes the activity of d-fenfluramine in most of the tests, suggests that 5-HT is more broadly involved than the catecholamines in the mechanisms controlling eating disorders.

Acknowledgement

We are grateful to Nathalie Devallan for her assistance in editing this manuscript.

References

Antelman, S. M. and Caggiula, A. R. (1978). Tails of stress-related behavior: a neuropharmacological model. In *Animal models in psychiatry and neurology*, (ed. I. Hanin and E. Udsin), pp. 227–45. Pergamon, New York.

Antelman, S. M., Rowland, N., and Kocan, D. (1981). Anorectics: lack of cross tolerance among serotoninergic drugs and sensitization of amphetamine's effect. In *Anorectic agents—mechanism of action and tolerance*, (ed. S. Garattini and R. Samanin), pp. 45–62. Raven Press, New York.

Blundell, J. and Hill, A. J. (1985). Effect of dextrofenfluramine on feeding and body weight. Relationship with food consumption and palatability. In *Metabolic complication of human obesities*, (ed. J. Vague *et al.*), pp. 199–206. Elsevier, Amsterdam.

Blundell, J. and Latham, C. (1980). Characterisation of adjustments to the structure of feeding behaviour following pharmacological treatment: effects of amphetamine and Fenfluramine and the antagonism produced by Pimozide and Metergoline. *Pharmacology Biochemistry and Behavior,* **12**, 717–22.

Borsini, F., Bendotti, C., Samanin, R. (1985). Salbutamol, d-amphetamine and d-fenfluramine reduce sucrose intake in freely fed rats by acting on different neurochemical mechanisms. *International Journal of Obesity*, **9**, 277–83.

Carruba, M. O., Ricciardi, S., Spano, P., and Mantegazza, P. (1985). Dopaminergic and serotoninergic agents differentially antagonize insulin and 2-DG induced hyperphagia. *Life Sciences*, **36**, 1739–49.

Curzon, G. (1991). 5-Hydroxytryptamine in the control of feeding and its possible implications for appetite disturbance. In *5-Hydroxytryptamine in psychiatry; a spectrum of ideas*, (ed. M. Sandler, A. Coppen, and S. Harnett), pp. 279–302. Oxford University Press.

Fantino, M. and Cabanac, M. (1980). Body weight regulation with a proportional hoarding response in the rat. *Physiology and Behavior*, **24**, 939–42.

Fantino, M., Boucher, A., Faion, F., and Mathiot, P. (1988). Dexfenfluramine in body weight regulation: experimental study with hoarding behaviour. *Clinical Neuropharmacology*, **11**, Suppl 1, S97-S104.

Garattini, S. (1986). Efects of d-fenfluramine on eating disorders. In *Disorders of eating behaviour—a psychoendocrine approach*, (ed E. Ferrari), pp. 327–41. Pergamon, Oxford.

Garattini, S., Bizzi, A., Cassia, S., Mennini, T., and Samanin, R. (1988). Progress in assessing the role of serotonin in the control of food intake. *Clinical neuropharmacology*, **11**, Suppl 1, S8–S32.

Guy-Grand, B., Apfelbaum, M., Crepaldi, G., Gries, A., Lefebvre, P., and Turner, P. (1989). International trial of long-term Dexfenfluramine in obesity. *Lancet* **ii**, 1142–4.

Hirsch, J.A., Goldberg, S., Wurtman, R.J. (1982). Effect of (+) or (−) enantiomers of fenfluramine or norfenfluramine on nutrient selection by rats. *Journal of Pharmacy and Pharmacology*, **34**, 18–21.

Hoebel, B. G., Hernandez, L., McClelland, R. C., and Schwartz, D. (1988). Dexfenfluramine and feeding reward. *Clinical Neuropharmacology*, **11**, Suppl 1, S72–S85.

Sclafani, A. and Springer, D. (1976). Dietary obesity in adult rats: simalarities to hypothalamic and human obesity syndromes. *Physiology and Behavior*, **17**, 461–71.

Thurbly, P. L. and Samanin, R. (1981). Effects of anorectic drugs and prior feeding on food rewarded runway behaviour. *Pharmacology Biochemistry and Behavior*, **14**, 799–804.

Wurtman, R. J. (1988). Effects of their nutrient precursors on the synthesis and release of serotonin, the catecholamines, and acetylcholine: implication of behavioural disorders. *Clinical Neuropharmacology*, **11**, Suppl. 1, S187–S193.

22. Disturbance of the 5-hydroxytryptamine metabolism in ageing and in Alzheimer's and vascular dementias

C. G. Gottfries

Introduction

Syndromes of cognitive, emotional, and psychomotor disturbance in the elderly that are of disabling severity are called dementias and are classified as idiopathic, vascular (VD), and secondary dementias. The main group of idiopathic dementias (primary degenerative or metabolic disturbances) are those of Alzheimer type. Originally Alzheimer's disease (AD) was the name of an early onset dementia with characteristic cortical lesions. However, similar neuropathological findings are made in the brains of patients with senile dementia; therefore, this group was named senile dementia of Alzheimer type (SDAT). The two forms are often brought into one group, Alzheimer-type dementia (AD/SDAT). Quantitatively this is the most important group, containing about 60 per cent of all patients with dementia.

Vascular dementia is diagnosed when there is an assumed causal relationship between vascular disorders and the appearance of dementia. Multi-infarct dementia (MID) is a subgroup of VD characterized by a temporary relationship between stroke attacks and the appearance of dementia. There are other subgroups of VD where hypoxic or haemodynamic disturbances or small vessel disorders are assumed to be of pathogenetical importance. According to our findings (Wallin *et al.* 1989), non-MID VD is a rather common disorder, possibly more common than MID.

It has long been agreed that disturbance of the 5-hydroxytryptamine (5-HT, serotonin) system may be part of the pathophysiology of affective disorders, panic, anxiety, feeding disorders, and uncontrolled aggressiveness. Now dementia disorders can be added to this list. The aim of this paper is to review data indicating disturbance of the 5-HT system in patients with AD/SDAT and non-MID VD. Data about changes in the 5-HT metabolism in ageing are also reported.

Disturbance of the 5-HT system in ageing

Post-mortem investigations

Most of the data on 5-HT metabolism in the human brain come from post-mortem investigations in which the concentrations of 5-HT and 5-hydroxyin-doleacetic acid (5-HIAA) are measured in discrete areas of the brain. The 5-HT concentration is assumed to be mainly a marker of the number of 5-HT neurones or terminals, and the concentration of 5-HIAA is assumed to be a marker of the metabolic activity in these neurones. The precursors to 5-HT, tryptophan and 5-hydroxytryptophan, are usually not measured because changes after death in these amino acids make interpretation of the results difficult.

In post-mortem investigations of the globus pallidus, hippocampal cortex (Bucht *et al.* 1981), caudate nucleus, putamen, and hypothalamus (Carlsson and Gottfries 1986; Gottfries *et al.* 1986), 5-HT has been found to be significantly reduced with age. The patients in these investigations were aged 60 or older. However, in some studies, for example from the frontal cortex and the basal ganglia, no significant reduction of 5-HT with age has been found (Carlsson *et al.* 1980; Bucht *et al.* 1981). A significant positive correlation between age and the concentration of 5-HT in the brainstem was found by Carlsson *et al.* (1980). In a study at our institute (C. G. Gottfries, unpublished work) negative correlations between age and 5-HT concentrations were found in seven of eight areas of the brain and the correlation was statistically significant ($p < 0.05$) in four areas (Fig. 22.1 and Table 22.1).

It is of interest that 5-HT is negatively correlated with age whereas the end metabolite 5-HIAA has continuously been found not to be significantly correlated with age (Table 22.1). As far as we know, no data on significant correlations between 5-HIAA and age have been published. This may indicate that, although the number of 5-HT neurones is reduced with age, as reflected in reduced 5-HT concentrations, this loss is compensated by an increased turnover rate of the remaining neurones, as reflected in the unchanged 5-HIAA concentration. This may be attributable to a compensatory mechanism of the neurones (Carlsson *et al.* 1988).

5-HT-sensitive imipramine binding is considered a marker of pre-synaptic 5-HT neurone terminals. A decrease ($p < 0.05$) in B_{max} with age was found in the cortex gyrus cinguli, whereas in the frontal cortex, hippocampus, amygdalae, and putamen no such correlation was found (Marcusson *et al.* 1987).

Although no significant correlations have been found between age and the concentrations of 5-HIAA in brain tissue, there is a significant positive correlation between the concentrations of 5-HIAA in cerebrospinal fluid (CSF) and age (Gottfries *et al.* 1971). There is as yet no answer to the question of whether this increase of 5-HIAA is caused by an increased

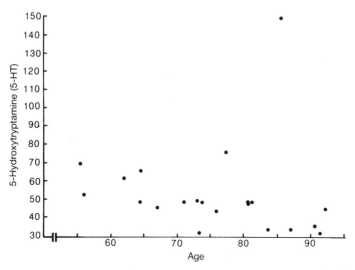

FIG. 22.1. The post-mortem concentration of 5-HT in hippocampus plotted against age for 21 non-demented subjects. Spearman correlation $= -0.52$, $p < 0.05$.

release of 5-HT in the brain or spinal cord, or by a reduced discharge of 5-HIAA from the liquor space.

Disturbance of the 5-HT system in AD/SDAT

There is evidence from several post-mortem studies on AD/SDAT that the concentrations of both 5-HT and 5-HIAA are reduced in brains of demented patients compared with age-matched controls (Gottfries *et al.* 1976; Arai *et al.* 1984; reviewed in Hardy *et al.* 1985 and Gottfries 1988). The reduced concentrations of 5-HT and 5-HIAA are found not only in cortical areas but also in basal ganglias and brainstem areas. Reduced concentrations of 5-HT have also been reported in biopsy studies of AD/SDAT patients (Bowen *et al.* 1988).

The 5-HT-sensitive imipramine binding in tissue from AD/SDAT brains shows an almost 50 per cent decrease in B_{max} when compared with age-matched controls (Marcusson *et al.* 1987) (Fig. 22.2).

The enzyme that synthesizes 5-HT, tryptophan hydroxylase (TPH), was investigated by Nagatsu and Iizuka (1989). TPH activity was found to be lower in various areas of the brain for patients with AD/SDAT and the differences were statistically significant in the lateral segments of the globus pallidus, in the locus caeruleus, and in the substantia nigra. Mann and Yates (1983) and Curcio and Kemper (1984) showed degenerative changes in the raphe nucleus in patients with this type of dementia.

TABLE 22.1. *The Spearman correlation coefficient for age against the concentrations of 5-HT or 5-HIAA in different areas of the brain*

Area of brain	5-HT	5-HIAA
Hypothalamus	0.32 $n=20$	0.27 $n=21$
Caudate nucleus	−0.62*** $n=21$	0.04 $n=21$
Left putamen	0.70*** $n=21$	0.17 $n=21$
Right putamen	−0.63*** $n=21$	0.08 $n=21$
Mesencephalon	−0.12 $n=21$	0.21 $n=21$
Hippocampus	−0.52* $n=21$	0.14 $n=21$
Cortex gyrus hippocampus	−0.17 $n=21$	0.20 $n=21$
Cortex lobus temporalis	−0.29 $n=20$	−0.02 $n=20$

*, $p < 0.05$; ***, $p < 0.005$.

Thus, there are several post-mortem markers for a disturbed 5-HT metabolism in brains from patients with AD/SDAT.

Investigations of the CSF in AD/SDAT patients

In 1969 we showed that the concentration of 5-HIAA in CSF was reduced in patients with SDAT (Gottfries *et al.* 1969). This was confirmed by probenecid loading tests which showed that the accumulation of 5-HIAA in CSF was reduced in patients with AD/SDAT compared with age-matched groups (Gottfries and Roos 1973), and several other investigations of CSF from patients with AD/SDAT have also shown reduced concentrations of 5-HIAA (Westenberg and Verhoeven 1988). We compared 123 patients with AD/SDAT with 57 age-matched controls (K. Blennow *et al.*, unpublished work). The concentration of 5-HIAA in CSF was 159 ± 63 nmol l^{-1} in the controls,

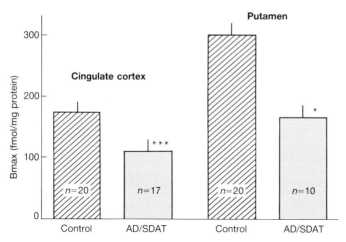

FIG. 22.2. Imipramine binding in cingulate cortex and putamen from age-matched controls and patients with AD/SDAT (after Marcusson *et al.* 1987). ***, $p < 0.001$; *, $p < 0.05$.

and 116 ± 49 nmol l^{-1} in the AD/SDAT group. The difference was significant; $p < 0.0001$.

It should also be mentioned that Forssell *et al.* (1989) found reduced concentrations of tryptophan in CSF when AD/SDAT patients were compared with age-matched controls.

Activity of monoamine oxidase in ageing and in AD/SDAT

Monoamine oxidase (MAO) is the main metabolizing enzyme of 5-HT. It exists in two forms, A and B. 5-HT is mainly the substrate for the A form. In normal ageing there is a significant increase in the activity of MAO-B in both grey and white matter (Adolfsson *et al.* 1981; Oreland and Gottfries 1986). Results from animal experiments indicate that this increased activity may arise from an increase in extraneuronal tissue in the aged brain. Thus, MAO-B seems to be a marker of gliosis. The increase in MAO-B activity is considerably greater in patients with AD/SDAT than in age-matched controls in both grey and white matter (Figures 22.3 and 22.4). This may indicate that there is a more pronounced gliosis in the demented brain than in the normal aged brain. It is difficult to speculate about the biological importance of increased MAO-B activity. As 5-HT is mainly the substrate of the A form, it can be assumed that the increase in activity of the B form is of no biological importance for the 5-HT system.

Platelets have only the B form of MAO, and increased MAO activity in platelets has been recorded in patients with AD/SDAT compared with age-matched controls (Adolfsson *et al.* 1980). This increase is difficult to explain

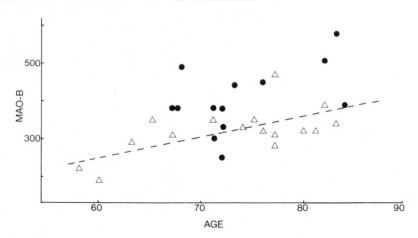

FIG. 22.3. The activity of monoamine oxidase B (MAO-B) in the hippocampus plotted against age. △, controls; ●, patients with dementia (AD/SDAT).

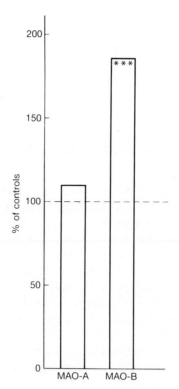

FIG. 22.4. Increased activity of monoamine oxidase B (MAO-B) in white matter from patients with AD/SDAT compared with that from controls (dotted line) (after Oreland and Gottfries 1986). ***, $p < 0.001$.

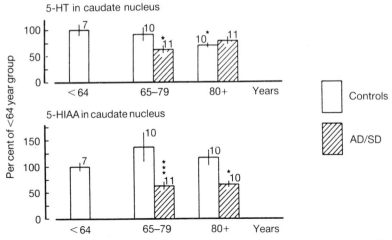

FIG. 22.5. Concentrations of 5-HT and 5-HIAA in the caudate nucleus in different age groups of controls and patients with AD/SDAT (after Carlsson *et al.* 1988). ***, $p < 0.001$; *, $p < 0.05$.

because it must be distinct from increased MAO-B activity in brain tissue. Regland *et al.* (1988) demonstrated that the increased activity of platelet MAO occurs mainly in SDAT patients, that is those with late onset of dementia. Vitamin B_{12} deficiency was also shown in this subgroup of Alzheimer-demented patients. The authors considered the high MAO activity in platelets to be attributable to immature platelets in these non-anaemic demented patients. Non-demented patients with pernicious anaemia also have extremely high MAO platelet activity (Glover *et al.* 1980; Regland *et al.* 1990). The high MAO activity in patients with pernicious anaemia, as well as in patients with dementia, rapidly normalizes when vitamin B_{12} is given.

Thomas *et al.* (1988) used platelet aggregation induced by 5-HT as a test of functional responsiveness of peripheral 5-HT receptors. There was no significant difference between the aggregative responses in the demented patients and controls.

Comparisons between ageing and AD/SDAT

There are both quantitative and qualitative differences between the changes in the 5-HT system in individuals with normal ageing and patients with AD/SDAT. As shown by Carlsson *et al.* (1988), the remaining 5-HT neurones in the normally aged brain seem to increase their metabolism and in this way compensate for the loss of neurones. No such compensatory increase in metabolism has been found in AD/SDAT-afflicted brains. The concentrations of 5-HT, as well as of the end metabolite of 5-HIAA, are reduced in demented brains (Fig. 22.5). This may indicate that the remaining 5-HT neurones in the brains of those suffering from Alzheimer-type dementia do not function properly.

Vascular dementia

Post-mortem investigations of brains from patients with non-MID VD have shown reduced concentrations of 5-HT and 5-HIAA in discrete areas of brain tissue, indicating a general disturbance of the 5-HT metabolism (Wallin *et al.* 1989). These reduced concentrations could not be related to the presence of infarcts or to Alzheimer encephalopathy.

Neuroendocrine disturbances and the 5-HT metabolism

The 5-HT system is important in neuroendocrine function; it seems to control activity in the hypothalamus. Behavioural disturbances such as symptoms of sleep disorders, eating disorders, and disturbed circadian rhythms are common in patients with dementias. These symptoms indicate a dysfunction of the hypothalamus. Several researchers have performed dexamethasone suppression tests (DST) in patients with AD/SDAT and VD (Balldin *et al.* 1983). The results vary, but 20 to 70 per cent of AD/SDAT patients, as well as VD patients, do not respond normally to the test. According to Balldin *et al.* (1988), it is a combination of stress factors and the dementing process that induces the pathological response to DST.

In post-mortem studies of the brains of patients with AD/SDAT and VD (Karlsson *et al.* 1988), the membrane components, phospholipids, cholesterol, gangliosides, and sialoglycoproteins, were found normal in the hypothalamus. The concentrations of 5-HT and 5-HIAA, however, were significantly ($p < 0.05$) reduced in the demented group compared with age-matched controls. Also, significantly ($p < 0.05$) increased concentrations of somatostatin, galanin, and arginine vasopressin (AVP) were found in the demented group when the neuropeptides in the hypothalamus were measured. The neuropeptide corticotropin-releasing factor (CRF) was also increased, although not significantly ($p > 0.05$). Widerlöv *et al.* (1988) reported that AVP is more potent than CRF in stimulating production of adrenocorticotropic hormone by the pituitary gland. According to these data, there seems to be hyperactivity in the hypothalamus in patients with AD/SDAT and VD, and this may explain the increased activity in the hypothalamo-pituitary-adrenal (HPA) axes, as marked by DST.

We studied the correlations between the concentrations of 5-HT and 5-HIAA and those of the neuropeptides in the hypothalamus (C. G. Gottfries, unpublished work). Between 5-HT and the neuropeptides there were negative correlations, with r varying between -0.27 and -0.29, but these results were not statistically significant. 5-HIAA, however, was significantly and negatively correlated with somatostatin ($r = -0.42, p < 0.01$) and

AVP ($r = -0.43$, $p < 0.05$). As it is assumed that 5-HT activity in the hippocampus is important in the control of the activity in the hypothalamus, we also studied the correlations between the 5-HT variables in the hippocampus and the concentrations of neuropeptides in the hypothalamus. The hippocampal 5-HT concentration and the concentrations of neuropeptides in the hypothalamus were not significantly correlated. However, the concentrations of somatostatin and galanin in the hypothalamus were negatively correlated with the hippocampal concentration of 5-HIAA ($p < 0.05$). AVP was also negatively correlated with 5-HIAA, but the correlation only bordered on significant ($p < 0.10$). Thus our data suggest a relationship between the 5-HT input in the hypothalamus and the activity in the HPA axes.

Treatment with selective 5-HT re-uptake blockers

To further study the possible relationship between 5-HT brain metabolism and HPA activity we treated patients with AD/SDAT with a selective 5-HT re-uptake blocker, citalopram (Balldin *et al.* 1988; Nyth *et al.* 1990). In a subgroup of these patients, CSF was drawn before and after four weeks of treatment and a significant decrease of 5-HIAA in the CSF was found. This was expected, because an increased amount of 5-HT is assumed to accumulate in the synaptic cleft and stimulate the autoreceptors which turn down the synthesis of 5-HT. However, it is thought that the total effect of the drug treatment is an up-regulation of the 5-HT system. DST were made before and after the four-week treatment and the citalopram significantly decreased the post-dexamethasone cortisol levels. Thus, the treatment seems to inhibit the activity in the HPA axes in patients with AD/SDAT. This study was done using the double-blind technique with placebo as the reference substance (Nyth *et al.* 1990). There were 98 patients in the trial and the drug treatment caused very few side-effects. No improvement was seen in motor performance or in intellectual capacities, but emotional disturbances, confusion, irritability, restlessness, and fear-panic were reduced, and the mood level was raised.

Acknowledgements

This study was supported by grants from the Swedish Medical Research Council (B90-21x-05002-14C); the Greta och Johan Kocks Stiftelser; the Konung Gustaf V:s och Drottning Victorias Stiftelse; the Torsten och Ragnar Söderbergs Stiftelser; Stiftelsen för Gamla Tjänarinnor; Lundbeckfonden.

References

Adolfsson, R., Gottfries, C. G., Oreland, L., Wiberg, Å., and Winblad, B. (1980). Increased activity of brain and platelet monoamine oxidase in dementia of Alzheimer type. *Life Sciences*, **27**, 1029–34.

Adolfsson, R., Gottfries, C. G., Roos, B. E., and Winblad, B. (1981). Monoamines in the human brain in normal aging and in senile dementia. In *Aging a challenge to science and social policy*, Vol. II, (ed. M. Marois), pp. 238–47. Oxford University Press.

Arai, H., Kosaka, K., and Iizuka, R. (1984). Changes of biogenic amines and their metabolites in postmortem brains from patients with Alzheimer-type dementia. *Journal of Neurochemistry*, **43**, 388–93.

Balldin, J. Gottfries, C. G., Karlsson, I., Lindstedt, G. Långström, G., and Wålinder, J. (1983). Dexamethasone suppression test and serum prolactin in dementia disorders. *British Journal of Psychiatry*, **143**, 277–81.

Balldin, J., Gottfries, C. G., Karlsson, I., Lindstedt, G., Långström, G., and Svennerholm, L. (1988). The clonidine growth hormone test in patients with dementia disorders: relation to clinical status and cerebrospinal fluid metabolite levels. *International Journal of Geriatric Psychiatry*, **3**, 115–23.

Bowen, D. M. *et al.* (1988). In *Aging and the brain*, (ed. R. D. Terry), Aging Series, Vol. 32. Raven Press, New York.

Bucht, G., Adolfsson, R., Gottfries, C. G., Roos, B. E., and Winblad, B. (1981). Distribution of 5-hydroxytryptamine and 5-hydroxyindoleacetic acid in human brain in relation to age, drug influence, agonal status, and circadian variations. *Journal of Neural Transmission*, **51**, 185–203.

Carlsson, A. and Gottfries, C. G. (1986). Neurotransmitter abnormalities in old age dementias. In *Proceedings of the Vth South-East European Neuropsychiatric Conference, Graz, 1983*, (ed. H. Leichner and A. Paraschos), pp. 634–45. University Studio Press, Tessaloniki, Greece.

Carlsson, A., Adolfsson, R., Aquilonius, S. M., Gottfries, C. G., Oreland, L., Svennerholm, L., *et al.* (1980). Biogenic amines in human brain in normal aging, senile dementia and chronic alcoholism. In *Ergot compounds and brain function: neuroendocrine and neuropsychiatric aspects*, (ed. M. Goldstein, D. B. Calne, A. Lieberman, and M. O. Thorner), pp. 295–304. Raven Press, New York.

Carlsson, A., Gottfries, C. G., Eckernås, S. Å., Alafuzoff, I., Winblad, B. (1988). Neurotransmitter changes in dementia: failure to demonstrate relation to histopathologic lesions or multiple infarctions. *Biogenic Amines*, **5**, 199–204.

Curcio, C. A. and Kemper, T. (1984). Nucleus raphe dorsalis in dementia of the Alzheimer type: neurofibrillary changes and neuronal packing density. *Journal of Neuropathology and Experimental Neurology*, **43**, 359–68.

Forssell, L. G., Eklöf, R., and Winblad, B. (1989). Early stages of late onset Alzheimer's disease. II. Derangements in protein metabolism with special reference to tryptophan, tyrosine and cystine. *Acta Neurologica Scandinavica*, **79**, Suppl. 121, 27–42.

Glover, V., Sandler, H., Hughes, A., Hoffbrand, A. V. (1980). Platelet monoamine oxidase activity in megaloblastic anaemia. *Journal of Clinical Pathology*, **33**, 963–5.

Gottfries, C. G. (1988). Alzheimer's disease. A critical review. *Comprehensive Gerontology C*, **2**, 47–62.

Gottfries, C. G. and Roos, B. E. (1973). Acid monoamine metabolites in cerebrospinal fluid from patients with presenile dementia (Alzheimer's disease). *Acta Psychiatrica Scandinavica*, **49**, 257–63.

Gottfries, C. G., Gottfries, I., and Roos, B. E. (1969). Homovanillic acid 5-hydroxyindoleacetic acid in the cerebrospinal fluid of patients with senile dementia, presenile dementia and Parkinsonism. *Journal of Neurochemistry*, **16**, 1341–45.

Gottfries, C. G., Gottfries, I., Johansson, B., Olsson, R., Persson, T., Roos, B. E., and Sjöström, R. (1971). Acid monoamine metabolites in human cerebrospinal fluid and their relations to age and sex. *Neuropharmacology*, **10**, 665–72.

Gottfries, C. G., Roos, B. E., and Winblad, B. (1976). Monoamine and monoamine metabolites in the human brain post mortem in senile dementia. *Aktuelle Gerontologie*, **6**, 429–35.

Gottfries, C. G., Bartfai, T., Carlsson, A., Eckernäs, S. Å., and Svennerholm, L. (1986). Multiple biochemical deficits in both gray and white matter of Alzheimer brains. *Progress in Neuro-Psychopharmacology and Biological Psychiatry*, **10**, 405–13.

Gottfries, C. G., Adolfsson, R., Aquilonius, S. M., Carlsson, A., Eckernäs. S. Å., Nordberg, A., *et al.* (1983). Biochemical changes in dementia disorders of Alzheimer type (AD/SDAT). *Neurobiology of Aging*, **4**, 261–71.

Hardy, J., Adolfsson, R., Alafuzoff, I., Bucht, G., Marcusson, J., Nyberg, P., *et al.* (1985). Review. Transmitter deficits in Alzheimer's disease. Critiques: Gottfries, C. G., Rossor, M. N. and Yates, C. M. *Neurochemistry International*, **7**, 545–63.

Karlsson, I., Ekman, R., Gottfries, C. G., Wallin, A., and Widerlöv, E. (1988). Hypothalamic neuropeptide increase in Alzheimer dementia. *Psychopharmacology*, **96**, Suppl.

Mann, D. M. A. and Yates, P. O. (1983). Serotonin nerve cells in Alzheimer's disease. *Journal of Neurology, Neurosurgery and Psychiatry*, **46**, 96.

Marcusson, J., Alafuzoff, I., Bäckström, I. T., Ericson, E., Gottfries, C. G., and Winblad, B. (1987). 5-Hydroxytryptamine-sensitive [^{3}H]imipramine binding of protein nature in the human brain. II. Effect of normal aging and dementia disorders. *Brain Research*, **425**, 137–45.

Nagatsu, T. and Iizuka, R. (1989). Tyrosine hydroxylase, tryptophan hydroxylase, and the biopterin k-factor in the brains from patients with Alzheimer's disease. *Journal of Neural Transmission*, **1**, 21.

Nyth, A. L., Gottfries, C. G., Elgen, K., Engedal, K., Harenko, A., Juhela, P., *et al.* (1990). The clinical efficacy of citalopram in the treatment of emotional disturbances in dementia disorders. A Nordic multi-centre study. *British Journal of Psychiatry*, in press.

Oreland, L. and Gottfries, C. G. (1986). Platelet and brain monoamine oxidase in aging and in dementia of Alzheimer's type. *Progress in Neuro-Psychopharmacology and Biological Psychiatry*, **10**, 533–40.

Regland, B., Gottfries, C. G., Oreland, L., and Svennerholm, L. (1988). Low B_{12} levels related to high activity of platelet MAO in patients with dementia disorders. A retrospective study. *Acta Psychiatrica Scandinavica*, **78**, 451–57.

Regland, B., Gottfries, C. G., and Oreland, L. (1990). Vitamin B_{12} induced reduction of platelet MAO activity in patients with dementia and pernicious anaemia. *European Archives of Psychiatry and Neurological Sciences*, in press.

Thomas, D. R., Jones, E., Warner, N., Harris, B., Williams, P., and Bentley, P. (1988). Peripheral serotoninergic receptor sensitivity in senile dementia of the Alzheimer type. *Biological Psychiatry*, **23**, 136–40.

Wallin, A., Alafuzoff, I., Carlsson, A., Eckernäs, S. Å., Gottfries, C. G., Karlsson, I., *et al.* (1989). Neurotransmitter deficits in a non-multi-infarct category of vascular dementia. *Acta Neurologica Scandinavica*, **79**, 397–406.

Westenberg, H. G. and Verhoeven, W. M. (1988). CSF monoamine metabolites in patients and controls: support for a bimodal distribution in major affective disorders. *Acta Psychiatrica Scandinavica*, **78**, 541–9.

Widerlöv, E., Ekman, R., Jensen, L., Borglund, L. and Nyman, K. (1988). Arginine vasopressin, but not corticotropin releasing factor, is a potent stimulator of adrenocorticotropic hormone following electroconvulsive treatment. *Journal of Neurotransmission*, **75**, 101–9.

Discussion

LINNOILA: When you did dexamethasone suppression tests, did you measure the dexamethasone concentrations? It is imperative to do this before and after administration of a drug, because the drug might induce or inhibit the metabolism of dexamethasone.

GOTTFRIES: You mean that after a four-week treatment with citalopram there might be a higher dexamethasone concentration because the drug reduces its metabolism?

LINNOILA: With fluoxetine that would probably be the case because it is a strong cytochrome *P*-450 inhibitor in addition to being a 5-hydroxytryptamine (5-HT, serotonin) re-uptake inhibitor. I am not sure what the effect would be with citalopram.

Chronic administration of any highly specific re-uptake inhibitor always affects both noradrenaline and 5-HT. That happens in human cerebrospinal fluid (CSF), plasma, and urine. Thus, one does not have to invoke a direct noradrenergic effect.

The behavioural changes with citalopram are not surprising. What has been loosely called 'emotional lability' in patients with Alzheimer's disease may be a problem of impulse control, possibly secondary to reduced serotonergic functioning. A drug that increases serotonergic functioning would be expected to dampen irritability and increase appropriate responses to various stimuli.

GOTTFRIES: I agree, but the effect is important for the patients. When we evaluate demented patients we focus on cognitive impairment. This may be a bad strategy, because these patients, especially when they are admitted to hospital, are emotionally unstable. They are sensitive to stress; they feel bad; they do not have major depression but they have depressive symptoms. Improvement of these symptoms will benefit the patients greatly. I have tried to rename citalopram an emotional stabilizer rather than an antidepressant.

LINNOILA: I was not belittling the importance of the finding. I was trying to offer a possible mechanistic way of looking at it which could then be translated into clinical instruments to quantify the response more accurately.

OXENKRUG: You show that the dexamethasone suppression test correlates with all items on the Hamilton scale, except cognitive impairment, in both depressed and demented patients. When depressed patients recover the dexamethasone test results normalize and cognitive function improves, but in demented patients citalopram normalizes the dexamethasone test results but does not affect the cognitive impairment. Therefore, although both depressed patients and demented patients have an abnormal response to dexamethasone, I think that the mechanism of dexamethasone non-suppression is different in these disorders.

GOTTFRIES: The data do not support that idea. The question is whether there is a causal relationship between the cognitive impairment and the dysfunction of the hypothalamus. There is a statistically significant correlation between these functions; if the brain has deteriorated severely, the hypothalamic dysfunction is severe. But a causal relationship is not proven. My data indicate that the hypothalamic dysfunction may arise from a disturbance in a monoaminergic system which is perhaps not as important for the cognitive impairment.

OXENKRUG: Wolkowitz and Weingartner (1989) studied the effect of acute and chronic dexamethasone and prednisolone on cognitive function in healthy people. They showed specific cognitive impairment, similar to that described in Alzheimer's disease. Those results strongly suggest that elevation of cortisol could cause or contribute to the cognitive impairment in Alzheimer's dementia.

MELTZER: Was platelet imipramine binding studied in conjunction with the citalopram study? There is a subgroup of patients, particularly those with severe agitation and dementia, who have low platelet imipramine binding, which would agree with your post-mortem findings. Perhaps that subgroup would be particularly responsive to citalopram.

GOTTFRIES: We have not done that. Nor have we measured monoamine oxidase (MAO) activity in platelets. We have other findings indicating that a subgroup of patients with dementia with vitamin B_{12} deficiency have large immature platelets. These platelets have increased MAO activity. This subgroup should be identified before we make further platelet studies.

MENDLEWICZ: There is an early onset, familial genetic form of senile dementia of Alzheimer type (SDAT) with a major gene on chromosome 21. Have the biochemical or neurochemical differences between this type of dementia and the non-familial type been studied?

GOTTFRIES: In clinical practice familial and early onset dementias are sampled into one group—Alzheimer's disease (AD). There are several differences between this group and the group with late onset SDAT. There are more severe disturbances in neurotransmitters in the AD group than in the SDAT group (Iizuka and Arai 1989). We found that there are also differences in the symptomatology and white matter disturbance, as measured by computer-assisted tomography. It is therefore not correct to sample these groups together.

MENDLEWICZ: Are there changes in both cholinergic and serotonergic systems?

GOTTFRIES: Yes, Iizuka and Arai found differences in both systems.

CARLSSON: Could there be a close relationship between the improvement of emotional lability and the improvement of confusion with citalopram? There has been speculation that during a confusional episode there is an increased release of glutamic acid and that the neurotoxic action of this glutamic acid is an important trigger for progression of the disorder. If this is so, it might be interesting to see whether the process is slowed by treatment with citalopram.

GOTTFRIES: The GBS rating scale includes one variable covering confusion which is divided into seven parts. The effect of citalopram on confusion was unexpected. Another factor incorporating symptoms of depression and anxiety improved during citalopram treatment. An 'intellectual factor' did not change, but a factor including confusion, slow tempo, and symptoms of reduced attention also improved. I cannot say if these factors improved to the same extent. In early onset Alzheimer dementia there is no confusion at the beginning of the disorder, although it may be present later; in late onset dementia there is much confusion. According to findings at our institute, confusion and white matter low attenuation in computed tomography scans are related.

LINNOILA: The best correlation between intellectual decline and the concentration of a neuromodulator or transmitter, at least in CSF, is observed for somatostatin. Were any changes in somatostatin associated with the treatment?

GOTTFRIES: We measured somatostatin only in the hypothalamus, where we found increased concentrations, which is opposite to the findings in CSF. I agree that in cortical areas and in CSF decreased concentrations of somatostatin can be correlated with cognitive impairment.

MELTZER: Studies of treatment of SDAT with other tricyclic antidepressants were negative. Was this also the case with zimelidine? Is this an area like obsessive-compulsive disorder in which the specific serotonin uptake blockers appear to be more effective than the mixed agents?

GOTTFRIES: The tricyclics are ineffective because patients with dementia cannot tolerate these drugs at therapeutic doses. Zimelidine was found to have some effects on depressive symptoms in demented elderly patients, but confusion and anxiety were not studied as extensively as in our work.

COPPEN: The results of your four-week trial are impressive. In an antidepressant trial one sees quite small changes at four weeks—the big differences are seen in the one-year trials of placebo versus active medication. Have you done any long-term studies? How do you see the use of these drugs in the long-term management of these large numbers of patients?

GOTTFRIES: This treatment seems to be of benefit and I look forward to confirmation of the results by another group. However, it is not the dementia syndrome *per se* that is the target. This remains a treatment for some symptoms which possibly arise from disturbance of the 5-HT system in patients with Alzheimer's disease. Long-term treatment in an open study is in progress at our institute. Perhaps we should consider a double-blind long-term study.   .

MURPHY: Using *m*-chlorophenylpiperazine (*m*-CPP) challenges, our group has evidence of altered serotonergic system responsivity in patients with Alzheimer's disease (Lawlor *et al.* 1989*a*). These patients were behaviourally hyper-responsive to *m*-CPP; they became irritable and agitated, and some of them suffered unusual perceptional distortions, even hallucinations. This was not seen in age-matched controls. Given the findings with *m*-CPP in schizophrenia, perhaps this kind of hallucination or perceptual distortion is the product of some unrecognized brain damage in schizophrenic individuals.

Lawlor *et al.* (1989*b*) also used *m*-CPP to study the effect of age on serotonergic responses. There were no differences in neuroendocrine responses, temperature responses or peak plasma *m*-CPP levels, but anxiety and other behavioural responses were significantly less in the older controls. Decreased serotonin receptors in brain have been found in older rodents and humans, but the study by Lawlor *et al.* provides the first evidence of a change in serotonergic function in older individuals.

GOTTFRIES: The psychotic symptoms may arise from an over-activity. With demented patients one must be very careful with the doses. We intend to use combinations of citalopram and L-DOPA. If L-DOPA alone is given to these patients they get confused but a low dose of L-DOPA with citalopram may give improvement.

OXENKRUG: Were there more female than male patients in your sample?

GOTTFRIES: There were more women than men. There were about 60 patients with Alzheimer's and 30 with vascular dementia. According to our statistical analysis, the sex distribution does not influence the results.

YOUDIM: Have you used a combination of citalopram and a cholinergic drug or phyostigmine?

GOTTFRIES: We plan to look at that, but do we have a good cholinergic drug? I would first use a combination of citalopram and L-DOPA.

INSEL: In the post-mortem brain studies, was there a correlation between the decrease in 5-HT and the decrease in cholinergic markers? Or are there two different groups—one that is more likely to show the 5-HT deficit and one that is more likely to show a cholinergic deficit?

GOTTFRIES: I have no data on that.

CARLSSON: In an earlier study there was no correlation. We could sort out different profiles among the individuals; some were low in the cholinergic, others in the serotonergic system (Carlsson 1981).

GOTTFRIES: The sum of the lesions in the different systems was correlated to the level of dementia.

INSEL: What clinical pattern were the serotonin-deficient patients more likely to have?

CARLSSON: That was not studied.

INSEL: Have any animal studies shown that cholinergic lesions lead to a change in serotonin content in some of those areas that you are studying? Is there any reason to consider an interaction?

DEAKIN: We did that in rats. Nucleus basalis lesions had no effects on 5-hydroxyindoleacetic acid content in higher centres. But we did find some evidence for a 5-HT$_1$ binding site on cholinergic terminals (Cross and Deakin 1985).

PEROUTKA: 5-HT$_{1B}$ receptors modulate acetylcholine release: there is definitely an interaction between 5-HT and cholinergic systems.

References

Carlsson, A. (1981). Aging and brain neurotransmitters. In *Funktionsstörungen des Gehirns in Alter*, (ed. D. Platt), pp. 67–81. F. K. Schattauer Verlag, Stuttgart.

Cross, A. J. and Deakin, J. F. W. (1985). Cortical serotonin receptor subtypes after lesion of ascending cholinergic neurones in rat. *Neuroscience Letters*, **60**, 261–5.

Iizuka, R. and Arai, H. (1989). Neurotransmitter changes in Alzheimer type dementia and its therapeutic strategies. In *Abstracts: Alzheimer's and Parkinson's Diseases*, p. 56. Kyoto, Japan.

Lawlor, B. A., Sunderland, T., Mellow, A. M., Hill, J. L., Molchan, S. E., and Murphy, D. L. (1989a). Hyperresponsivity to the serotonin agonist m-chlorophenylpiperazine in Alzheimer's disease: a controlled study. *Archives of General Psychiatry*, **46**, 542–9.

Lawlor, B. A., Sunderland, T. Hill, J. L., Mellow, A. M., Molchan, S. E., Mueller, E. A. *et al.* (1989b). Evidence for a decline with age in behavioral responsivity to the serotonin agonist, m-chlorophenylpiperazine in healthy subjects. *Psychiatry Research*, **29**, 1–10.

Wolkowitz, O. M. and Weingartner, H. (1989). Defining cognitive changes in a depression and anxiety: a psychobiological analysis. *Psychiatrie and Psychobiologie*, **3**, 131S–138S.

23. 5-HT$_3$ receptor antagonists and their potential in psychiatric disorders

Michael G. Palfreyman, Stephen M. Sorensen, Albert A. Carr, Hsien C. Cheng, and Mark W. Dudley

Gaddum and Picarelli's (1957) classification of 5-hydroxytryptamine (5-HT, serotonin) receptors in the guinea pig ileum into 'D' receptors located on smooth muscle cells and those located on intramural cholinergic neurones of the myenteric plexus (M type) has been superseded by the classification into '5-HT$_1$-like', 5-HT$_2$, and 5-HT$_3$ by Bradley *et al.* (1986). Pharmacological analysis of the 5-HT$_2$ receptor suggested that it was identical to Gaddum's 'D' receptor. The 5-HT$_3$ receptor appears to be the acceptor component of a ligand-gated cation channel which bears comparison with the nicotinic acetylcholine-operated ion channel. Serotonergic activation causes a rapid depolarizing response associated with an increase in the membrane conductance to Na$^+$ and K$^+$ ions. Desensitization occurs rapidly, as shown by Derkach *et al.* (1989). The 5-HT$_3$ receptor was not identified in the central nervous system (CNS) until Kilpatrick *et al.* (1987) demonstrated binding of the selective 5-HT$_3$ antagonist [^{3}H]GR 65630 to various brain membrane preparations.

The explosion of interest in this receptor subtype and the plethora of new and very selective 5-HT$_3$ antagonists owe much of their origin to pioneer studies undertaken in the late 1970s by John R. Fozard (Fozard 1989), and then by Brian Richardson and his colleagues at Sandoz (Richardson and Buchheit 1988). Very few selective agonists are available. 2-Methyl-5-HT is a potent agonist at 5-HT$_3$ receptors, but it also has high affinity for 5-HT$_{1D}$ receptors and appreciable affinity for 5-HT$_{1A}$ and 5-HT$_{1C}$ sites (Fozard 1990). Phenylbiguanide, on the other hand, appears to be a much more selective 5-HT$_3$ agonist. In the rabbit heart preparation it has about 5 per cent of the potency of 5-HT but is a full agonist. The 5-HT$_3$ antagonist, MDL 73147, gave pA$_2$ values against 5-HT and phenylbiguanide of 9.9 and 9.8 respectively, with slope factors not significantly different from unity. However, phenylbiguanide does cause carrier-mediated release of dopamine from slices of rat caudate (Schmidt and Black 1989) which bodes caution in interpretation of its effects in intact tissues.

Radioligand-binding assays using a variety of tritiated 5-HT$_3$ antagonists to brain membranes or slices have been used to identify 5-HT$_3$ receptors in the

CNS. Of relevance to a potential therapeutic use of 5-HT$_3$ antagonists in psychiatric disorders is the demonstration by Waeber *et al.* (1989) of specific binding of [^{3}H]ICS 205-930 to a number of regions of human brain. Of particular note were high levels of binding in discrete nuclei of the lower brainstem, dense labelling of the substantia gelatinosa of the spinal cord, and low, but specific, binding in forebrain regions which was concentrated in parts of the limbic system. The area postrema was a binding 'hot spot' in human brain, as in other species, and doubtlessly forms the anatomical basis for part of the potent antiemetic activity of this class of 5-HT antagonist (Fozard 1989).

The euphoric component of many drugs of abuse is thought to involve activation of mesolimbic dopaminergic systems, and several studies have suggested that nicotine, morphine, amphetamines, and cocaine increase dopamine (DA) release in the nucleus accumbens. Dialysis and biochemical studies support this contention (Di Chiara *et al.* 1987) and show that the nicotine- and morphine-induced release of dopamine from the nucleus accumbens can be attenuated by pretreatment with the 5-HT$_3$ antagonists MDL 72222 and ICS 205-930 (Carboni *et al.* 1989*a*; Imperato and Angelucci 1989). Moreover, the drug-reinforcing properties of morphine and nicotine, determined in a place-preference procedure, were blocked in a dose-dependent manner by the aforementioned 5-HT$_3$ antagonists. In contrast, the reinforcing properties of amphetamines were *not* modified (Carboni *et al.* 1989*b*).

The initial observations by Costall and co-workers (1987) that very small doses of the 5-HT$_3$ antagonist GR 38032F injected into the nucleus accumbens (0.01–1 ng) or intraperitoneally (0.01–1 mg kg^{-1}) could block the hyperlocomotion induced by intra-accumbens injection of amphetamine or dopamine stimulated considerable interest in the possible antipsychotic activity of this class of antagonist. These 5-HT$_3$ antagonists are obviously 'atypical' in their pharmacological profiles as antipsychotics because they do not work in a wide variety of animal models that are used to screen for 'neuroleptics' (F. P. Miller, personal communication). It is interesting to note that two atypical antipsychotics, clozapine, and a close analogue, MDL 81582 (Young and Meltzer 1980), are antagonists of 5-HT$_3$ receptors in the rabbit heart preparation (pA$_2$ 7.6 and 7.3, respectively) and are both reasonably potent at antagonizing the suppressant action of the 5-HT$_3$ agonist, 2-methylserotonin, on firing of medial prefrontal cortical cells (Ashby *et al.* 1989; C. Ashby and R. Y. Wang, personal communication).

It is clear that 5-HT$_3$ antagonists have no acute effects on the basal release of dopamine, nor on the firing of dopamine neurones in the A9 or A10 cell body regions of the CNS under resting conditions (Koulu *et al.* 1989; Sorensen *et al.* 1989). However, 5-HT$_3$ antagonists do appear able to antagonize certain, but not all, activators of the limbic dopamine system when determined in biochemical or electrophysiological experiments.

Injection of the stable neurokinin analogue DiMe-C7 into the A10 region activates limbic dopaminergic systems and this activation can be attenuated, but not blocked, by systemic administration of a 5-HT$_3$ antagonist (Hagan *et al.* 1987). Likewise, nicotine, morphine or haloperidol activation of limbic dopamine pathways following systemic administration can be attenuated by 5-HT$_3$ antagonists (Carboni *et al.* 1989*a*), whereas activation by systemically administered amphetamine is not blocked. Taken together, these data imply that 5-HT$_3$ antagonists may decrease the activity of the limbic dopamine system under certain conditions of activation, possibly at a pre-synaptic site.

To test this hypothesis a number of experiments were conducted with the potent and highly selective 5-HT$_3$ antagonist MDL 73147EF (Gittos and Fatmi 1989). We have already shown that acute administration of MDL 73147EF was without effect on the firing rate of dopamine neurones in the substantia nigra and ventral tegmental area of anaesthetized rats but that chronic (21-day) administration significantly decreased the firing rates in both dopamine cell body regions, with the greatest effect in the A10 cell group (Sorensen *et al.* 1989). A similar dosing protocol was employed in biochemical experiments (Dudley *et al.* 1989). Acute administration of MDL 73147EF (5 mg kg^{-1} i.p.) did not affect the concentrations of dopamine, or its metabolites, in the striatum (Table 23.1). More strikingly, chronic pretreatment with MDL 73147EF (5 mg kg^{-1} i.p. × 21 days) or clozapine (10 mg kg^{-1} i.p. × 21 days) significantly enhanced the increase in striatal *and* nucleus accumbens DOPAC concentrations to a challenge dose of haloperidol (0.1 mg kg^{-1} i.p.). This was in marked contrast to the situation in haloperidol-pretreated animals (1.0 mg kg^{-1} i.p. × 21 days) where the challenge with haloperidol on the twenty-second day produced a markedly attenuated DOPAC elevation in the striatum (Table 23.1). In the accumbens, the haloperidol challenge elevated DOPAC levels in the haloperidol-pretreated animals, but not to the extent seen in the MDL 73147EF- or clozapine-pretreated animals (Table 23.1). As expected, chronic treatment with haloperidol increased the number of DA$_2$ receptors (as measured with [^{3}H]spiroperidol) in the striatum from 981 ± 21 to 1400 ± 33 fmol per mg protein, whereas MDL 73147EF and clozapine treatment were without effect (977 ± 34 and 924 ± 32 fmol per mg protein, respectively).

By inhibiting cell firing in the nigrostriatal pathway with γ-aminobutyrolactone (GBL) it is possible to study the pre-synaptic effects of apomorphine (Walters and Roth 1976). In rats pretreated with GBL (750 mg kg^{-1}) and the decarboxylase inhibitor NSD 1015 (100 mg kg^{-1}), apomorphine produced a dose-related suppression of the striatal DOPA content. In rats pretreated with haloperidol (1.0 mg kg^{-1} i.p. × 21 days) the DOPA-suppressing effect of apomorphine was accentuated, an effect not seen following chronic MDL 73147EF (5 mg kg^{-1}) or clozapine (10 mg kg^{-1}). Therefore, the enhanced response to haloperidol following chronic MDL 73147EF or clozapine does

TABLE 23.1. *Effect of acute and chronic treatment with MDL 73147EF, clozapine, and haloperidol on rat striatal and accumbens dopamine metabolism*

Treatment		DOPAC concentration	
		Striatum (μg per g tissue)	Accumbens (ng per mg protein)
A. Single Dose			
Saline		2.80 ± 0.15	36.4 ± 2.1
MDL 73147EF		2.15 ± 0.18	48.4 ± 3.1
Clozapine		2.46 ± 0.10	43.5 ± 4.4
Haloperidol		$5.35 \pm 0.18^*$	$109.2 \pm 12.0^*$
B. Multiple dose			
Days 1–21	*Day 22*		
Saline	Saline	2.80 ± 0.15	31.6 ± 1.9
Saline	Haloperidol	$4.18 \pm 0.21^*$	$41.2 \pm 4.3^*$
Haloperidol	Saline	2.43 ± 0.15	31.3 ± 2.7
Haloperidol	Haloperidol	2.87 ± 0.21	$43.4 \pm 3.5^*$
MDL 73147EF	Saline	2.93 ± 0.11	36.5 ± 7.8
MDL 73147EF	Haloperidol	$5.46 \pm 0.45^{*\dagger}$	$52.7 \pm 5.2^{*\dagger}$
Clozapine	Saline	2.33 ± 0.29	35.3 ± 3.1
Clozapine	Haloperidol	$5.59 \pm 0.62^{*\dagger}$	$59.1 \pm 3.8^{*\dagger}$

* $p < 0.05$ vs saline.
† $p < 0.05$ vs haloperidol (Day 22).
Rats were killed 1 h after last treatment. Animals received MDL 73147EF (5 mg kg^{-1} i.p.), clozapine (10 mg kg^{-1} i.p.) or haloperidol (1 mg kg^{-1} i.p.) in the acute study and on Days 1–21 of the multiple dose study. A challenge dose of haloperidol (0.1 mg kg^{-1} i.p.) was given on Day 22 in the latter study. Values are mean $\pm$ S.E.M., $n = 8$–12.

not appear to reflect a change in sensitivity of the pre-synaptic dopamine autoreceptor or the post-synaptic DA$_2$ receptor. Taken together these data suggest that MDL 73147EF interacts with the limbic and striatal dopaminergic systems in a manner similar to clozapine and different from haloperidol. Further work will be needed to unravel the molecular and neuronal basis for these interactions.

5-HT$_3$ antagonists with high potency and exceptional selectivity are now available (Fig. 23.1). Considerable preclinical evidence suggests that they may have efficacy in anxiety, drug abuse, and schizophrenia. To date, no clinical data related to these indications have been reported, even though their therapeutic efficacy against chemotherapy and radiotherapy-induced nausea and vomiting has been demonstrated in numerous clinical studies. So far no obvious side-effects in the CNS have been reported. Since 5-HT$_3$ receptors are unquestionably present in the CNS and potent and safe

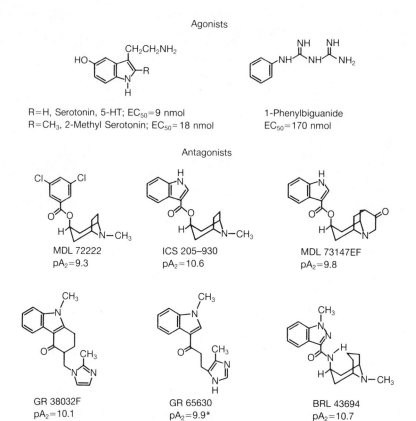

FIG. 23.1. 5-HT$_3$ agonists and antagonists. EC$_{50}$ and pA$_2$ values were obtained from the rabbit heart preparation (Fozard 1989*b*; H. C. Cheng and M. G. Palfreyman, unpublished), except * where pA$_2$ was obtained in isolated rat vagus (Kilpatrick *et al.* 1987).

antagonists are available, it will be of great interest to see what evolves from future clinical evaluation of this important new class of serotonin antagonists.

References

Ashby, C. R., Jr., Edwards, E., Harkins, K. L., and Wang, R. Y. (1989). Differential effect of typical and atypical antipsychotic drugs on the suppressant action of 2-methylserotonin on medical prefrontal cortical cells: a microiontophoretic study. *European Journal of Pharmacology*, **166**, 583–4.

Bradley, P. B., Engel, G., Feniuk, W., Fozard, J. R., Humphrey, P. B. A., Middlemiss, D. N., *et al.* (1986). Proposals for the classification and nomenclature of functional receptors for 5-hydroxytryptamine. *Neuropharmacology*, **25**, 563–76.

Carboni, E., Acquas, E., Frau, R., and Di Chiara, G. (1989*a*). Differential inhibitory effects of a 5-HT₃ antagonist on drug-induced stimulation of dopamine release. *European Journal of Pharmacology*, **164**, 515–9.

Carboni, E., Acquas, E., Leone, P., and Di Chiara, G. (1989*b*). 5-HT₃ receptor antagonists block morphine- and nicotine- but not amphetamine-induced reward. *Psychopharmacology*, **97**, 175–8.

Costall, B., Domeney, A. M., Naylor, R. J., and Tyers, M. B. (1987). Effects of the 5-HT₃ receptor antagonist, GR 38032F, on raised dopaminergic activity in the mesolimbic system of the rat and marmoset brain. *British Journal of Pharmacology*, **92**, 881–94.

Derkach, V., Surprenant, A., and North, R. A. (1989). 5-HT₃ receptors are membrane ion channels. *Nature*, **339**, 706–9.

Di Chiara, G., Imperato, A., and Saint-Marc, M. (1987). Preferential stimulation of dopamine release in the mesolimbic system: a common feature of drugs of abuse. In *Neurotransmitter interaction in the basal ganglia*, (ed. M. Sandler, C. Feuerstein, and B. Scatton), pp. 171–82. Raven Press, New York.

Dudley, M., Sorensen, S., and Ogden, A. (1989). The 5-HT₃ antagonist MDL 73,147 resembles clozapine, not haloperidol, in its effect on DA autoreceptor supersensitivity in rat striatum. *Society for Neuroscience*, **15**, 6.10 (Abstract).

Fozard, J. R. (1989). The development and early clinical evaluation of selective 5-HT₃ receptor antagonists. In *The peripheral actions of 5-hydroxytryptamine*, (ed. J. R. Fozard), pp. 354–76. Oxford University Press.

Fozard, J. R. (1990). Agonists and antagonists of 5-HT₃ receptors. In *Cardiovascular pharmacology of 5-hydroxytryptamine*, (ed. P. R. Saxena, D. I. Wallis, W. Wouters, and P. Bevang), pp. 101–15. Kluwer, Dordrecht.

Gaddum, J. H. and Picarelli, Z. P. (1957). Two kinds of tryptamine receptors. *British Journal of Pharmacology*, **12**, 323–8.

Gittos, M. W. and Fatmi, M. (1989). Potent 5-HT₃ antagonists incorporating a novel bridged pseudopelletierine ring system. *Actualite Chimie Therapeutiques*, **16**, 187–98.

Hagan, R. M., Butler, A., Hill, J. M., Jordan, C. C., Ireland, S. J., and Tyers, M. B. (1987). Effect of the 5-HT₃ receptor antagonist, GR 38032F, or responses to injection of a neurokinin agonist into the ventral tegmental area of the rat brain. *European Journal of Pharmacology*, **138**, 303–5.

Imperato, A. and Angelucci, L. (1989). 5-HT₃ receptors control dopamine release in the nucleus accumbens of freely moving rats. *Neuroscience Letters*, **101**, 214–7.

Kilpatrick, G. J., Jones, B. J., and Tyers, M. B. (1987). Identification and distribution of 5-HT₃ receptors in rat brain using radioligand binding. *Nature*, **330**, 746–8.

Koulu, M., Sjöholm, B., Lappolainen, J., and Virtanen, R. (1989). Effects of acute GR 38032F (Odansetron), a 5-HT₃ receptor antagonist, on dopamine and serotonin metabolism in mesolimbic and nigrostriatal dopaminergic neurons. *European Journal of Pharmacology*, **169**, 321–4.

Richardson, B. P. and Buchheit, K. H. (1988). The pharmacology, distribution and function of 5-HT₃ receptors. In *Neuronal serotonin*, (ed. N. N. Osborne and M. Hamon), pp. 465–504. Wiley, Chichester.

Schmidt, C. J. and Black, C. K. (1989). The putative 5-HT₃ agonist phenylbiguanide induces carrier-mediated release of [³H]dopamine. *European Journal of Pharmacology*, **167**, 309–10.

Sorensen, S. M., Humphreys, T. M., and Palfreyman, M. G. (1989). Effect of acute and chronic MDL 73,147EF, a 5-HT₃ receptor antagonist, on A9 and A10 dopamine neurons. *European Journal of Pharmacology*, **163**, 115–18.

Waeber. C., Hoyer, D., and Palacios, J. M. (1989). 5-Hydroxytryptamine$_3$ receptors in the human brain: autoradiographic visualization using[^{3}H]ICS 205–930. *Neuroscience*, **31**, 393–400.

Walters, J. R. and Roth, R. H. (1976). Dopaminergic neurons: an *in vivo* system for measuring drug interactions with presynaptic receptors. *Naunyn-Schmiedeberg's Archives of Pharmacology*, **296**, 5–14.

Young, M. A. and Meltzer, H. Y. (1980). RMI-81,582, a novel antipsychotic drug. *Psychopharmacology*, **67**, 101–6.

24. Atypical antipsychotic drugs: the 5-HT$_2$/DA$_2$ ratio

Herbert Y. Meltzer

There has been considerable interest in clozapine, an atypical antipsychotic drug which has not been reported to produce tardive dyskinesia, produces fewer extrapyramidal symptoms, and is a more effective antipsychotic drug in decreasing positive and negative symptoms than any of the typical neuroleptic drugs (Meltzer 1989*b*). Clozapine has been reported to have superior efficacy in treatment-resistant schizophrenia as well as typical schizophrenia (Kane *et al.* 1988; Claghorn *et al.* 1987). Along with those benefits, it also does not produce serum prolactin elevations in man (Meltzer *et al.* 1979).

A common mechanism may explain the many clinical differences between clozapine and typical antipsychotic drugs. It has been proposed that clozapine produces depolarization inactivation of the dopamine (DA) neurones in the striatum but not the nucleus accumbens (Chiodo and Bunney 1983). The ability of clozapine to block DA$_2$ receptors *in vitro* is in accord with its clinical potency (Seeman and Lee 1975), which suggests that DA$_2$ receptor blockade is not involved in its clinical advantages. However, Fardé *et al.* (1988) suggested that in man clinically effective doses of clozapine occupy fewer DA$_2$ receptors in the basal ganglia than typical antipsychotic drugs. Subsequently, Fardé *et al.* (1989) indicated that clozapine occupies more DA$_1$ receptors in the basal ganglia than typical antipsychotic drugs. This suggests that relative effects at the DA$_1$ versus the DA$_2$ receptor may be important. The DA$_1$ receptor-blocking effects of clozapine were also emphasized by Andersen and Braestrup (1986). The 5-HT$_3$ agonist effects of clozapine were also suggested to be important (Ashby *et al.* 1989).

We have proposed that the ability of clozapine to block serotonin$_2$ (5-HT$_2$) receptors or possibly to promote the indirect stimulation of 5-HT$_{1A}$ receptors may be important factors in its action (Meltzer 1989*a*). There is much evidence that clozapine *in vivo* produces significant 5-HT$_2$ receptor blockade. Early studies did not examine selective effects of clozapine on 5-HT receptor subtypes, but more recent studies have done so. Drescher and Hetey (1988) reported that *in vivo* clozapine enhances 5-HT release at the nerve terminal autoreceptor in the rat nucleus accumbens. We have shown that *in vitro* and *in vivo* it can function as a potent 5-HT$_2$ antagonist (Meltzer 1989*b*). In rats, temperature and neuroendocrine studies demonstrate *in vivo* 5-HT$_2$ antagonism by clozapine (Nash *et al*. 1988). Chronic schizophrenic patients treated with clozapine compared to untreated schizophrenic patients and patients treated with typical neuroleptics (including those treated with chlorpromazine, which *in vitro* is a potent 5-HT$_2$ antagonist) had a decreased cortisol response to 5-HT agonists such as 5-hydroxytryptophan and MK 212. Clozapine markedly increases human platelet 5-HT$_2$ receptors (R. C. Arora and H. Y. Meltzer, unpublished data), although in rodent brain it is a very potent 5-HT$_2$ down-regulator in the frontal cortex (Matsubara *et al*. 1989).

To further clarify the relative importance of DA$_1$ and DA$_2$ versus 5-HT$_2$ receptor-blocking properties of clozapine, we compared the pK$_1$ values of ten typical and seven atypical antipsychotic drugs on these parameters using membranes from rat striatum for DA$_1$ and DA$_2$ and cortex for 5-HT$_2$ binding (Meltzer *et al*. 1989). We were able to develop a discriminant function which clearly separated the typical from the atypical drugs. The DA$_2$ affinity and, to a lesser extent, the 5-HT$_2$ affinity served to discriminate the typical from the atypical antipsychotic compounds. The typical antipsychotic compounds are much more potent DA$_2$ antagonists than they are 5-HT$_2$ antagonists. The critical factor in the model proved to be the ratio of the DA$_2$ to the 5-HT$_2$ affinities, which was significantly higher in the atypical compounds. We confirmed this model in another group of 20 antipsychotic drugs (Meltzer *et al*. 1989). We also noted a striking correlation between the *in vitro* 5-HT$_2$ and DA$_2$ affinities in this group of atypical compounds. We are collecting *in vivo* binding data to see if this differentiation will hold up. It may be possible to predict the atypical nature of a putative antipsychotic drug by virtue of its DA$_2$ and 5-HT$_2$ affinities (Meltzer *et al*. 1989).

Palfreyman *et al*. (this volume) suggest that the action of clozapine at 5-HT$_3$ receptors may be important. There is not enough data on the effect of other atypicals at 5-HT$_3$ receptors to know whether that characteristic is shared by other atypical compounds. A crucial characteristic of clozapine is its many neurochemical effects. A good way to determine which of these effects are important is to compare the compounds that appear to be clozapine-like clinically and see what characteristics they share. This is how Arvid Carlsson identified the relevance of DA$_2$ antagonism to the action of the typical neuroleptic drugs. The 5-HT$_2$ antagonism may be relevant to the decreased frontal cortical activity that is thought to be relevant to negative symptoms in schizophrenia. There is evidence for hypofrontality in schizophrenia from a variety of brain-imaging techniques. It appears that 5-HT$_2$ antagonism is important to metabolic activity and blood flow in the frontal cortex, such that 5-HT$_2$ agonists can enhance the electrical activity of prefrontal cortical neurones (Ashby and Wang 1990).

Clozapine has been shown by several groups, for example Drescher and Hetey (1988), using synaptosomes, and Compton and Johnson (1989), using slices, to enhance DA or 5-HT release, apparently by one or both of the following mechanisms: (a) by blocking DA autoreceptors; and (b) by blocking DA or 5-HT heteroreceptors on 5-HT and DA neurones that inhibit 5-HT or DA release. In this manner, clozapine could enhance the synaptic levels of 5-HT and DA, at least in some areas. Clozapine has been shown to increase DA release in frontal cortex (Imperato and Angelucci 1988) as well as in striatum and nucleus accumbens (Ichikawa and Meltzer 1990) by use of *in vivo* microdialysis in freely moving rats. Studies are under way in our laboratory to determine the effect of clozapine on 5-HT release in striatum and motor cortex. At the same time that it enhances DA and 5-HT release, clozapine blocks the post-synaptic DA_1, DA_2, and $5\text{-}HT_2$ receptors. It also up-regulates DA_1 receptors and down-regulates $5\text{-}HT_2$ receptors. Under these circumstances, there is every reason to expect clozapine could increase the stimulation of post-synaptic $5\text{-}HT_{1A}$ receptors as well as other pre- and post-synaptic 5-HT receptors. It may also increase DA_1 receptor stimulation. Thus, the $5\text{-}HT_2/5\text{-}HT_{1A}$, as well as the $5\text{-}HT_2/DA_2$ balance, may be relevant to the action of clozapine and perhaps some aspects of schizophrenia.

In summary, it appears that 5-HT may be of major importance to the action of atypical antipsychotic drugs via a variety of mechanisms. This further supports a role of 5-HT in schizophrenia and other psychotic illnesses (Meltzer 1989*a*).

Acknowledgements

The research reported here was supported in part by USPHS MH 41684, MH 41594, GGRC MO1RR0080, and grants from the Cleveland Foundation, The John Pascal Sawyer Memorial Foundation, and NARSAD. H. Y. M. is the recipient of a USPHS Research Scientist Award MH 47808.

References

Andersen, P. H. and Braestrup, C. (1986). Evidence for different states of the dopamine D1 receptor: clozapine and fluperlapine may preferentially label an adenylate cyclase-coupled state of the D1 receptor. *Journal of Neurochemistry*, **47**, 1830–1.

Ashby, C. R. and Wang, R. Y. (1990). Effect of antipsychotic drugs on $5\text{-}HT_2$ receptors in the medial prefrontal cortex: microiontophoretic studies. *Brain Research*, **506**, 346–8.

Ashby, C. R., Edwards, E., Harkins, K. L., and Wang, R. Y. (1989). Differential effect of typical and atypical antipsychotic drugs on the suppressant action of 2-methylserotonin on medial prefrontal cortical cells: a microiontophoretic study. *European Journal of Pharmacology*, **166**, 583–4.

Chiodo, L. A. and Bunney, B. S. (1983). Typical and atypical neuroleptics: differential effects of chronic administration on the activity of A9 and A10 midbrain dopaminergic neurons. *Journal of Neuroscience*, **3**, 1607–9.

Claghorn, J., Honigfeld, G., Abuzzahab, F. S., Wang, R., Steinbook, R., Tuason, V., and Klerman, G. (1987). The risks and benefits of clozapine versus chlorpromazine. *Journal of Clinical Psychopharmacology*, **7**, 377–84.

Compton, D. R. and Johnson, K. M. (1989). Effects of acute and chronic clozapine and haloperidol on *in vitro* release of acetylcholine and dopamine from striatum and nucleus accumbens. *Journal of Pharmacology and Experimental Therapeutics*, **248**, 521–30.

Drescher, K. and Hetey, L. (1988). Influence of antipsychotics and serotonin antagonists on presynaptic receptors modulating the release of serotonin in synaptosomes of the nucleus accumbens of rats. *Neuropharmacology*, **27**, 31–6.

Fardé, L., Wiesel, F.-A., Halldin, C., and Sedvall, G. (1988). Central D2-dopamine receptor occupancy in schizophrenic patients treated with antipsychotic drugs. *Archives of General Psychiatry*, **45**, 71–6.

Fardé, L., Wiesel, F.-A., Nordstrom, A.-L., and Sedvall, G. (1989). D1- and D2-dopamine receptor occupancy during treatment with conventional and atypical neuroleptics. *Psychopharmacology*, **99**, S28–S31.

Ichikawa, J. and Meltzer, H.Y. (1990). Differential effects of repeated treatment with clozapine and haloperidol on DA release and metabolism in rat striatum and nucleus accumbens in freely moving rats studied by microdialysis. *European Journal of Pharmacology*, **176**, 371–4.

Imperato, A. and Angelucci, L. (1988). Effects of the atypical neuroleptics clozapine and fluperlapine on the *in vivo* DA-release in the dorsal striatum and in the prefrontal cortex. *Psychopharmacology*, Suppl. **96**, 79.

Kane, J., Honigfeld, G., Singer, J., Meltzer, H. Y. and the Clozaril Collaborative Study Group (1988). Clozapine for the treatment-resistant schizophrenic: a double-blind comparison with chlorpromazine. *Archives of General Psychiatry*, **45**, 789–96.

Matsubara, S. and Meltzer, H. Y. (1989). Effect of typical and atypical antipsychotic drugs on 5-HT$_2$ receptor density in rat cerebral cortex. *Life Sciences*, **45**, 1397–406.

Meltzer, H. Y. (1989*a*). Clinical studies on the mechanism of action of clozapine: the dopamine-serotonin hypothesis of schizophrenia. *Psychopharmacology*, **99**, S13–S17.

Meltzer, H. Y. (1989*b*). Clozapine: clinical advantages and biological mechanisms. In *Schizophrenia: scientific progress*, (ed. S. C. Schulz and C. A. Tamminga), pp. 302–9. Oxford University Press.

Meltzer, H. Y., Goode, D. J., Schyve, P. M., Young, M., and Fang, V. S. (1979). Effect of clozapine on human serum prolactin levels. *American Journal of Psychiatry*, **136**, 1550–5.

Meltzer, H. Y., Matsubara, S., and Lee, J. C. (1989). Classification of typical and atypical antipsychotic drugs on the basis of Dopamine D-1, D-2 and serotonin$_2$ pK$_1$ values. *Journal of Pharmacology and Experimental Therapeutics*, **251**, 238–46.

Nash, J. F., Jr., Meltzer, H. Y., and Gudelsky, G. A. (1988). Antagonism of serotonin receptor mediated neuroendocrine and temperature responses by typical neuroleptics in the rat. *European Journal of Pharmacology*, **151**, 463–9.

Palfreyman, M. G., Sorenson, S. M., Carr, A. A., Cheng, H. C., and Dudley, M. W. (1991). 5-HT$_3$ receptor antagonists and their potential in psychiatric disorders. In *5-Hydroxytryptamine in psychiatry: a spectrum of ideas*, (ed. M. Sandler, A. Coppen, and S. Harnett), pp. 324–330. Oxford University Press.

Seeman, P. and Lee, T. (1975). Antipsychotic drugs: direct correlation between clinical potency and presynaptic action on dopamine neurons. *Science*, **188**, 1217–19.

Discussion

BRILEY: Blockade of 5-HT_{1A} autoreceptors has been proposed as a way of getting antidepressant drugs. Has clozapine any antidepressant activity?

MELTZER: We treated a few people who had psychotic depression and tardive dyskinesia with clozapine. The depression cleared up along with the tardive dyskinesia. But there are no controlled studies of clozapine as an antidepressant.

DEAKIN: What is the incidence of post-psychotic depression in the trials of clozapine in schizophrenia?

MELTZER: One most often sees a brightening of mood with clozapine. Depression can occur, however. The improvement in negative symptoms influences the outcome. It is often difficult to sort out depression from negative symptoms.

LINNOILA: Sven Ove Ogren at the Karolinska Institute has evidence that in the relevant concentration range clozapine is also a serotonin re-uptake inhibitor. Is that simply an artefact of autoreceptor blockade?

MELTZER: Not knowing his methodology, I cannot comment on that. But such a finding would certainly be consistent with my suggestion that making serotonin available is important.

PALFREYMAN: Your cluster analysis of 5-HT_2 versus DA_2 affinities is a useful approach. Have you tried to do the same with 5-HT_{1C} versus DA_2 effects?

MELTZER: That did not work as well as the 5-HT_2 blockade, but I would like to see more 5-HT_{1C} data.

COWEN: We have also shown changes in platelet 5-HT_2 receptor binding in patients receiving fluphenazine and flupenthixol (Schachter *et al.* 1985). This implies that these drugs also block 5-HT_2 receptors, at least in the platelet.

MELTZER: We saw that also with the typical antipsychotic drugs, but not to the same extent as with clozapine; a 25–35 per cent increase occurred with the typical drugs versus almost a doubling with clozapine.

Reference

Schachter, M., Geaney, D. P., Grahame-Smith, D. G., Cowen, P. J., and Elliott, J. M. (1985). Increased platelet membrane [^{3}H]-LSD binding in patients on chronic neuroleptic treatment. *British Journal of Clinical Pharmacology*, **19**, 453–7.

25. Summary

Arvid Carlsson

The theme of this volume goes back to Alec Coppens's pioneering work 30 years ago. It must be gratifying for him to witness the events of the past decade that have confirmed his work and the views he expressed on the role of serotonin (5-hydroxytryptamine, 5-HT) in affective disorders.

We began with overviews of pre- and post-synaptic aspects of the serotonergic system (Peroutka and Schmidt; Murphy, this volume) which emphasized its complexity and heterogeneity. This complexity is to be expected, given that the serotonergic system is phylogenetically probably the oldest of the monoaminergic systems. We must talk now about receptor families rather than subtypes. There is also considerable heterogeneity at the pre-synaptic level; the nerve fibres that terminate in the hypothalamus, for example, have much coarser varicosities than those terminating in the cerebral cortex. This has consequences for sensitivity and for vulnerability to neurotoxins.

In 1968 I proposed that the hypothalamic and the cortical cerebral systems antagonize each other, and that this might account for some pharmacological discrepancies that are still unresolved (Carlsson 1968). For example, Jouvet (1968) showed that treatment with p-chlorophenylalanine (p-CPA) or destruction of the raphe system leads to insomnia. On the other hand, stimulation of the serotonergic system leads to an arousal reaction. It is possible that there are two antagonistic systems—a hypothalamic one which favours sleep, and a cerebral system, which favours arousal (Carlsson *et al.* 1980). The finding that slow-wave sleep is increased when 5-HT$_2$ receptors in the cerebral cortex are blocked supports this idea.

In future, interaction between molecular biology and medicinal chemistry will lead to further differentiation and characterization of the serotonin receptor families. We shall obtain more selective tools. However, perhaps we shall not pay equal attention to each of the receptor subtypes. Evolution does not result from careful planning; not everything occurring in our brains is likely to be functionally relevant. We run the risk of spending a lifetime on some redundant vestige. We should work on the systems that are essential for our survival and we may have to be more critical about the importance of various receptors and mechanisms in the brain. We must do the crucial experiments to demonstrate the functional consequences of eliminating a certain mechanism. For example, if serotonin is removed from the brain there are some, albeit undramatic, behavioural changes, such as increased irritability and reduced pain threshold.

We should like to have specific receptor antagonists to see what functional deficit occurs when we block a particular receptor. We have no good specific and potent antagonists for 5-HT$_{1A}$ receptors. Ritanserin was thought to be a reasonably specific 5-HT$_2$ receptor antagonist, but now we hear that it blocks 5-HT$_{1C}$ receptors. However, 5-HT$_{1C}$ receptors are in the 5-HT$_2$ family. Jose Leysen (personal communication) thinks that the behavioural consequences of blocking these receptors with ritanserin are so subtle that there is not likely to be any impressive tonic stimulation on the 5-HT$_2$ receptors. Are these receptors relevant behaviourally? They might even be working against us. Paul Janssen tells us that ritanserin increases the quality of sleep in healthy people. This implies that we can benefit from blocking 5-HT$_2$ receptors. This improvement in sleep might explain the alleged effect of ritanserin on dysthymia. We should consider such things more seriously.

However, we are just at the beginning. In future there might be many findings that demonstrate the necessity of 5-HT$_2$ receptors for brain function and survival. It is becoming increasingly clear that interactions between receptors can have dramatic consequences, even when manipulation of a particular receptor alone does not have a marked effect. We should investigate this further.

To the list of clinical aspects of 5-HT we should now add obsessive-compulsive disorder, which is a highly specific disorder (Insel, this volume). Curzon (this volume) has shown that we must also pay more attention to appetite disorders. I am pleased that schizophrenia has also entered this area. It does not matter on which of these disturbances or neurotransmitters we focus; in each case, each of the major transmitters is involved. I wonder whether 5-HT$_{1A}$ agonists should be investigated in relation to schizophrenia, especially in view of the findings that the 5-HT uptake inhibitors may be anticonfusional (Gottfries, this volume). In pharmacology almost every agent that is anticonfusional is also antipsychotic. Compounds that induce psychosis and confusion are similarly linked. Work on schizophrenia will be important in future.

Important information has been presented on affective disorders, suicidal behaviour, aggressiveness, impulsivity, sexual dysfunction, anxiety disorders, panic disorders, ageing, and dementias. The evidence that serotonin is involved fundamentally in these is very compelling. For basic research as well as clinically the advent of the selective serotonin uptake inhibitors has been a significant advance. We must discover which receptor is involved. It is clear that these uptake inhibitors are indirect agonists. Thus, we must look for agonists on one or more of the 5-HT receptors. As we have heard, apart from at the 5-HT$_1$ receptor, it is antagonists that are being discussed as therapeutic agents. The progression from 5-HT uptake inhibitors to 5-HT$_{1A}$ receptor agonists was a logical one. I have been engaged in this development, starting with the tricyclics where we found that not only noradrenaline uptake but also serotonin uptake is inhibited. We found that clomipramine was especially active on the serotonin system. From there we went to zimelidine and found its antidepressant actions (for review, see Carlsson 1981). We developed 8-hydroxy-*N*,*N*-dipropyl-2-aminotetralin (8-OH-DPAT), a very potent serotonergic agonist (for review and discussion, see Hjorth *et al.* 1987; Carlsson 1987). When buspirone was developed as a dopaminergic agonist, we found that it is a serotonergic agonist (Hjorth and Carlsson 1982). This has made our group very interested in the serotonergic system, especially the 5-HT$_{1A}$ receptors.

What problems are we facing? There are many elusive matters. For example, in feeding and sexual behaviour we have a discrepancy between the actions of 5-hydroxytryptophan and 5-HT$_{1A}$ receptor agonists (Curzon, this volume). We could be dealing either with an autoreceptor agonist or action at the post-synaptic level when the partial agonist becomes an antagonist at certain synaptic sites. It is difficult to analyse that but this area is extremely important for the further development of this subject.

This field of research sprang out of pharmacology several decades ago and has initiated much work in biological psychiatry to discover biochemical disturbances in various mental disorders. We have heard of post-mortem brain studies, neuroendocrine strategies, and the work on platelet serotonin. Here we face problems that are even more difficult than the pharmacological issues which we have discussed. Nevertheless, progress has been made, especially in the area of affective disorders and geriatrics. We have reason to hope that ultimately the biochemical lesions underlying the various forms of mental illness will be precisely defined.

References

Carlsson, A. (1968). Reporter's remarks. In *Advances in Pharmacology*, Vol. 6, Part B, pp. 115–22. Academic Press, New York.

Carlsson, A. (1981). Some current problems related to the mode of action of antidepressant drugs. *Acta Psychiatrica Scandinavica*, Suppl. 290, **63**, 63–6.

Carlsson, A. (1987). Introduction. In *Brain 5-HT-1A receptors*, (ed. C. T. Dourish, S. Ahlenius, and P. H. Hutson), pp. 15–18. Ellis Horwood, Chichester.

Carlsson, A., Svennerholm, L., and Winblad, B. (1980). Seasonal and circadian monoamine variations in human brains examined post mortem. *Acta Psychiatrica Scandinavica*, Suppl. 280, **61**, 75–82.

Curzon, G. (1991). 5-Hydroxytryptamine in the control of feeding and its possible implications for appetite disturbance. In *5-Hydroxytryptamine in psychiatry: a spectrum of ideas*, (ed. M. Sandler, A. Coppen, and S. Harnett), pp. 279–302. Oxford University Press.

Gottfries, C. G. (1991). Disturbance of the 5-hydroxytryptamine metabolism in ageing and in Alzheimer's and vascular dementias. In *5-Hydroxytryptamine in psychiatry: a spectrum of ideas*, (ed. M. Sandler, A. Coppen, and S. Harnett), pp. 310–323. Oxford University Press.

Hjorth, S., Carlsson, A., Magnusson, T., and Arvidsson, L.-E. (1987). In vivo biochemical characterization of 8-OH-DPAT: evidence of 5-HT receptor selectivity and agonist action in the rat CNS. In *Brain 5-HT-1A receptors*, (ed. C. T. Dourish, S. Ahlenius, and P. H. Hutson), pp. 94–105. Ellis Horwood, Chichester.

Insel, T. R. (1991). Serotonin in obsessive-compulsive disorder: a causal connection or more monomania about a major monoamine? In *5-Hydroxytryptamine: a spectrum of ideas*, (ed. M. Sandler, A. Coppen, and S. Harnett), pp. 228–257. Oxford University Press.

Jouvet, M. (1968). Insomnia and decrease of cerebral 5-hydroxytryptamine after destruction of the raphe system in the cat. In *Advances in Pharmacology*, Vol. 6, Part B, pp. 265–79. Academic Press, New York.

Murphy, D. L. (1991). An overview of serotonin neurochemistry and neuroanatomy. In *5-Hydroxytryptamine in psychiatry: a spectrum of ideas*, (ed. M. Sandler, A. Coppen, and S. Harnett), pp. 23–36. Oxford University Press.

Peroutka, S. J. and Schmidt, A. W. (1991). An overview of 5-hydroxytryptamine receptor families. In *5-Hydroxytryptamine in psychiatry: a spectrum of ideas*, (ed. M. Sandler, A. Coppen, and S. Harnett), pp. 2–22. Oxford University Press.

Index

effects of chronic treatment with 148, 150
(*table*)
corticotropin-releasing hormone (factor) 129,
213, 272, 316
cortisol 60, 125, 128–9, 132
psychosocial difficulties, effect on 148
response to fenfluramine in suicidal patients
170 (*fig.*)
cyanopindolol 6, 200 (*table*)
cyclic adenosine monophosphate (cAMP)
dependent endogenous phosphorylation
120
phosphorylation system 117–20, 121 (*figs*)
microtubules preparation 117
phosphorylation *in vitro* 118
photoaffinity labelling with 8-N$_3$-
[^{32}P]cAMP 117
protein assay 118
cyproheptadine 9, 178, 283, 284
effect on inhibition of social interaction by
m-CPP 200 (*table*)

degenerative diseases 19
dementia 309
idiopathic *see* Alzheimer's disease
multi-infarct 309
secondary 309
vascular 309, 316
dexamethasone suppression test 316
male:female ratio 322
deprenyl (selegiline) 184 (*table*), 192
depression 21, 225
abnormal 5-HT neuroendocrine function in
124–35
abnormal hypothalamo-pituitary-adrenal
function in 129
abnormalities of serotonergic processes 50
animal models 20
anxiety symptoms 143
'atypical' 208 (*table*)
classification 154
depressive delusions in 164
desynchronization of circadian rhythm as
cause 110
glucose metabolism in 264–5
growth hormone response to clonidine 130
5-hydroxyindoleacetic acid in cerebrospinal
fluid 88
5-HT$_1$ receptor family in 148–9, 150–1
(*figs*)
5-HT$_2$ binding in platelets 73
indoleamine hypothesis 124
melancholic subtype 164
paroxetine binding 72
platelet 5-HT uptake in 58–60
platelet imipramine binding in 61–3, 71
prolactin response to fenfluramine 132–3

psychotic bipolar 88
serotonergic system in hypothalamus,
underactivity of 196
sex distribution 225
social aetiology 152
subgroups, continuous spectrum of distinct
diseases? 174
tryptophan availability in brain 34
unipolar 154–5
V_{max} as trait marker 58
desipramine 46, 110, 118, 196, 231
serotonin uptake inhibition 254
desmethylclomipramine 171, 231–2
dexamethasone 155
suppression test 316, 320
suppressors/non-suppressors 155–6
diazepam 102
amitriptyline compared 164
hippocampal injection effect on 5-HT
synthesis 201
suppressant effects of intraperitoneal
administration 211 (*fig.*)
5,7-dichlorokynurenic acid 209
dieting 131, 141
branched chain amino acids during 141
5,6-dihydroxytryptamine 179
5,7-dihydroxytryptamine 180
distress cries (separation-induced
vocalizations) 209
dopamine 26, 39
release 10
dopamine$_2$ receptors 16, 38, 331–3

eating, *see* feeding
eating disorders 284–90
fenfluramine and animal models 303–7
Ecstasy (3,4-methylene
dioxymethamphetamine (MDMA)) 20,
24, 155, 223
electroconvulsive shock, rat pineal melatonin
synthesis stimulation 110–14
methods 111
results 111–12
electroconvulsive therapy (ECT) 58, 110, 164
eltoprazine 164, 272
enkephalin 26
enuresis 71
ergots 16

fawn-hooded rat 299
fear 143
feeding 279–300
behaviour structure 305
glucoprivic 306
macronutrient selection 288–9
motivation 303–5